COLOR ATLAS of
CLINICAL
EMBRYOLOGY

COLOR ATLAS of
CLINICAL EMBRYOLOGY

KEITH L. MOORE, BA, MSc, PhD, FIAC, FRSM

Professor Emeritus of Anatomy and Cell Biology
Faculty of Medicine, University of Toronto
Toronto, Ontario, Canada
Visiting Professor of Clinical Anatomy
Department of Human Anatomy and Cell Science
University of Manitoba
Winnipeg, Manitoba, Canada

T.V.N. PERSAUD, MD, PhD, DSc, FRC Path (Lond)

Professor Emeritus and Former Head
Department of Human Anatomy and Cell Science
Professor of Pediatrics and Child Health
Associate Professor of Obstetrics, Gynecology, and Reproductive Sciences
University of Manitoba, Faculties of Medicine and Dentistry
Consultant in Pathology and Clinical Genetics
Health Sciences Centre
Winnipeg, Manitoba, Canada

KOHEI SHIOTA, MD, D Med Sc

Professor and Chairman
Department of Anatomy and Developmental Biology
Director of Congenital Anomaly Research Center
Graduate School of Medicine
Kyoto University
Kyoto, Japan

SECOND EDITION

W.B. SAUNDERS COMPANY
A Harcourt Health Sciences Company
Philadelphia   London   New York   St. Louis   Sydney   Toronto

W. B. SAUNDERS COMPANY
A Harcourt Health Sciences Company

The Curtis Center
Independence Square West
Philadelphia, PA 19106

Acquisitions Editor: William Schmitt
Project Manager: Patricia Tannian
Senior Production Editor: Melissa Lastarria
Book Design Manager: Gail Morey Hudson
Cover Designer: Teresa Breckwoldt

COLOR ATLAS OF CLINICAL EMBRYOLOGY, 2ND EDITION   ISBN 0-7216-8263-4

Printed in the United States of America.

Last digit is the print number: 9   8   7   6   5   4   3   2   1

*Dedicated to a greater understanding of life
and to our*
wives and children

Illustrations
Sari O'Sullivan, B.F.A., B.Sc., AAM
Valda Glennie, B.A., B.Sc., AAM
Heinz Loth, B.Sc., AAM
David Mazierski, B.Sc., AAM
Hans Neuhart
Glenn Reid, B.Sc., AAM

Photographs
Paul Schwartz, B.A.
Stephen Epstein
Toshiaki Nagai
Roy Simpson

Keyboarding
Marion Moore, B.A.
Barbara Clune

Microdissection
Chigako Uwabe, B.Sc.

Preface

The reproductive revolution in the last decade has resulted in rapid advances in our understanding of human embryology and in readily accessible techniques for assessing the status of developing humans. Human embryos and fetuses have become medicine's newest patients.

This thoroughly revised color atlas is designed to give a well-illustrated and systematic overview of life before birth. The color photographs, drawings, scanning electron micrographs, sonograms, MRIs, and pen and ink sketches give an appreciation of embryos and fetuses at various stages of development and indicate periods when the formation of the tissues and organs may be affected by teratogenic agents (e.g., drugs, viruses, and radiation). Some photographs have been color-enhanced to show the natural appearance of the embryos, fetuses, and their associated membranes. This edition of the *color atlas* contains numerous new full-color illustrations and an increased coverage of common birth defects.

*The atlas provides a **visual summary of human development** and an outline of the most important developmental concepts. It should be useful to all health care professionals, but it will likely be most helpful to clinical geneticists, dysmorphologists, embryologists, embryopathologists, maternity nurses, medical students, medicolegal experts, obstetricians, pediatricians, and perinatologists. The introductory text at the beginning of each chapter has been expanded and with the legends to the illustrations provides an overview of the main stages and crucial events of life before birth. The principal systems involved in congenital anomalies are also illustrated, and photomicrographs of various tissues and organs are described. Selected serial sections of embryos during the period when most defects originate are also included.

We have been most fortunate in the expert assistance we have received from several medical photographers: Paul Schwartz and Stephen Epstein in Creative Communications, Instructional Media Services, Faculty of Medicine, University of Toronto; Toshiaki Nagai in the Department of Anatomy, Faculty of Medicine, Kyoto University, Kyoto, Japan; and Roy Simpson, Department of Human Anatomy and Cell Science, Faculty of Medicine, University of Manitoba. Our principal medical illustrators were Sari O'Sullivan, David Mazierski, Valda Glennie, and Hans Neuhart. Without their expert skill and desire to achieve excellence in their art, the quality of this atlas could not have been attained. We are also most grateful to Ms. Chigako Uwabe of the Congenital Anomaly Research Center, Faculty of Medicine, Kyoto University. She examined most of the embryos in the collection and performed the microdissections of the embryos illustrated in this atlas. We are very grateful to Marion Moore and Barbara Clune, who typed the manuscript, and to Gisela Persaud who proofread drafts of it and also helped with the bibliography.

Dr. Albert E. Chudley, Professor of Pediatrics and Child Health and Professor of Human Genetics in the Faculty of Medicine, University of Manitoba, and Head of Genetics and Metabolism, Children's Hospital, Winnipeg, Manitoba, Canada, and Dr. Dagmar K. Kalousek, Program Head, Cytogenetics/Embryopathology Laboratory and Professor of Pathology and Laboratory Medicine in the University of British Columbia, British Columbia Children's and Women's Hospital, Vancouver, B.C., Canada, provided many of the photographs of embryos, fetuses, and neonates with congenital anomalies. Barbara Paradice in Dr. Kalousek's laboratory was also most helpful. Dr. Albert E. Chudley assisted us considerably with the revision of Chapter 5 *(Congenital Anomalies and Birth Defects)*. We are grateful to Dr. Raymond F. Gasser, Professor of Anatomy at Louisiana State University, Medical Center, New Orleans, Louisiana, for help with the presentation of the serial sections of human embryos. His expertise in this area is widely recognized. We are also grateful to many other colleagues who kindly provided illustrations for the atlas. Their contributions are acknowledged in the legends for the figures.

Finally, we would like to thank Mr. William Schmitt, Medical Editor, and the staff of W.B. Saunders for their invaluable support in the preparation of this work.

Keith L. Moore
T.V.N. Persaud
Kohei Shiota

Contents

1

The First Two Weeks of Human Development

Human development begins at fertilization (conception) when an oocyte (ovum) from a woman is fertilized by a sperm (spermatozoon) from a man. *The sperm and oocyte, the male and female gametes, are highly specialized sex cells.* They contain half the number of chromosomes (haploid number) that is present in somatic (body) cells. The number of chromosomes is reduced during **meiosis,** a special type of cell division that occurs during gametogenesis. This maturation process is called **spermatogenesis** in males and **oogenesis** in females (Fig. 1-1). Disturbances of meiosis during gametogenesis, for example, **nondisjunction,** result in the formation of *chromosomally abnormal gametes* (Fig. 1-2). If involved in fertilization, these gametes with numerical chromosome abnormalities cause abnormal development such as occurs in infants with *Down syndrome* (see Chapter 5).

Oocytes are produced in the ovary *(oogenesis)* and expelled from it during *ovulation.* The fimbriae of the uterine tube sweep the oocyte into the ampulla where it may be fertilized. Sperms are produced in the seminiferous tubules of the testes *(spermatogenesis)* and are stored in the epididymis. Ejaculation of semen during sexual intercourse results in the deposit of millions of sperms in the vagina around the external uterine os. Several hundred sperms pass through the uterus and enter the uterine tubes. At the ampulla of the uterine tube, many of them surround the secondary oocyte if it is present. When the sperm enters the oocyte, a second polar body is formed; the nucleus of the mature oocyte constitutes the *female pronucleus,* and the head of the sperm separates from the tail and enlarges to become the *male pronucleus.* Fertilization is complete when the pronuclei unite and the maternal and paternal chromosomes intermingle during metaphase of the first mitotic division of the *zygote,* the cell that is the primordium of a human being (Figs. 1-4 and 1-5).

Formation of the zygote normally occurs in the ampulla of the uterine tube (fallopian tube), the longest and widest part of the tube (Fig. 1-4). *In vitro fertilization* (IVF) of an oocyte in a Petri dish (Fig. 1-5) and the more recently developed technique of intracytoplasmic sperm injection (ICSI) provide the opportunity to alleviate infertility resulting from blocked uterine tubes or oligospermia (reduced number of spermatozoa). *Text continued on p. 6*

NORMAL GAMETOGENESIS

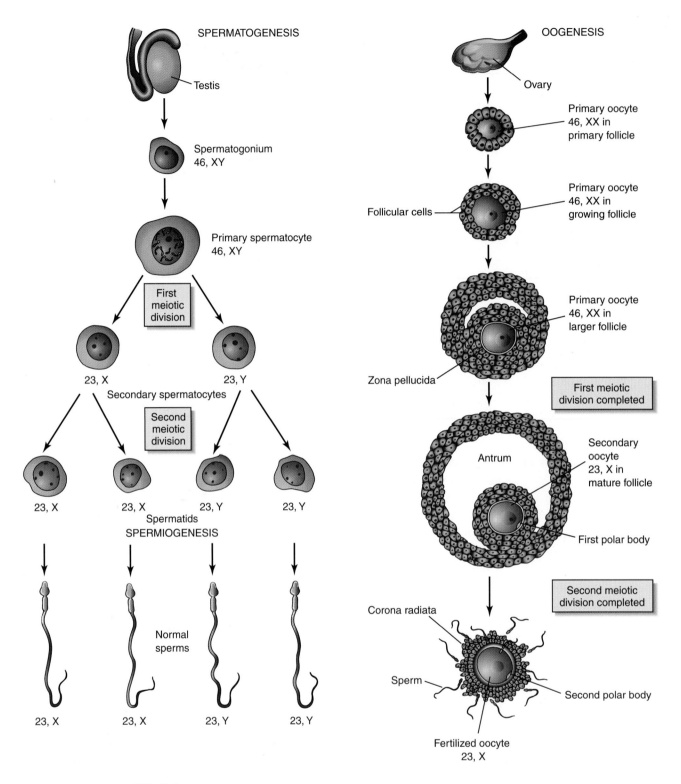

FIG. 1-1

Gametogenesis—conversion of germ cells into gametes. The drawings compare spermatogenesis and oogenesis. Oogonia are not shown in this figure because they differentiate into primary oocytes before birth. The chromosome's complement of the germ cells is shown at each stage. The number designates the total number of chromosomes, including the sex chromosome(s) shown after the comma. Note: (1) following the two meiotic divisions, the diploid number of chromosomes, 46, is reduced to the haploid number, 23; (2) four sperms form from one primary spermatocyte, whereas only one mature oocyte results from maturation of a primary oocyte; and (3) the cytoplasm is conserved during oogenesis to form one large cell, the mature oocyte or ovum. The polar bodies are small nonfunctional cells that eventually degenerate.

ABNORMAL GAMETOGENESIS

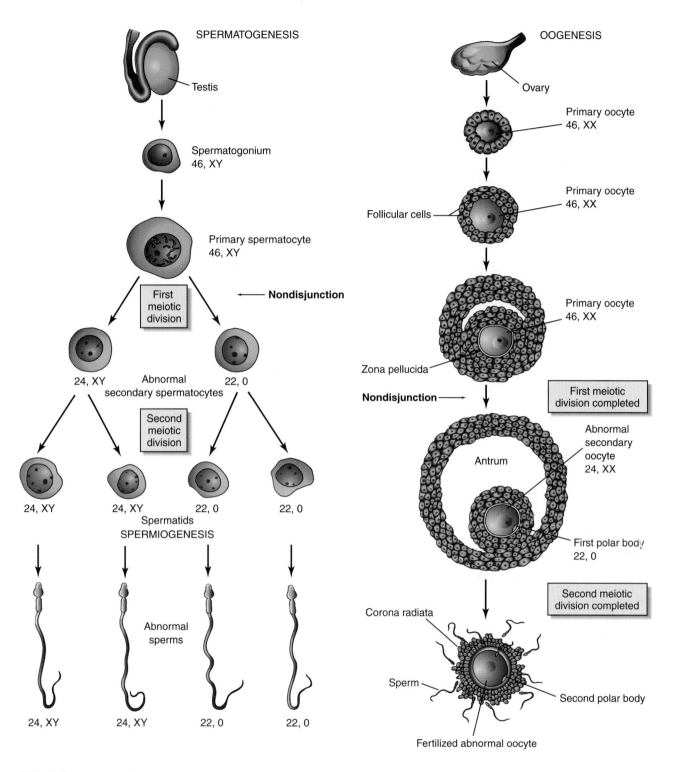

FIG. 1-2

Abnormal gametogenesis. The drawings show how nondisjunction, an error in cell division, results in an abnormal chromosome distribution in germ cells. Although nondisjunction of sex chromosomes is illustrated, a similar defect may occur during the division of autosomes. When nondisjunction occurs during the first meiotic division of spermatogenesis, one secondary spermatocyte contains 22 autosomes plus an X and a Y chromosome, and the other one contains 22 autosomes and no sex chromosome. Similarly, nondisjunction during oogenesis may give rise to an oocyte with 22 autosomes and two X-chromosomes (as shown) or may result in one with 22 autosomes and no sex chromosomes.

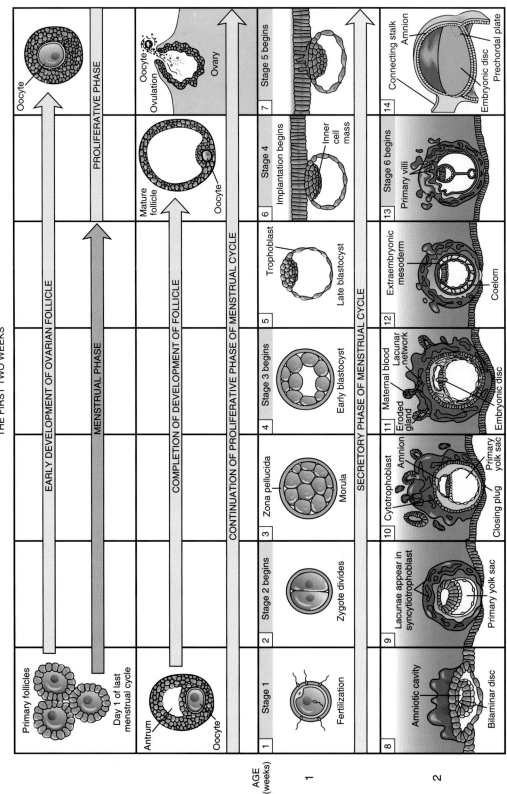

FIG. 1-3

Gestational age is calculated from day 1 of the last normal menstrual period (LNMP); however, the embryo does not begin to develop until fertilization of the oocyte occurs about 14 days later. Development of an ovarian follicle and ovulation of the oocyte occur during the first two weeks of the menstrual cycle. Stage 1 of development begins when the oocyte (ovum) is fertilized to form a zygote, about 14 days after LNMP. Cleavage of the zygote occurs during stage 2. The morula enters the uterus on day 3 and the blastocyst forms during stage 3. During stages 4 and 5 the blastocyst attaches to and implants in the endometrium. Stage 6 occurs at the end of the second week when the bilaminar embryonic disc forms and primary chorionic villi appear. (Modified from Moore KL, Persaud TVN: *The developing human*, ed 6, Philadelphia, 1998, Saunders.)

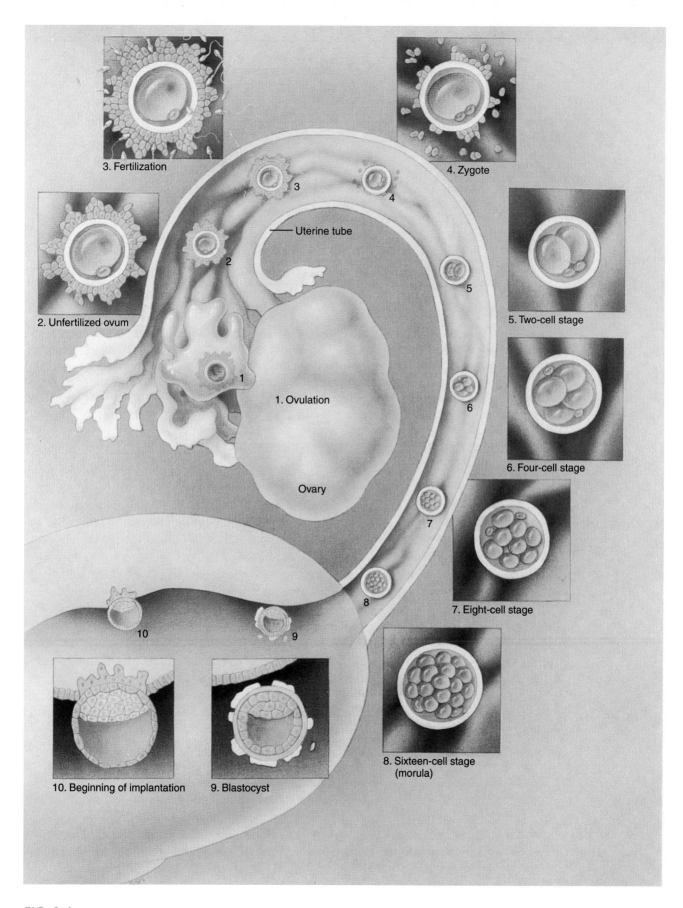

3. Fertilization

4. Zygote

2. Unfertilized ovum

Uterine tube

1. Ovulation

Ovary

5. Two-cell stage

6. Four-cell stage

7. Eight-cell stage

8. Sixteen-cell stage
(morula)

10. Beginning of implantation

9. Blastocyst

FIG. 1-4

Illustration of the first week of human development showing ovulation, fertilization, and cleavage of the zygote. Observe that the first two stages of development occur in the uterine tube. The morula enters the uterus on day 3 and the blastocyst forms on day 4, stage 3 of development (see Fig. 1-3). After floating in the uterus for about two days, the blastocyst begins to implant in the endometrium of the uterus.

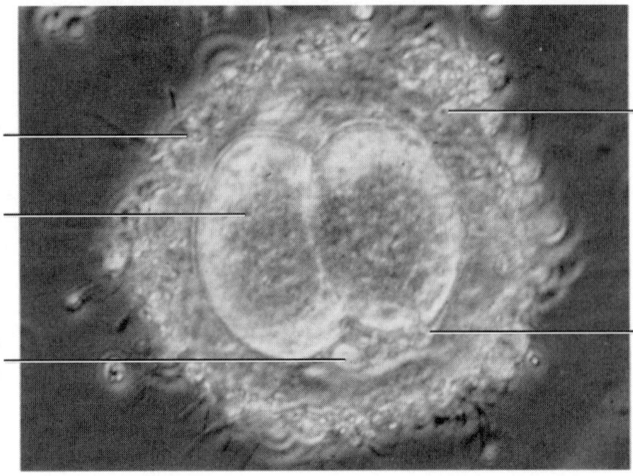

Corona radiata (composed of follicular cells)

Blastomere

Polar body (nonfunctional cell)

Degenerating sperm

Zona pellucida

FIG. 1-5

Illustration of a two-cell cleaved zygote at Carnegie stage 2, developing in vitro. Observe that it is surrounded by many sperms. Each blastomere has the potential to develop into an embryo. The polar body is a nonfunctional cell. The dividing zygote is observed until the four-to-eight-cell stage and is then placed in the uterus. To increase the chances of pregnancy, three or four cleaved zygotes are inserted into the uterine tube or uterine cavity. (Courtesy of Drs. Maria T. Zenzes and Peng Wang, In Vitro Fertilization Program, Toronto Hospital, Toronto, Ontario, Canada.)

Fertilization initiates embryonic development by stimulating the zygote to undergo a series of mitotic cell divisions called **cleavage.** Within 24 hours after fertilization the zygote divides into two cells called *blastomeres* (Figs. 1-3 to 1-5). These primordial cells soon divide to form four blastomeres, eight blastomeres, and so on. Cleavage normally occurs as the zygote passes along the uterine tube toward the uterus (Fig. 1-4). During cleavage the blastomeres change their shape and size and tightly align themselves against each other to form a compact ball of blastomeres known as a morula (L. *morus,* mulberry). The **morula,** a cluster of 12 to 16 blastomeres, *forms about three days after fertilization,* just before entering the uterus (Figs. 1-3 and 1-4). Shortly after *the morula enters the uterus,* fluid-filled spaces appear between its central blastomeres. Soon the cells are separated into two parts: (1) a thin outer cell layer called the *trophoblast,* which forms the fetal part of the placenta; and (2) a group of centrally located blastomeres, which forms the **inner cell mass** or *embryoblast,* the primordium of the embryo. The conceptus is now known as a blastocyst (Figs. 1-3 and 1-4).

The **blastocyst** floats freely in the uterine cavity for about two days. While floating in the uterus, the blastocyst derives its nourishment from the secretions of the uterine glands (Figs. 1-6 and 1-7). About six days after fertilization (day 20 of a 28-day menstrual cycle),* *the blastocyst attaches to the endometrial epithelium* (Figs. 1-3 and 1-4). As this occurs, **the trophoblast proliferates** to form two layers: (1) an inner *cytotrophoblast* (cellular trophoblast) and (2) an outer *syncytiotrophoblast* (syncytial trophoblast). Fingerlike processes of the syncytiotrophoblast extend through the endometrial epithelium by secreting substances that erode the endometrial tissues. By the end of the first week, the blastocyst is superficially implanted in the endometrium (Figs. 1-3 and 1-4), and derives its nourishment and oxygen from the maternal endometrial tissues.

At eight to nine days, the **amniotic cavity** appears as a space between the cytotrophoblast and embryoblast (Fig. 1-7). *Amnioblasts* derived from the epiblast soon line the amniotic cavity and form the **amnion.** As the amniotic sac forms, the *yolk* sac lined by endodermal cells develops and spaces called *lacunae* form in the syncytiotrophoblast.

Text continued on p. 12

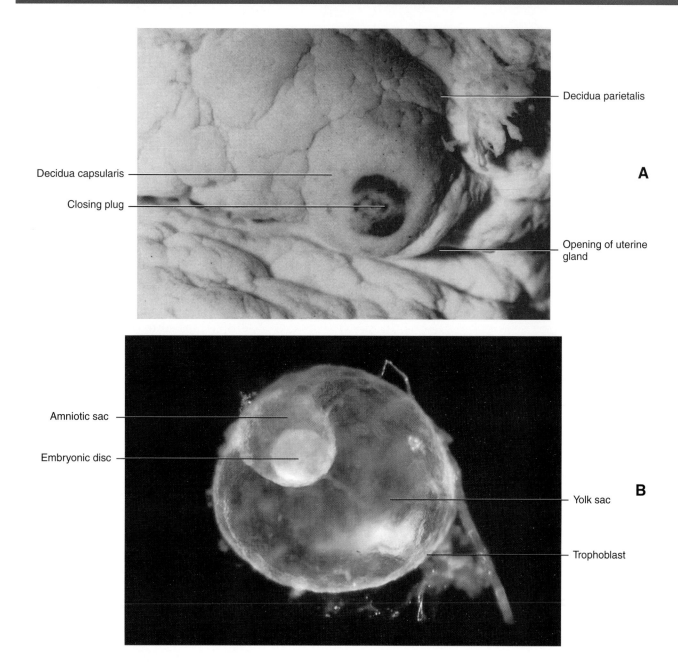

FIG. 1-6

A, Photograph showing a surface view of an implantation site of a human conceptus at an estimated fertilization age of 14 days. The implanted blastocyst produces a swelling of the endometrium (decidua capsularis) that bulges into the uterine cavity (see Fig. 4-1). The closing plug forms where the blastocyst entered the endometrium. **B,** Photograph of a blastocyst during Carnegie stage 6 of development, about 14 days. (**A,** From Nishimura H [editor]: *Atlas of human prenatal histology,* Tokyo, 1983, Igaku-Shoin. **B,** From Nishimura, et al: *Prenatal development of the human with special reference to craniofacial structures: an atlas,* Bethesda, 1977, US Department of Health, Education and Welfare, NIH.)

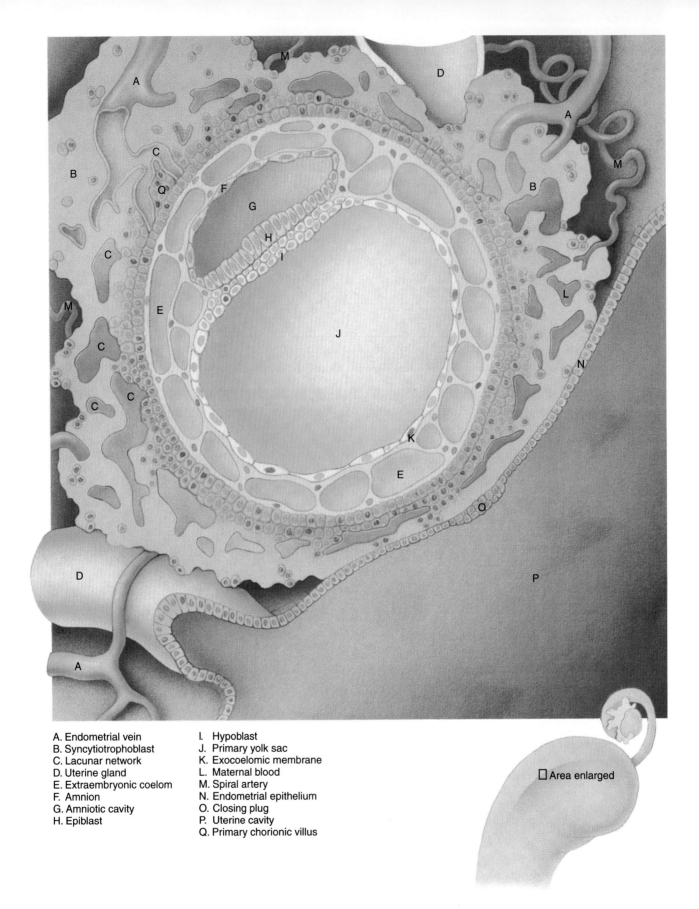

A. Endometrial vein
B. Syncytiotrophoblast
C. Lacunar network
D. Uterine gland
E. Extraembryonic coelom
F. Amnion
G. Amniotic cavity
H. Epiblast

I. Hypoblast
J. Primary yolk sac
K. Exocoelomic membrane
L. Maternal blood
M. Spiral artery
N. Endometrial epithelium
O. Closing plug
P. Uterine cavity
Q. Primary chorionic villus

☐ Area enlarged

FIG. 1-7

Drawing of a 14-day human blastocyst completely implanted in the endometrium. Lacunar networks (C) have developed in the external layer of the trophoblast known as the syncytiotrophoblast (B). Observe that maternal blood is entering the deepest lacunar network (top left). The embryo appears as the bilaminar embryonic disc. Observe that coelomic spaces appear in the extraembryonic mesoderm (E). These spaces fuse to form the extraembryonic coelom (primordium of the chorionic cavity.)

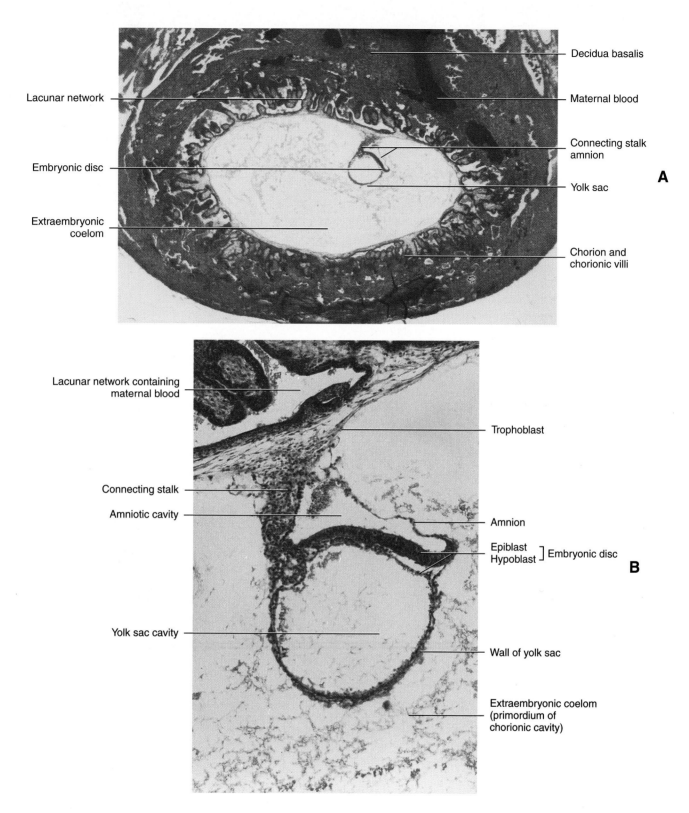

Lacunar network

Embryonic disc

Extraembryonic
coelom

Decidua basalis

Maternal blood

Connecting stalk
amnion

Yolk sac

Chorion and
chorionic villi

A

Lacunar network containing
maternal blood

Connecting stalk

Amniotic cavity

Yolk sac cavity

Trophoblast

Amnion

Epiblast ⎤ Embryonic disc
Hypoblast ⎦

Wall of yolk sac

Extraembryonic coelom
(primordium of
chorionic cavity)

B

FIG. 1-8

Photomicrographs of longitudinal sections of an implanted embryo at Carnegie stage 6, about 14 days. Note the large size of the extraembryonic coelom. A, Low-power view (×18). B, High-power view (×95). The embryo is represented by the bilaminar embryonic disc composed of epiblast and hypoblast (see also Fig. 1-7). (From Nishimura H [editor]: *Atlas of human prenatal histology,* Tokyo, 1983, Igaku-Shoin.)

FIG. 1-9

Drawings of sections through implanted human embryos, based mainly on Hertig et al, 1956. Observe: (1) the defect in the surface epithelium of the endometrium has disappeared; (2) a small secondary yolk sac has formed; (3) a large cavity, the extraembryonic coelom, now surrounds the yolk sac and amnion, except where the amnion is attached to the chorion by the connecting stalk; and (4) the extraembryonic coelom splits the extraembryonic mesoderm into two layers: extraembryonic somatic mesoderm lining the trophoblast and covering the amnion, and the extraembryonic splanchnic mesoderm around the yolk sac. A, 13 days, illustrating decrease in relative size of the primary yolk sac and the early appearance of primary chorionic villi. B, 14 days, showing the newly formed secondary yolk sac and the location of the prechordal plate in its roof. C, Detail of the prechordal plate area outlined in B.

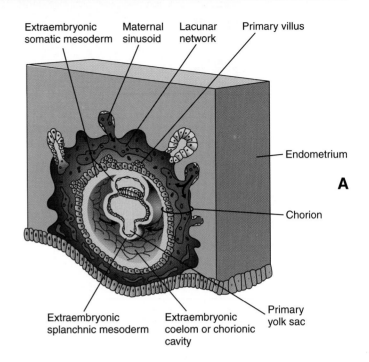

A

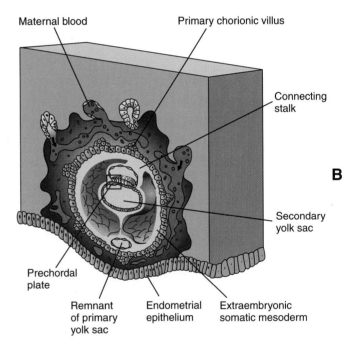

B

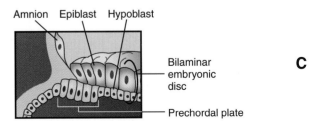

C

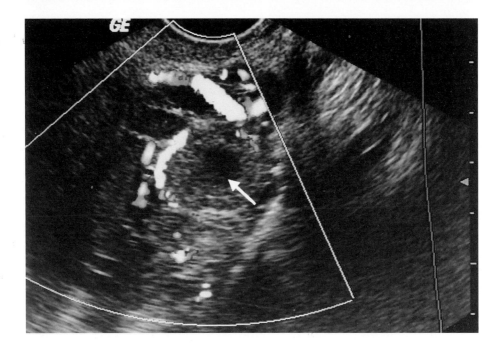

FIG. 1-10

Ectopic tubal pregnancy. This axial sonogram through the left adnexa of a 6-week pregnant patient shows a small gestational sac *(arrow)* in the left uterine tube with prominent vascularity in its periphery. This is characteristic of an ectopic tubal pregnancy. The incidence of tubal pregnancy ranges from 1 in 80 to 1 in 250 pregnancies. Most ectopic implantations (95% to 97%) occur in the uterine tube, usually in the isthmus or ampulla. (Courtesy of Dr. E.A. Lyons, Department of Radiology, Health Sciences Centre, University of Manitoba, Winnipeg, Manitoba, Canada.)

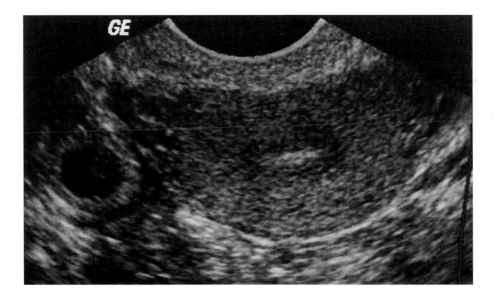

FIG. 1-11

Axial sonogram through the uterine fundus and right adnexa. The uterus is empty, and a rounded sac (2-cm diameter), with a small yolk sac within it, can be seen in the adnexa. This is diagnostic of a right ectopic pregnancy at 7-weeks' menstrual age. Other extrauterine implantation sites include the peritoneal cavity (abdominal pregnancy) and the ovary (ovarian pregnancy), but these are far less common than in the uterine tube (tubal pregnancy). (Courtesy of Dr. E.A. Lyons, Department of Radiology, Health Sciences Centre, University of Manitoba, Winnipeg, Manitoba, Canada.)

Fusion of lacunae forms **lacunar networks** that contain maternal blood. Flow of blood through the lacunar networks establishes a primordial *uteroplacental circulation.*

Implantation of the blastocyst is completed by the end of the second week (Figs. 1-6 and 1-7). As this process takes place, changes occur in the embryoblast that produce a **bilaminar embryonic disc,** composed of two layers, *epiblast* and *hypoblast* (Figs. 1-8 and 1-9). As the blastocyst implants in the endometrium, the syncytiotrophoblast produces *human chorionic gonadotropin* (hCG), which enters the maternal blood. This hormone maintains the endometrium and forms the basis for pregnancy testing.

Ectopic pregnancies occur when blastocysts implant outside the uterus, most often in the uterine tube (Figs. 1-10 and 1-11). There are several causes of ectopic pregnancy, but *abnormal sites of implantation* are often related to factors that delay or prevent transportation of the zygote to the uterus. **Spontaneous abortions** are common during the first two weeks resulting from abnormalities of the blastocysts and problems associated with their implantation. The early *spontaneous abortion rate* is thought to be about 45%. Many of such early spontaneous abortions occur without the knowledge of the mother (unrecognized abortion or subclinical abortion).

Throughout this atlas, references are made to the developmental stages of embryonic development. These numerical stages are based on the **Carnegie Embryonic Classification System** proposed by O'Rahilly and Müller (1987), which is outlined in Table 5-1 and described in Chapter 5. The Carnegie Collection of Embryos is in the Human Developmental Anatomy Center in the National Museum of Health and Medicine, Armed Forces Institute of Pathology, Washington, DC.

---

*This atlas uses the estimated date of fertilization as the beginning of pregnancy. To obtain *gestational age* (calculated from the last normal menstrual period [Fig. 1-3]), add 14 days to the estimated *fertilization age.*

2

The Third to Eighth Weeks of Human Development

The primordia, or beginnings, of all major external and internal structures are established during this period. By the end of the eighth week all main organ systems have begun to develop, but the function of most of them is minimal. As the organs form, the shape of the embryo changes so that by 56 days (the end of the eighth week) it has a distinctly human appearance.

THE THIRD WEEK

Rapid development of the embryo from the embryonic disc formed during the second week is characterized by the appearance of the primitive streak, formation of the notochord, and differentiation of three **germ layers** from which all tissues and organs develop (Fig. 2-1). The *beginning of morphogenesis* (development of body form) is the most significant event occurring during the third week. Gastrulation, the process that establishes the three germ layers (ectoderm, mesoderm, and endoderm), begins with formation of the **primitive streak** in the epiblast (Figs. 2-1 to 2-3). At 15 days the disclike embryo is oval to round.

The primitive streak has a narrow primitive groove with slightly bulging folds on each side. It appears at the beginning of the third week as a localized thickening of the epiblast at the caudal end of the embryonic disc. The primitive streak results from migration of epiblastic cells to the median plane of the embryonic disc. As it elongates by addition of cells to its caudal end, its cranial end proliferates to form a **primitive node** with a small depression in it, the primitive pit. Invagination of epiblastic cells from the primitive streak gives rise to mesenchymal cells (see Fig. 2-2, *A* and *B*) that migrate ventrally, laterally, and cranially between the epiblast and hypoblast. Mesenchymal cells produced by the primitive streak soon organize into a third germ layer, the *intraembryonic mesoderm.* As soon as the primitive streak begins to produce mesenchymal cells, the epiblast layer is known as the embryonic ectoderm. Some cells of the epiblast displace the hypoblast and form the embryonic endoderm. Thus the cells of the epiblast give rise to all three germ layers in the embryo, the primordia of all its tissues and organs.

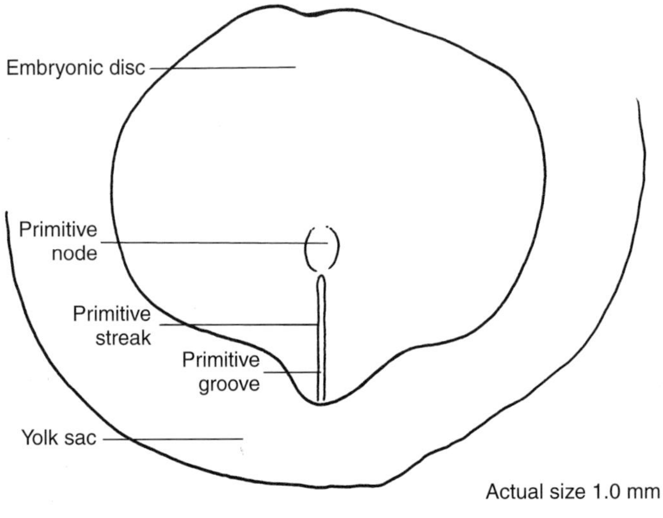

FIG. 2-1
A, Dorsal view of a presomite embryo at Carnegie stage 7, about 16 days. **B,** Diagram indicating the structures shown in *A*. The primitive streak extends caudally from the primitive node (knot) as a zone of ectodermal proliferation in the embryonic disc, the caudal part of which is disrupted. A shallow sulcus, called the primitive groove, is visible, especially in the caudal part of the streak. (From Nishimura H, Tanimura T: *Clinical aspects of the teratogenicity of drugs,* Excerpta Medica/American, 1976, Elsevier.)

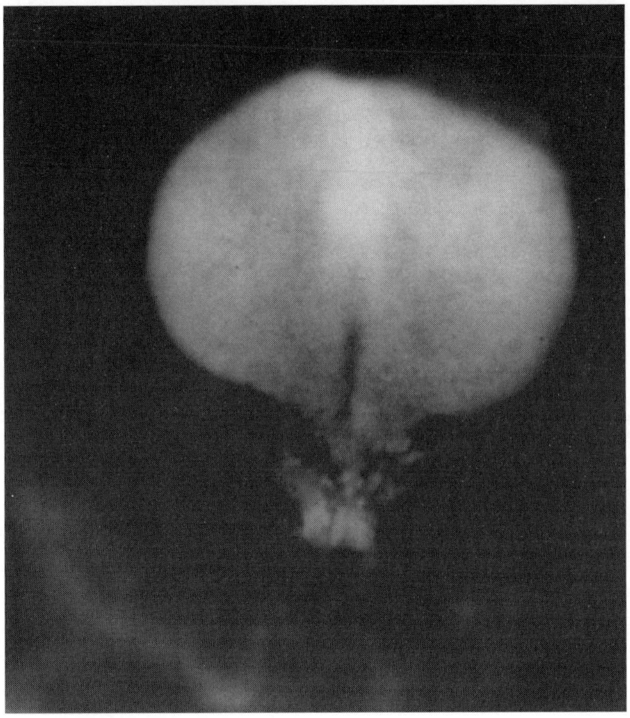

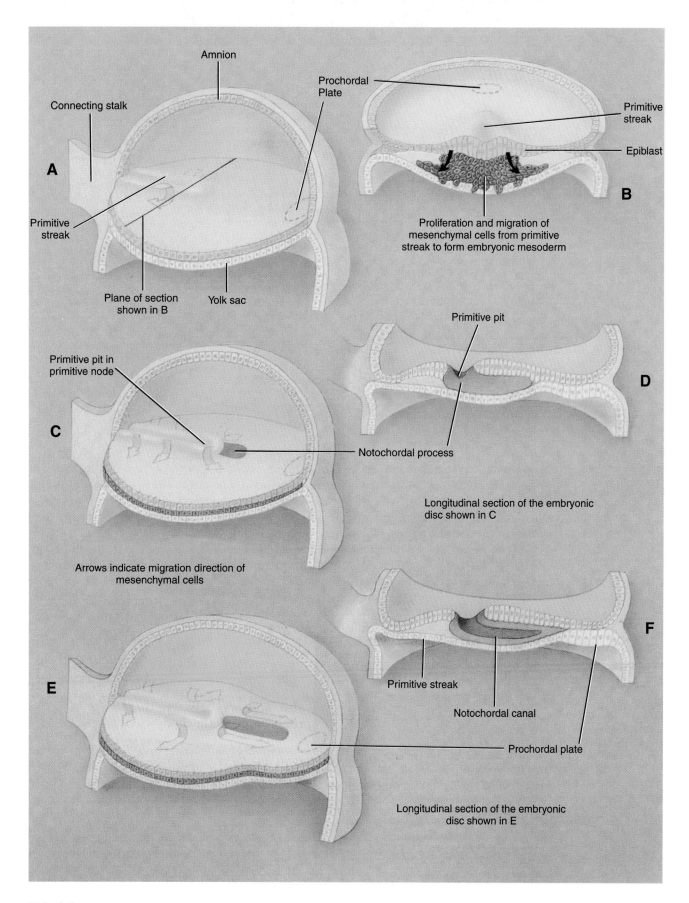

FIG. 2-2

Schematic drawings of the embryonic disc during the third week. Its associated membranes (amnion and yolk sac) have been cut away to show the developmental features of the embryonic disc. In *B,* note that mesenchyme (embryonic connective tissue) arises from the primitive streak. The prochordal plate, an organizer of the head region, indicates the future site of the mouth. The notochordal process is soon transformed into the notochord (see Fig. 2-3), which forms the axis of the embryo.

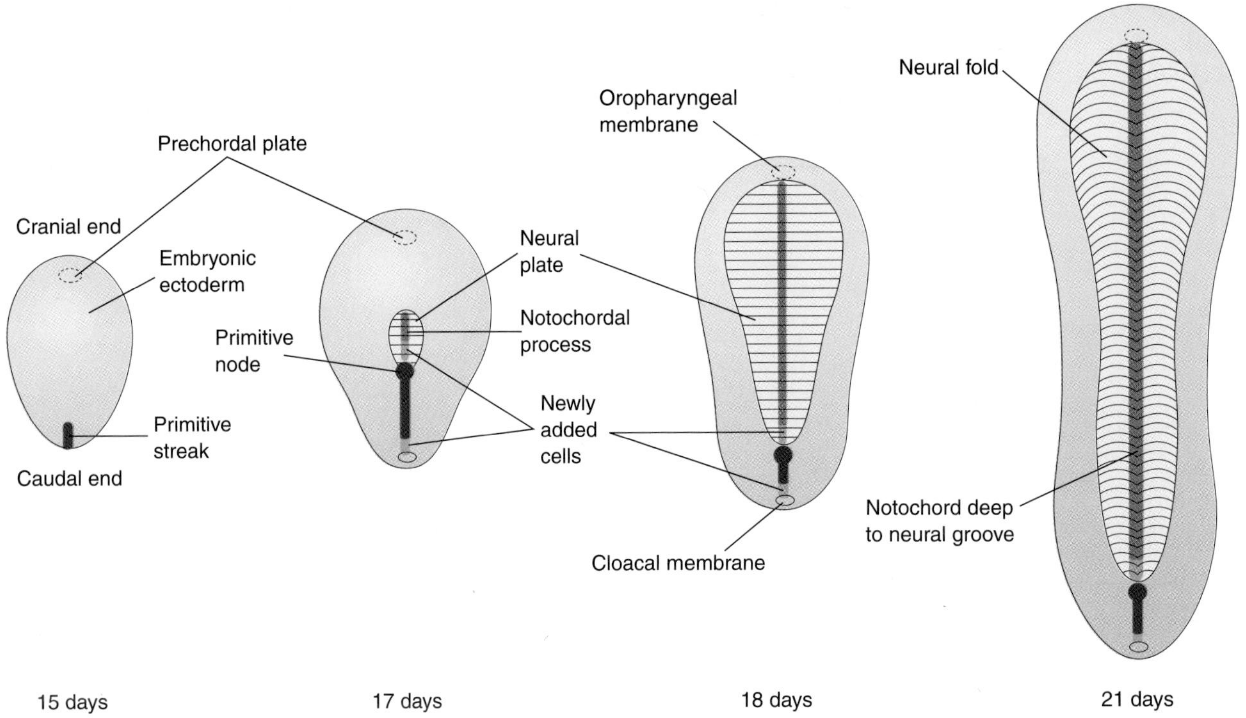

15 days   17 days   18 days   21 days

FIG. 2-3

Diagrammatic sketches of dorsal views of the embryonic disc showing how it lengthens and changes shape during the third week. The primitive streak lengthens by addition of cells at its caudal end, and the notochordal process lengthens by migration of cells from the primitive node. The notochordal process and adjacent mesoderm induce the overlying embryonic ectoderm to form the neural plate, the primordium of the central nervous system. Observe that as the notochordal process elongates, the primitive streak shortens. At the end of the third week the notochordal process is transformed into the notochord. Note that the embryonic disc is originally egg-shaped but soon becomes pear-shaped and then slipperlike as the notochord develops. (From Moore KL, Persaud TVN: *The developing human,* 6 ed, Philadelphia, 1998, Saunders.)

Cells of the intraembryonic mesoderm migrate to the edges of the embryonic disc, where they join the *extraembryonic mesoderm* covering the amnion and yolk sac. By the end of the third week mesoderm exists between the ectoderm and endoderm everywhere except at the oropharyngeal membrane, in the median plane occupied by the notochord, and at the cloacal membrane.

Normally the primitive streak diminishes in size and becomes an insignificant structure in the future sacrococcygeal region of the embryo. Remnants of the primitive streak may persist and give rise to a large tumor known as a *sacrococcygeal teratoma* (Fig. 2-4).

Early in the third week, mesenchymal cells arising from the primitive node of the primitive streak form the **notochordal process,** which extends cranially from the primitive node as a rod of cells between the embryonic ectoderm and endoderm. The primitive pit extends into the notochordal process and forms a *notochordal canal.* When fully developed, the notochordal process extends from the primitive node to the prechordal plate. Openings develop in the floor of the notochordal canal and soon coalesce, leaving a *notochordal plate.* The notochordal plate infolds to form the **notochord,** the primordial axis of the embryo around which the vertebral column forms (Fig. 2-5). The notochord functions as the primary inductor in the early embryo.

Neurulation is a major event that begins at the end of the third week. It involves the formation of the neural plate and its infolding to form the neural tube. The **neural plate**

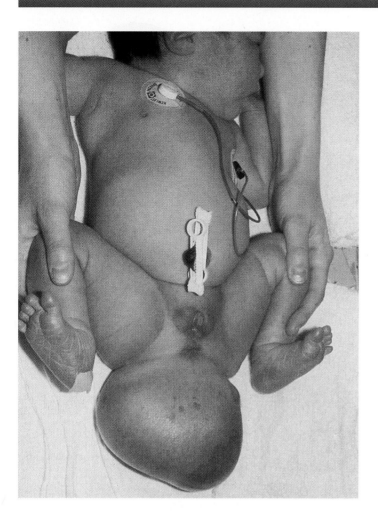

FIG. 2-4

Female infant with a large sacrococcygeal teratoma that developed from remnants of the primitive streak. The tumor, a neoplasm made up of several different types of tissue, was surgically removed. About 75% of infants with these tumors are female; the reason for this preponderance is unknown. (Courtesy of Dr. A.E. Chudley, Department of Pediatrics and Child Health, University of Manitoba, Children's Hospital, Winnipeg, Canada.)

appears as a thickening of the embryonic ectoderm, cranial to the primitive node. The neural plate is induced to form by the developing notochord. A longitudinal **neural groove** develops in the neural plate, which is flanked by *neural folds*. Fusion of the folds forms the neural tube, the primordium of the central nervous system. As the neural folds fuse to form the neural tube, neuroectodermal cells at the lateral margins of the neural plate migrate dorsolaterally to form a neural crest between the surface ectoderm and the neural tube. The neural crest soon divides into two cell masses that give rise to the sensory ganglia of the cranial and spinal nerves. Other neural crest cells migrate from the neural tube and give rise to various other structures (Figs. 2-6 and 2-7).

As the **neural tube,** the primordium of the central nervous system, is developing, the intraembryonic mesoderm proliferates to form columns of *paraxial mesoderm* lateral to the neural plate. Each column is continuous laterally with the *intermediate mesoderm* (Fig. 2-6), which gradually thins laterally into a layer of *lateral mesoderm*. By the end of the third week the cranial ends of the paraxial columns of mesoderm have begun to divide into two to three pairs of cuboidal bodies called **somites** (Figs. 2-6 and 2-7). The somites give rise to most of the axial skeleton, trunk and limb musculature, and the dermis of the skin. The formation and specification of somitic segments are controlled by a unique combination of Hox genes (Hox code). The **intraembryonic coelom** arises as isolated spaces or vesicles between the layers of lateral mesoderm (see Fig. 2-7, *D*), which is the primordium of the body cavities. The coelomic vesicles subsequently coalesce to form a single, horseshoe-shaped cavity that eventually gives rise to the pericardial, pleural, and peritoneal cavities.

Early development of the cardiovascular system also occurs during the third week. Blood vessels first appear in the wall of the yolk sac, allantois, and in the chorion. They develop

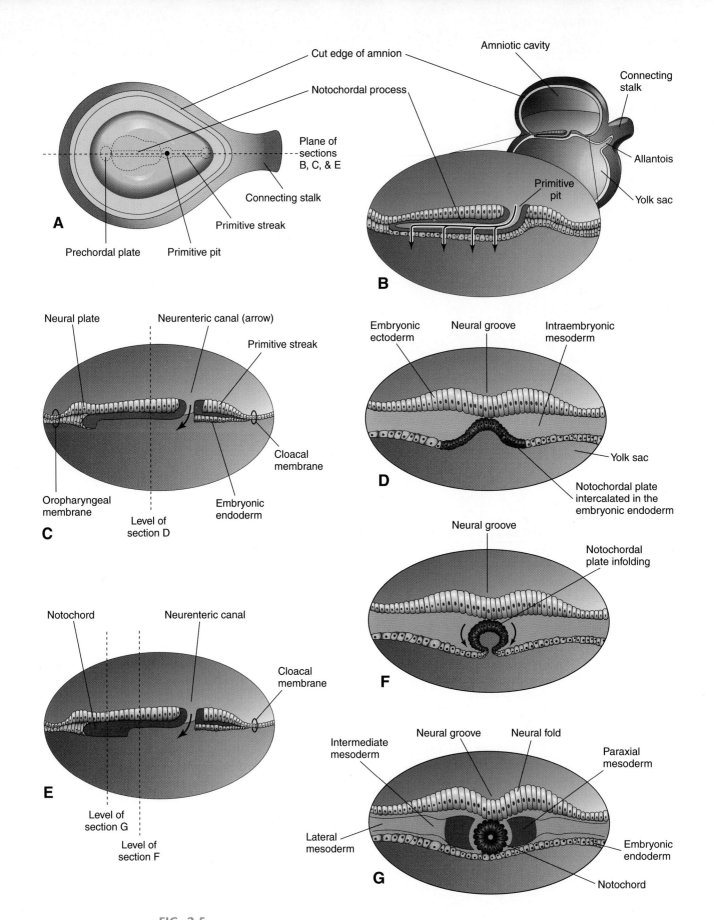

FIG. 2-5

Drawings illustrating further development of the notochord by transformation of the notochordal process. **A,** Dorsal view of the embryonic disc (about 18 days), exposed by removing the amnion. **B,** Three-dimensional median section of the embryo. **C** and **E,** Similar sections of slightly older embryos. **D, F,** and **G,** Transverse sections of the trilaminar embryonic disc at the levels shown in *C* and *E.* (From Moore KL, Persaud TVN: *The developing human,* 6 ed, Philadelphia, 1998, Saunders.)

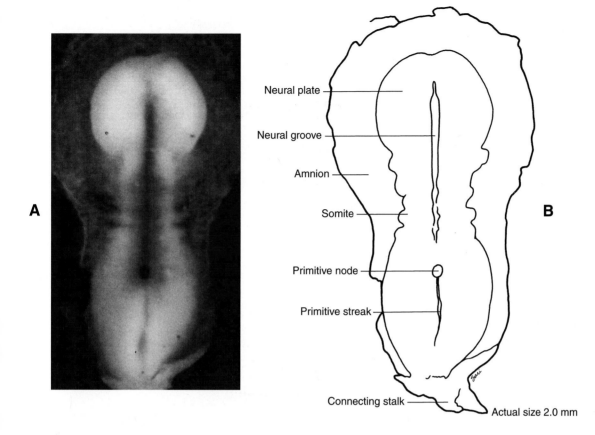

Neural plate

Neural groove

Amnion

Somite

Primitive node

Primitive streak

Connecting stalk

Actual size 2.0 mm

A

B

FIG. 2-6

A, Dorsal view of an embryo during the early period of somite formation. Carnegie stage 9, about 19 days. Most of the amnion has been removed to expose the embryo. B, Diagram indicating the structures shown in A. The mesoderm along the axis of the embryo (paraxial mesoderm) has just begun to divide to produce somites, the primordia of the dermis, subcutaneous tissue, musculature, and cartilage and bones of the axial skeleton.

within the embryo shortly thereafter. Spaces appear within aggregations of mesenchyme and are known as *blood islands*. The spaces soon become lined with endothelium derived from the mesenchymal cells. These primordial vessels unite with other vessels to form a *primordial cardiovascular system*. Toward the end of the third week, the heart is represented by paired endothelial heart tubes that are joined to blood vessels in the embryo and in the extraembryonic membranes (yolk sac, umbilical cord, and chorionic sac). By the end of the third week, the endothelial heart tubes have fused to form a tubular heart that is joined to vessels in the embryo, yolk sac, chorion, and connecting stalk to form a *primordial cardiovascular system*. The primordial blood cells—hemocytoblasts—are derived mainly from the endothelial cells of blood vessels in the walls of the yolk sac and allantois. Fetal and adult erythrocytes probably develop from different hematopoietic precursors.

Chorionic villi, which started to develop at the end of the second week, differentiate into secondary and, later, tertiary villi (primordia of stem villi), which contain *arteriocapillary networks* (see Chapter 4). *Primary chorionic villi* become *secondary chorionic villi* as they acquire mesenchymal cores. Before the end of the third week capillaries develop in the *secondary chorionic villi*, transforming them into *tertiary chorionic villi*. Cytotrophoblastic extensions from these stem villi join to form a **cytotrophoblastic shell** that anchors the chorionic sac to the endometrium. The rapid development of chorionic villi during the third week greatly increases the surface area of the chorion for the exchange of oxygen and nutrients and other substances between the maternal and embryonic circulations.

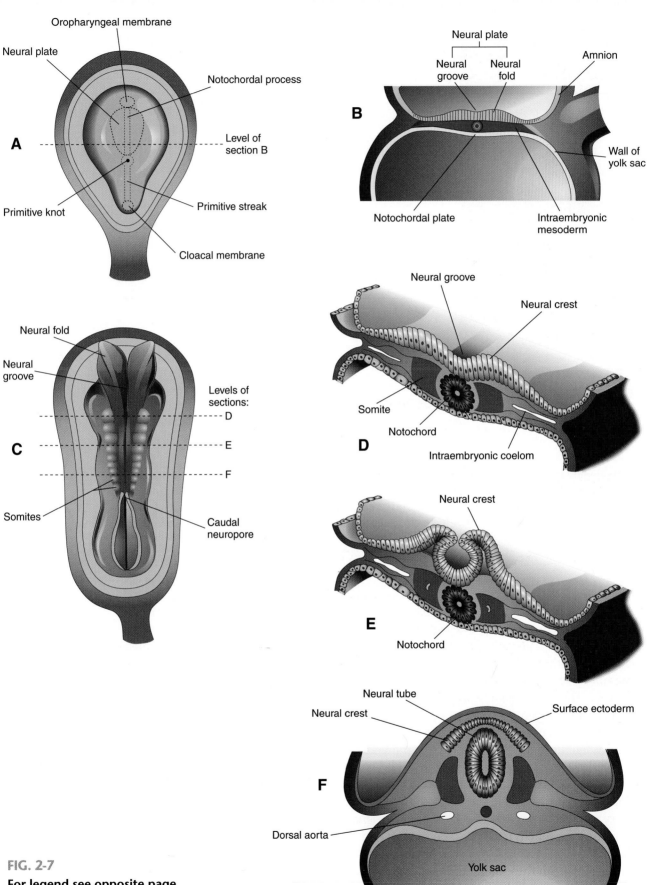

FIG. 2-7
For legend see opposite page.

FIG. 2-7

Diagrams illustrating folding of the neural plate into the neural tube and formation of the neural crest. **A,** Dorsal view of an embryo of about 18 days, exposed by removing the amnion. **B,** Transverse section of this embryo, showing the neural plate and early development of the neural groove. The developing notochord is also shown. **C,** Dorsal view of an embryo of about 22 days. The neural folds have fused opposite the somites but are widely spread out at both ends of the embryo. The rostral and caudal neuropores are indicated. **D** through **F,** Transverse sections of this embryo at the levels shown in C, illustrating formation of the neural tube and its detachment from the surface ectoderm. Note that some neuroectodermal cells are not included in the neural tube but remain between it and the surface ectoderm as the neural crest. Neural crest cells are the major source of connective tissue components, including cartilage, bone, and ligaments of the orofacial region. (From Moore KL, Persaud TVN: *The developing human,* 6 ed, Philadelphia, 1998, Saunders.)

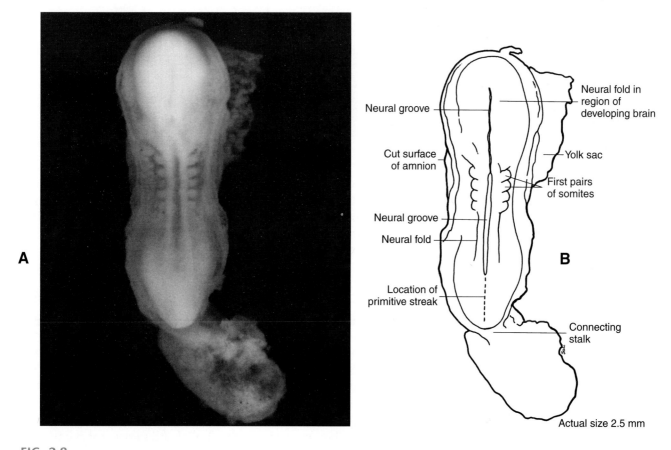

A

B

Neural groove

Neural fold in region of developing brain

Cut surface of amnion

Yolk sac

First pairs of somites

Neural groove

Neural fold

Location of primitive streak

Connecting stalk

Actual size 2.5 mm

FIG. 2-8

A, Dorsal view of a four-somite embryo at Carnegie stage 10, about 21 days. **B,** Diagram indicating the structures shown in A. Most of the amniotic and chorionic sacs have been cut away to expose the embryo. Observe the neural folds and the deep neural groove. The neural folds in the cranial region have thickened to form the primordium of the brain.

THE FOURTH WEEK

At the beginning of the fourth week, the embryo is almost straight, and the **somites** form conspicuous surface elevations (Figs. 2-8 and 2-9). A significant event occurring during the fourth week is folding of the flat trilaminar embryonic disc into an embryo (Figs. 2-7, *F,* 2-9, and 2-10).

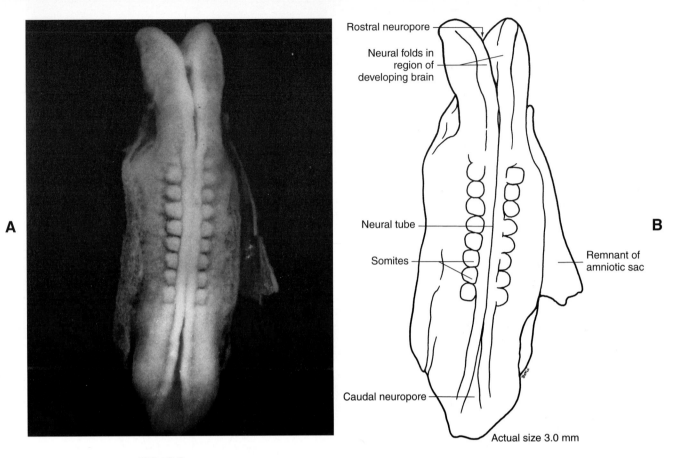

Rostral neuropore

Neural folds in region of developing brain

Neural tube

Somites

Remnant of amniotic sac

Caudal neuropore

Actual size 3.0 mm

FIG. 2-9

A, Dorsal view of an eight-somite embryo at Carnegie stage 10, about 22 days. **B**, Diagram indicating the structures shown in *A*. The neural folds have fused opposite the somites to form the neural tube (primordium of the spinal cord in this region). The neural tube is in open communication with the amniotic cavity at the cranial and caudal ends by way of the rostral and caudal neuropores, respectively.

Embryonic folding occurs in both the median and horizontal planes and results from the rapid growth of the embryo, particularly the central nervous system (CNS), that is, the brain and spinal cord. Folding of the embryo produces *head and tail folds* that result in the cranial and caudal regions moving ventrally (see Fig. 2-10). Folding of the embryo in the horizontal plane produces right and left *lateral folds*. Each fold moves toward the median plane, rolling the embryonic disc ventrally and forming a roughly cylindrical embryo (see Fig. 2-12; see also Fig. 6-2).

Fusion of the neural folds in the fourth week forms the **neural tube** (see Figs. 2-7 and 2-8), the primordium of the CNS. The *neural folds* at the cranial end of the embryo thicken to form the primordium of the brain (see Figs. 2-7 to 2-9). By the middle of the fourth week, the neural tube is formed opposite the somites, but it is widely open at the rostral and caudal **neuropores** (see Figs. 2-7 and 2-9). The rostral (anterior) neuropore normally closes on days 24 to 26, and the caudal (posterior) neuropore closes by 28 days. The embryo is now slightly curved as a result of the head and tail folds, and the heart produces a large ventral prominence (see Fig. 2-10).

As the neural tube separates from the surface ectoderm, the **neural crest** forms (see Fig. 2-7). It forms an irregular, flattened cellular mass between the neural tube and the surface ectoderm. *Neural crest cells* migrating from this crest give rise to spinal ganglia (dorsal root ganglia), autonomic ganglia, and the ganglia of certain cranial nerves. These

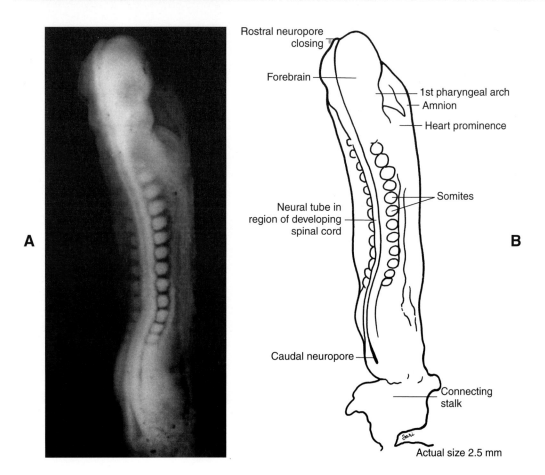

FIG. 2-10

A, Dorsal view of a 13-somite embryo at Carnegie stage 11, about 24 days. **B,** Diagram indicating the structures shown in *A*. The embryo is curved due to folding at the cranial and caudal ends. The rostral neuropore is almost closed, but the caudal neuropore is widely open.

cells also form the sheaths of peripheral nerves, the meninges covering the CNS, and various other structures, such as skeletal and muscular components in the head and neck (see Chapter 7).

Three pairs of *pharyngeal (branchial) arches* are visible by 26 days (Figs. 2-11 and 2-12), and the rostral neuropore is closed. Failure of this neuropore to close results in meroanencephaly (anencephaly [see Fig. 13-12]) or meningoencephalocele (see Fig. 13-10). Failure of the caudal neuropore to close results in *spina bifida* (see Fig. 13-15). The *forebrain* now produces a prominent elevation of the head, and folding of the embryo in the median plane has given the embryo a characteristic C-shaped curvature.

Limb buds appear as swellings on the ventrolateral body walls by the end of the fourth week (see Fig. 2-12). The *otic pits,* the primordia of the internal ears, are also clearly visible. Four pairs of **pharyngeal arches** are also visible by the end of the fourth week (see Fig. 2-12). They are involved with the formation of the head and neck (see Chapter 7). Ectodermal thickenings called *lens placodes,* indicating the future lenses of the eyes, are visible on the sides of the head. By the end of the fourth week, the *attenuated tail* is a characteristic feature (Figs. 2-12 and 2-13).

Because the CNS, heart, limbs, eyes, and ears are in their critical stages of development during the fourth week, teratogenic agents may cause severe congenital anomalies (e.g., absence of the limbs and congenital cataracts; see Chapter 5).

Text continued on p. 32

FIG. 2-11

A, Lateral view of a 27-somite embryo at Carnegie stage 12, about 26 days. **B,** Diagram indicating the structures shown in *A.* Not all the somites are visible in this photograph. The rostral neuropore is closed and three pairs of pharyngeal arches are present. The mandibular prominence of the first arch (primordium of the lower jaw) forms the caudal boundary of the stomodeum (primordium of the mouth). The embryo is very curved, especially its long tail. Observe the lens placode (primordium of the lens) and the otic pit indicating early development of the internal ear (see Chapter 14). (From Nishimura H, et al: *Prenatal development of the human with special reference to craniofacial structures: an atlas,* Washington, DC, 1977, National Institutes of Health.)

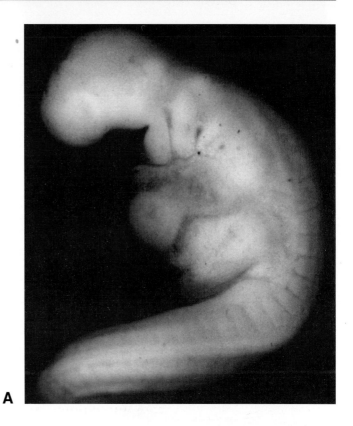

A

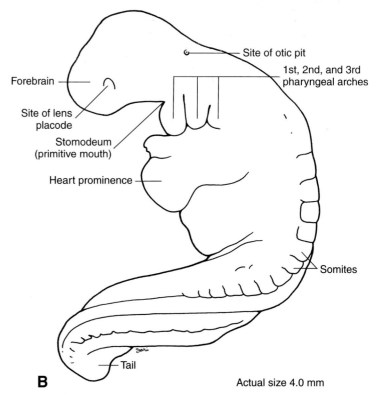

B

Actual size 4.0 mm

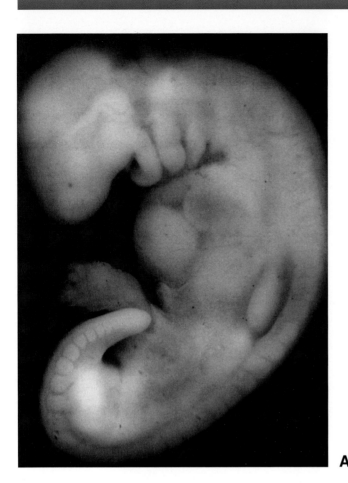

A

FIG. 2-12
A, Lateral view of an embryo at Carnegie stage 13, about 28 days. **B,** Drawing indicating the structures shown in A. The embryo has a characteristic C-shaped curvature, four pharyngeal arches, and upper and lower limb buds. The heart is large and its division into a primitive atrium and ventricle is visible. The rostral and caudal neuropores are closed. (From Nishimura H, et al: *Prenatal development of the human with special reference to craniofacial structures: an atlas,* Washington, DC, 1977, National Institutes of Health.)

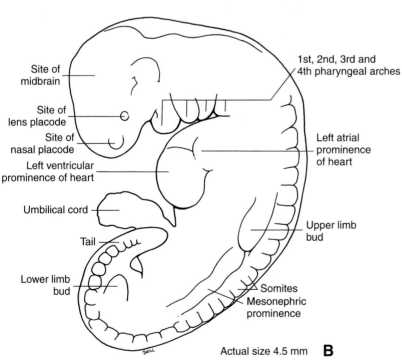

Site of midbrain

Site of lens placode

Site of nasal placode

Left ventricular prominence of heart

Umbilical cord

Tail

Lower limb bud

1st, 2nd, 3rd and 4th pharyngeal arches

Left atrial prominence of heart

Upper limb bud

Somites
Mesonephric prominence

Actual size 4.5 mm **B**

FIG. 2-13

Selected serial sections of an embryo at Carnegie stage 13, about 28 days. The level of each section is indicated on the small sketch of the embryo. **A,** The thin-walled roof of the hindbrain (rhombencephalon). **B,** The thicker, dorsal part of the hindbrain and the otic vesicles (primordia of the membranous labyrinth of the internal ear).

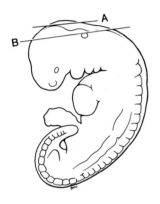

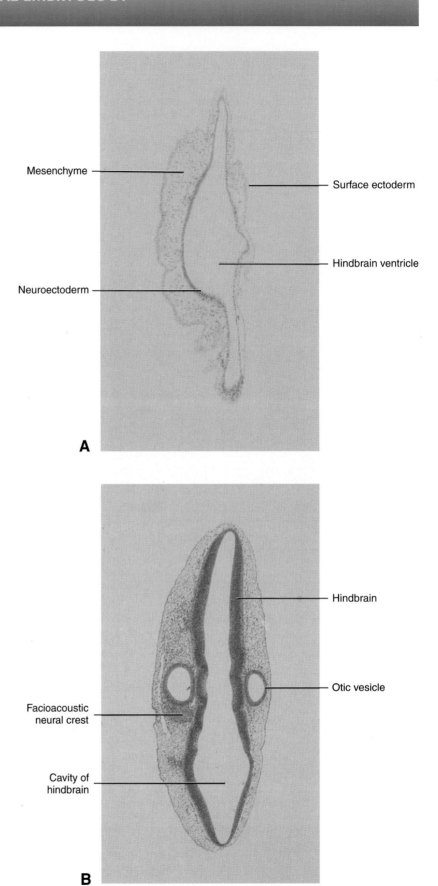

Mesenchyme

Surface ectoderm

Hindbrain ventricle

Neuroectoderm

A

Hindbrain

Otic vesicle

Facioacoustic neural crest

Cavity of hindbrain

B

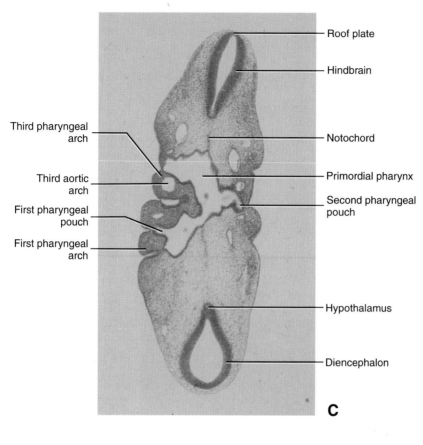

Roof plate

Hindbrain

Third pharyngeal arch

Notochord

Third aortic arch

Primordial pharynx

First pharyngeal pouch

Second pharyngeal pouch

First pharyngeal arch

Hypothalamus

Diencephalon

C

FIG. 2-13, cont'd

C, The diencephalon, hindbrain, and the primordial pharynx. Observe the first three pharyngeal arches and the first and second pharyngeal pouches. **D,** The forebrain, spinal cord, primordial pharynx, edge of the optic vesicle, and the truncus arteriosus of the embryonic heart.   *Continued*

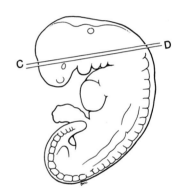

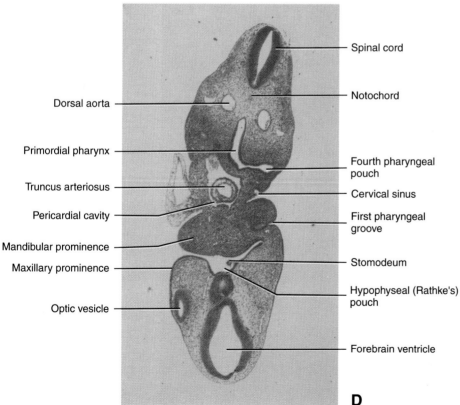

Spinal cord

Dorsal aorta

Notochord

Primordial pharynx

Fourth pharyngeal pouch

Truncus arteriosus

Cervical sinus

Pericardial cavity

First pharyngeal groove

Mandibular prominence

Stomodeum

Maxillary prominence

Hypophyseal (Rathke's) pouch

Optic vesicle

Forebrain ventricle

D

FIG. 2-13, cont'd

E, The diencephalon, spinal cord, embryonic heart, and optic vesicle. **F,** The forebrain, spinal cord, heart, esophagus, tracheal bifurcation, and the communication between the forebrain and the optic vesicle.

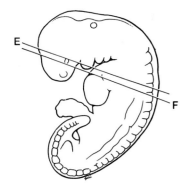

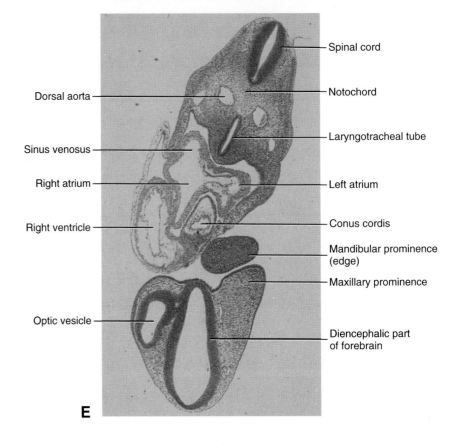

Dorsal aorta

Sinus venosus

Right atrium

Right ventricle

Optic vesicle

Spinal cord

Notochord

Laryngotracheal tube

Left atrium

Conus cordis

Mandibular prominence (edge)

Maxillary prominence

Diencephalic part of forebrain

E

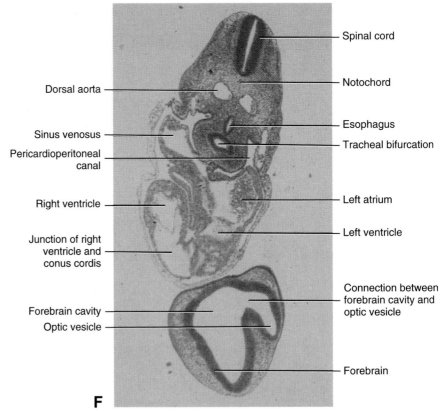

Dorsal aorta

Sinus venosus

Pericardioperitoneal canal

Right ventricle

Junction of right ventricle and conus cordis

Forebrain cavity

Optic vesicle

Spinal cord

Notochord

Esophagus

Tracheal bifurcation

Left atrium

Left ventricle

Connection between forebrain cavity and optic vesicle

Forebrain

F

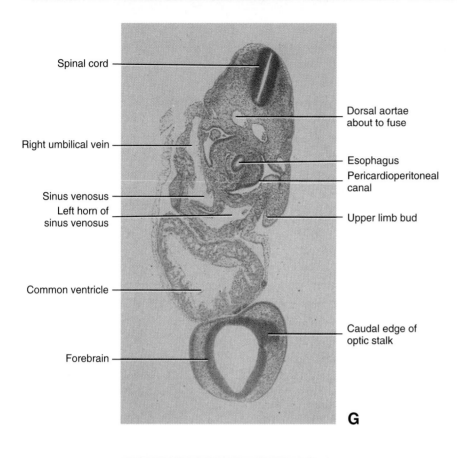

Spinal cord

Right umbilical vein

Sinus venosus

Left horn of sinus venosus

Common ventricle

Forebrain

Dorsal aortae about to fuse

Esophagus

Pericardioperitoneal canal

Upper limb bud

Caudal edge of optic stalk

G

FIG. 2-13, cont'd

G, The forebrain, caudal edge of the optic stalk, the heart, and the esophagus. Observe the pericardioperitoneal canal that connects the pericardial and peritoneal cavities (see Chapter 6). **H,** The common ventricle, sinus venosus, upper limb bud, primitive stomach, and spinal cord. *Continued*

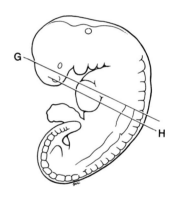

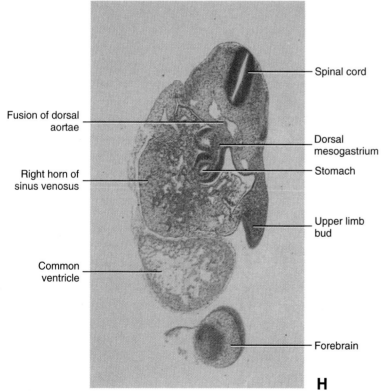

Fusion of dorsal aortae

Right horn of sinus venosus

Common ventricle

Spinal cord

Dorsal mesogastrium

Stomach

Upper limb bud

Forebrain

H

FIG. 2-13, cont'd

I, The common ventricle of the heart, upper limb bud, duodenum, liver, and spinal cord. **J,** The caudal end of the embryo showing the lower limb bud, hindgut, urogenital sinus, and umbilical arteries.

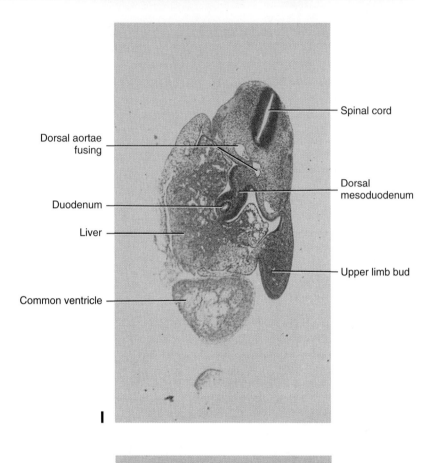

Spinal cord

Dorsal aortae fusing

Dorsal mesoduodenum

Duodenum

Liver

Upper limb bud

Common ventricle

I

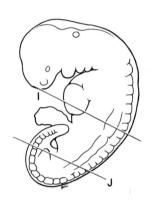

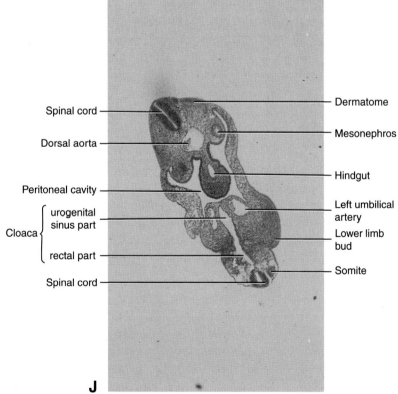

Dermatome

Spinal cord

Mesonephros

Dorsal aorta

Hindgut

Peritoneal cavity

Left umbilical artery

Cloaca { urogenital sinus part

Lower limb bud

rectal part

Spinal cord

Somite

J

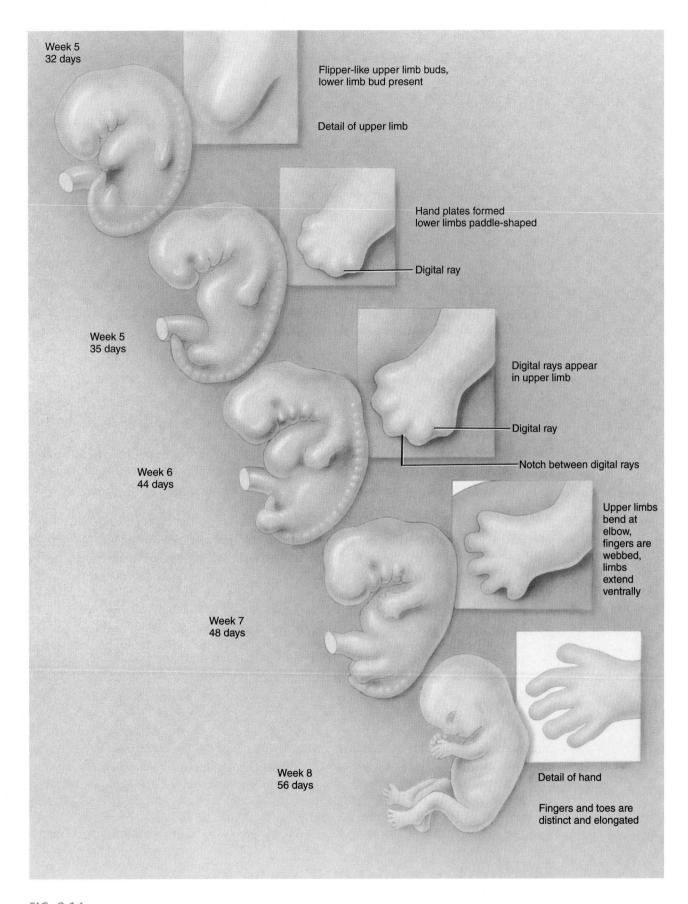

Week 5
32 days

Flipper-like upper limb buds,
lower limb bud present

Detail of upper limb

Hand plates formed
lower limbs paddle-shaped

Digital ray

Week 5
35 days

Digital rays appear
in upper limb

Digital ray

Notch between digital rays

Week 6
44 days

Upper limbs
bend at
elbow,
fingers are
webbed,
limbs
extend
ventrally

Week 7
48 days

Detail of hand

Week 8
56 days

Fingers and toes are
distinct and elongated

FIG. 2-14

**Drawings of lateral views of embryos ranging in age from 32 to 56 days. Development of
the upper limbs is highlighted because their appearance is a reliable guide to stages 13 to 23
of development (see Table 2-1).**

THE FIFTH TO EIGHTH WEEKS

The Fifth Week

Changes in body form are minor during this week compared with those that occurred during the fourth week, but growth of the head exceeds that of other regions because of the rapid development of the brain (Figs. 2-14, 2-15, *A*, and 2-16). The face soon contacts the heart prominence. The second pharyngeal arch has overgrown the third and fourth arches, forming an ectodermal depression known as the **cervical sinus** (Fig. 2-16). The distal ends of the upper limbs become paddle-shaped. It has been reported that embryos show spontaneous movements in the fifth week, such as twitching of the trunk and limbs.

The Sixth Week

The upper limbs show rapid regional differentiation during the sixth week (Figs. 2-17 to 2-20). The elbow and wrist regions are clearly identifiable and **digital rays,** indicating the future digits, are clearly visible by the end of the sixth week (see Fig. 2-20). Development of the lower limbs occurs about two days later than that of the upper limbs (see Fig. 2-14). Six small swellings develop around the pharyngeal groove between the first two pharyngeal arches (see Figs. 2-18 and 2-20). This groove becomes the *external acoustic meatus* and the swellings around it fuse to form the auricle (pinna) of the external ear. Largely because *retinal pigment* has formed, the eye is now obvious (see Figs. 2-15, *B*, 2-18, and 2-20). The head is now much larger relative to the trunk and is more bent over the **heart prominence.** This head position results from bending of the brain in the cervical region.

The Seventh and Eighth Weeks

The limbs undergo considerable change during the seventh week (Figs. 2-21 and 2-22). Notches appear between the digital rays in the hand plates, clearly indicating the future digits. At the beginning of the eighth week, the digits of the hand are short and noticeably webbed (Fig. 2-23). Notches are now clearly visible between the digital rays of the feet, and the tail is still present but stubby (Fig. 2-23). The **scalp vascular plexus** soon appears and forms a characteristic band around the head (Figs. 2-23 to 2-25). By the end of the eighth week, all regions of the limbs are apparent, and the digits have lengthened and are separated (see Figs. 2-14, 2-15, *C*, and 2-25). *Purposeful limb movements* first occur during the eighth week. All evidence of the tail disappears by the end of the eighth week. The scalp vascular plexus is now located near the vertex of the head (Fig. 2-26).

By the end of the eighth week, the embryo has distinct human characteristics; however, the head is still disproportionately large, constituting almost half of the embryo. The neck region is established and the eyelids are more obvious. Early in the eighth week the eyes are open but, toward the end of the week, the eyelids move toward each other. The auricles of the external ears begin to assume their final shape but are still low-set on the head. Although sex differences exist in the appearance of the external genitalia (Fig. 2-27), they are not distinct enough to permit accurate sexual identification by lay people.

METHODS OF MEASURING EMBRYOS

Because embryos early in the fourth week are straight, measurements of them indicate the greatest length (GL). The sitting height, or *crown rump length* (CRL), is most frequently used for older embryos. Standing height, or crown heel length (CHL), is sometimes mea-

Text continued on p. 48

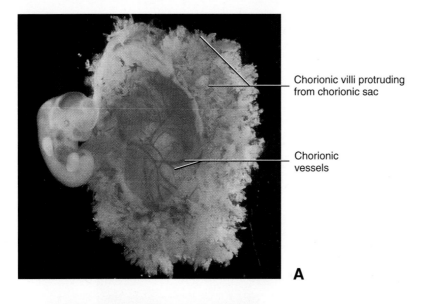

Chorionic villi protruding from chorionic sac

Chorionic vessels

A

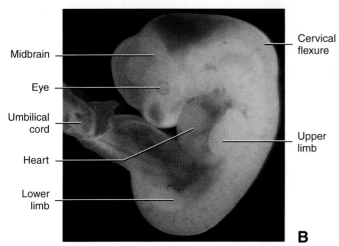

Midbrain

Eye

Umbilical cord

Heart

Lower limb

Cervical flexure

Upper limb

B

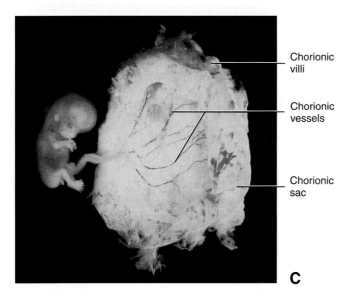

Chorionic villi

Chorionic vessels

Chorionic sac

C

FIG. 2-15

Photographs of embryos during the fifth to eighth weeks. The embryos have been removed from their amniotic and chorionic sacs. **A**, Lateral view of an embryo at Carnegie stage 14, about 32 days (see also Fig. 2-16). Observe that the chorionic sac is completely covered by chorionic villi. **B**, Lateral view of an embryo at Carnegie stage 15, about 36 days (see also Fig. 2-17). Pigment in the retina makes the eye clearly visible. **C**, Lateral view of an embryo at Carnegie stage 23, about 56 days (see also Figs. 2-26 and 2-27). Observe its human appearance. (From Nishimura H, et al: *Prenatal development of the human with special reference to craniofacial structures: an atlas,* Washington, DC, 1977, National Institutes of Health.)

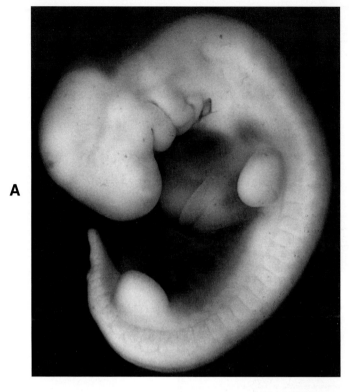

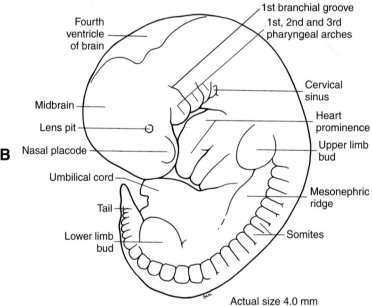

FIG. 2-16

A, Lateral view of an embryo at Carnegie stage 14, about 32 days. **B,** Drawings indicating the structures shown in *A*. The upper limb buds are paddle-shaped and the lower limb buds are flipperlike. The second pharyngeal arch has overgrown the third arch forming an ectoderm depression known as the cervical sinus. The mesonephric ridge indicates the site of the mesonephric kidney, and interim kidney (see Chapter 10). (From Nishimura H, et al: *Prenatal development of the human with special reference to craniofacial structures: an atlas,* Washington, DC, 1977, National Institutes of Health.)

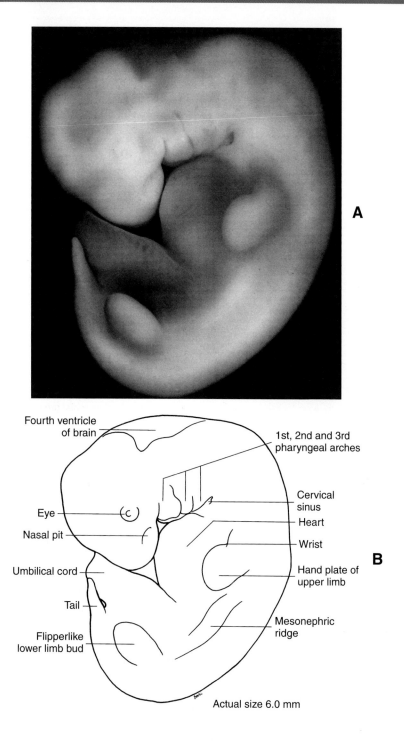

Fourth ventricle of brain

1st, 2nd and 3rd pharyngeal arches

Cervical sinus

Eye

Heart

Nasal pit

Wrist

Umbilical cord

Hand plate of upper limb

Tail

Mesonephric ridge

Flipperlike lower limb bud

Actual size 6.0 mm

FIG. 2-17

A, Lateral view of an embryo at Carnegie stage 15, about 36 days. **B,** Drawings indicating the structures shown in *A.* The nasal pit (primordium of the nasal aperture and cavity) is now visible, as is the wrist region. The third and fourth pharyngeal arches are indistinct as a result of overgrowth of them by the second arch. The fourth arch is in the cervical sinus. (From Nishimura H, et al: *Prenatal development of the human with special reference to craniofacial structures: an atlas,* Washington, DC, 1977, National Institutes of Health.)

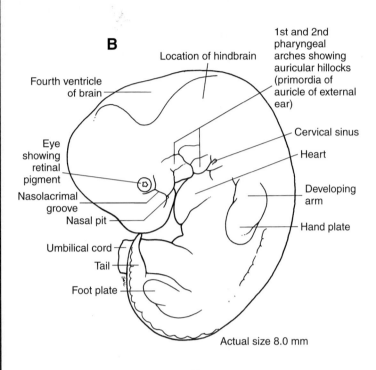

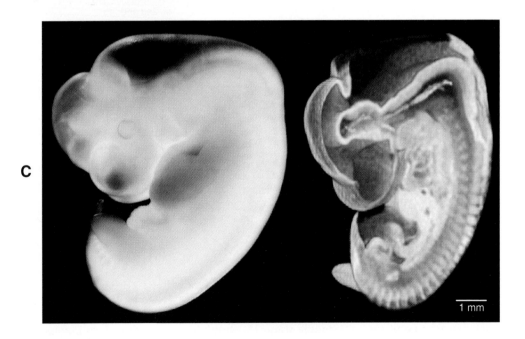

FIG. 2-18

A, Lateral view of an embryo at Carnegie stage 16, about 40 days. **B,** Drawing indicating the structures shown in *A*. The eye is distinct, as are the nasal pit and nasolacrimal groove (primordium of the nasolacrimal duct). The hand plate is more distinct and the foot plate has formed. Small swellings, called auricular hillocks, have developed around the first branchial groove (primordium of the external acoustic meatus). The auricular hillocks fuse to form the auricle of the external ear (see Chapter 14). **C,** A Carnegie stage 16 human embryo about 37 days postovulation, imaged with optical microscopy *(left)* and magnetic resonance microscopy (MRM) *(right)*. The three-dimensional data set from MRM has been edited to reveal anatomical detail from a midsagittal plane. (Courtesy of Dr. Bradley R. Smith, Center for In Vivo Microscopy, Duke University Medical Center, Durham, North Carolina.)

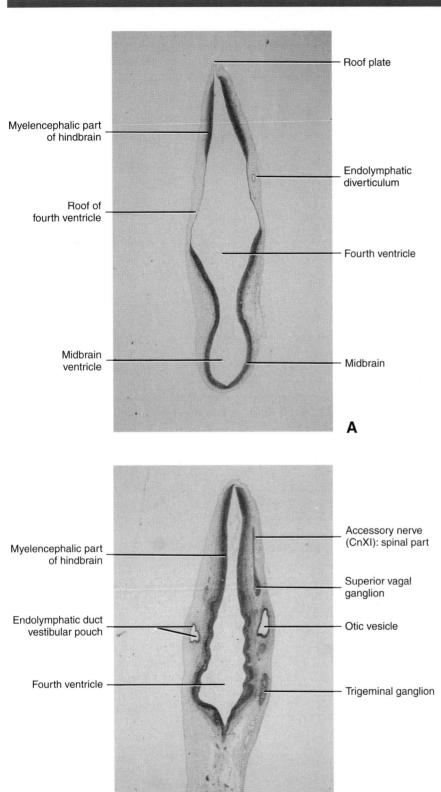

Roof plate

Myelencephalic part
of hindbrain

Endolymphatic
diverticulum

Roof of
fourth ventricle

Fourth ventricle

Midbrain
ventricle

Midbrain

A

Myelencephalic part
of hindbrain

Accessory nerve
(CnXI): spinal part

Superior vagal
ganglion

Endolymphatic duct
vestibular pouch

Otic vesicle

Fourth ventricle

Trigeminal ganglion

Midbrain

B

FIG. 2-19

Selected serial sections of an embryo at Carnegie stage 16, about 40 days. The level of each section is indicated on the small sketch of the embryo. A, The midbrain and the roof of the fourth ventricle. B, The cephalic flexure, midbrain, fourth ventricle, otic vesicle, and trigeminal ganglion.

Continued

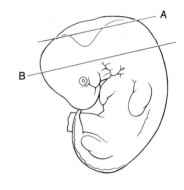

FIG. 2-19, cont'd

C, The third ventricle, spinal cord, primordial pharynx, stomodeum (primordial mouth), developing tongue, optic cup, and lens vesicle. Observe the first and second pharyngeal arches. **D,** The cerebral vesicle, lateral ventricle, ventricles of the heart, esophagus, and trachea.

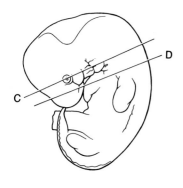

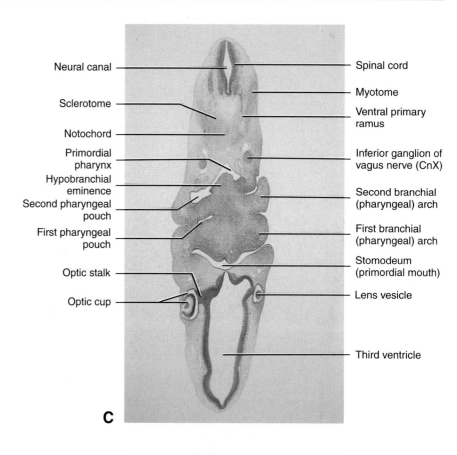

Neural canal — Spinal cord

Sclerotome — Myotome

— Ventral primary ramus

Notochord

Primordial pharynx — Inferior ganglion of vagus nerve (CnX)

Hypobranchial eminence

Second pharyngeal pouch — Second branchial (pharyngeal) arch

First pharyngeal pouch — First branchial (pharyngeal) arch

— Stomodeum (primordial mouth)

Optic stalk

Optic cup — Lens vesicle

— Third ventricle

C

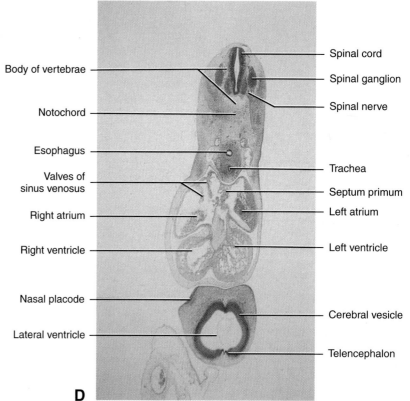

Body of vertebrae — Spinal cord

— Spinal ganglion

Notochord — Spinal nerve

Esophagus

Valves of sinus venosus — Trachea

Right atrium — Septum primum

— Left atrium

Right ventricle — Left ventricle

Nasal placode

Lateral ventricle — Cerebral vesicle

— Telencephalon

D

Spinal cord

Roof plate

Spinal ganglion

Basal plate

Upper limb bud

Left dorsal aorta

Esophagus
Superior lobar bud

Left primary brondius

Right horn of sinus venosus

Liver

Liver

Left ventricle

Umbilical cord

E

Vertebral arch

Spinal cord

Spinal ganglion

Body of vertebra

Upper limb

Mesonephros

Liver

Stomach

Serosa of liver

Ductus venosus

Umbilical coelom

Right umbilical artery

Allantois

Umbilical cord

Umbilical vein

Spinal cord in tail of embryo

F

FIG. 2-19, cont'd

E, The liver, left primary bronchus, heart, esophagus, and upper limb bud. **F,** The tail of the embryo, umbilical cord, liver, stomach, mesonephros, upper limb, and spinal cord.   *Continued*

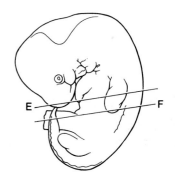

FIG. 2-19, cont'd

G, The lower limb buds, mesonephros, and spinal cord. **H,** The caudal end of the embryo.

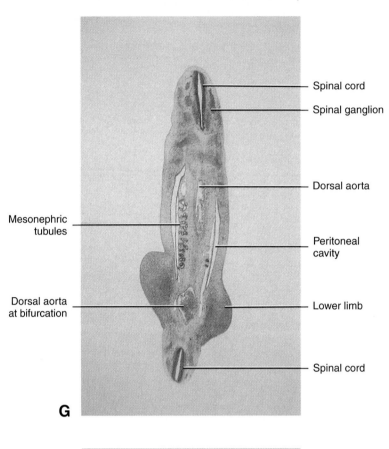

Spinal cord

Spinal ganglion

Dorsal aorta

Mesonephric tubules

Peritoneal cavity

Dorsal aorta at bifurcation

Lower limb

Spinal cord

G

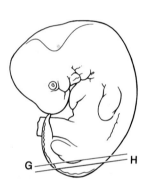

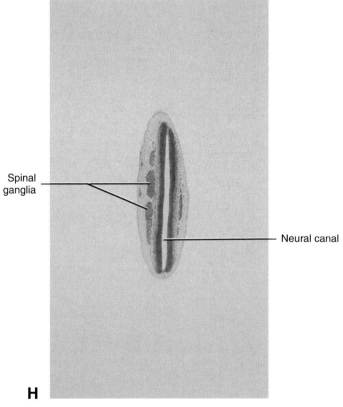

Spinal ganglia

Neural canal

H

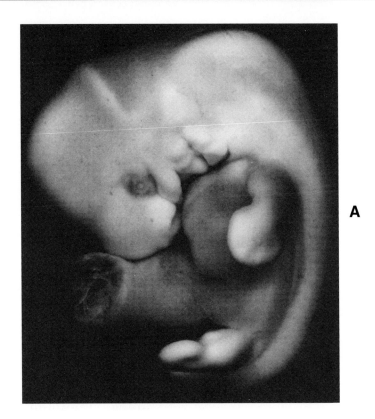

A

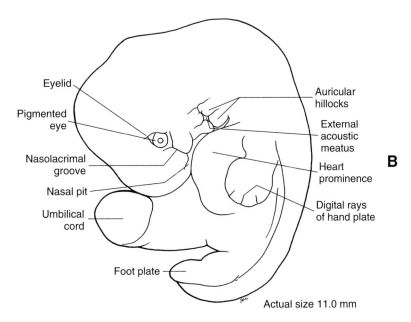

Eyelid

Pigmented eye

Nasolacrimal groove

Nasal pit

Umbilical cord

Foot plate

Auricular hillocks

External acoustic meatus

Heart prominence

Digital rays of hand plate

B

Actual size 11.0 mm

FIG. 2-20

A, Lateral view of an embryo at Carnegie stage 17, about 42 days. **B,** Drawing indicating the structures shown in *A*. The eye, auricular hillocks (primordia of external ear), and external acoustic meatus (auditory canal) are now more obvious. Digital rays in the large hand plate, indicating the future site of the digits, are now clearly visible.

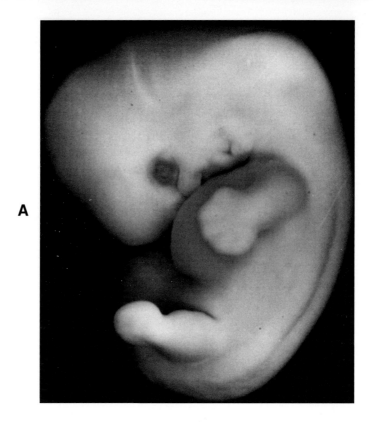

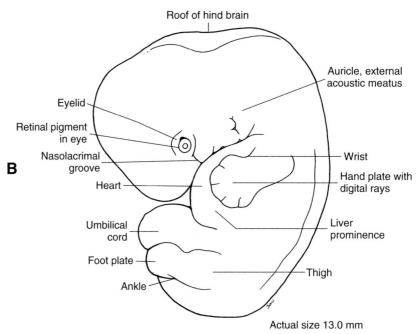

Roof of hind brain

Auricle, external
acoustic meatus

Eyelid

Retinal pigment
in eye

Nasolacrimal
groove

Wrist

Hand plate with
digital rays

B

Heart

Umbilical
cord

Liver
prominence

Foot plate

Thigh

Ankle

Actual size 13.0 mm

FIG. 2-21

A, Lateral view of an embryo at Carnegie stage 18, about 44 days. **B,** Drawing indicating the structures shown in *A*. The eye is prominent as a result of the presence of retinal pigment. The hand plate is very large and the digital rays are distinctive. The foot plate is well formed and the ankle region is visible. The auricle of the external ear is now distinguishable. The branchial (pharyngeal) arches are no longer distinct and the cervical sinus (visible in Fig. 2-16) has disappeared. (From Nishimura H, et al: *Prenatal development of the human with special reference to craniofacial structures: an atlas,* Washington, DC, 1977, National Institutes of Health.)

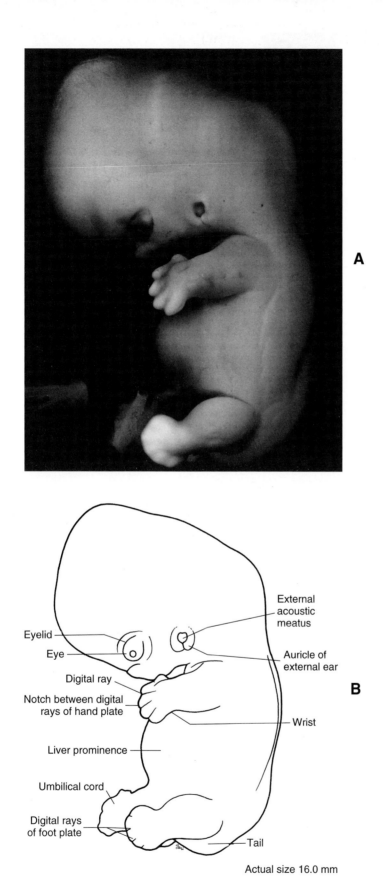

Actual size 16.0 mm

FIG. 2-22

A, Lateral view of an embryo at Carnegie stage 19, about 48 days. **B,** Drawing indicating the structures shown in *A*. The notches between the digital rays in the hand clearly indicate the developing digits. The auricle and external acoustic meatus are now clearly visible. Note the low position of the ear at this stage. Digital rays are now visible in the foot plate. The prominence of the abdomen is caused mainly by the large size of the liver.

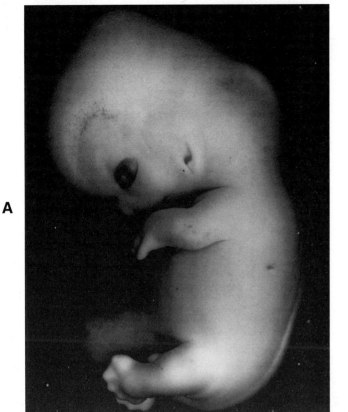

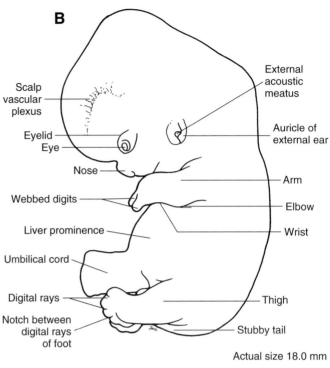

B

Scalp vascular plexus

External acoustic meatus

Eyelid
Eye

Auricle of external ear

Nose

Arm

Webbed digits

Elbow

Liver prominence

Wrist

Umbilical cord

Digital rays

Thigh

Notch between digital rays of foot

Stubby tail

Actual size 18.0 mm

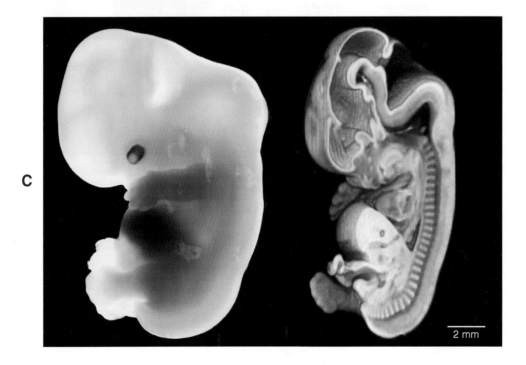

2 mm

FIG. 2-23

A, Lateral view of an embryo at Carnegie stage 20, about 51 days. **B,** Drawing indicating the structures shown in *A*. The limbs now extend ventrally. The fingers are well formed but are short and webbed. The upper limb is bent at the elbow. Notches have now appeared between the digital rays of the foot. The scalp vascular plexus is now visible. A stubby tail is still present. **C,** A Carnegie stage 20 human embryo, about 50 days postovulation, imaged with optical microscopy (left) and magnetic resonance microscopy (MRM) (right). The three-dimensional data set from MRM has been edited to reveal anatomical detail from a mid-sagittal plane. (**A** and **B,** From Nishimura H, et al: *Prenatal development of the human with special reference to craniofacial structures: an atlas,* Washington, DC, 1977, National Institutes of Health. **C,** Courtesy of Dr. Bradley R. Smith, Center for In Vivo Microscopy, Duke University Medical Center, Durham, North Carolina.)

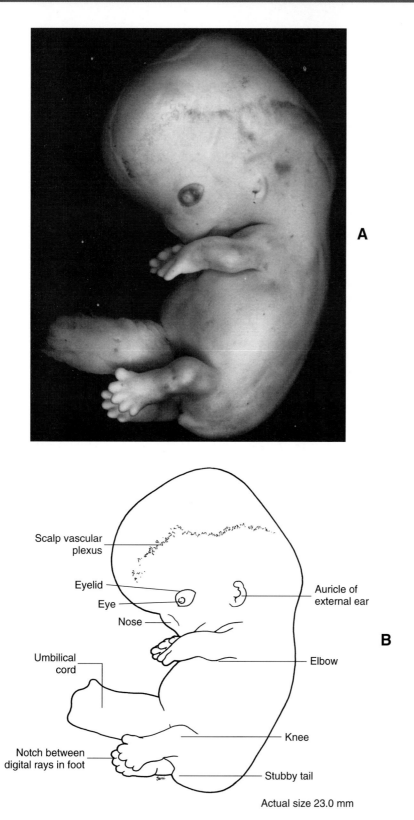

Scalp vascular plexus

Eyelid

Eye

Nose

Auricle of external ear

Umbilical cord

Elbow

Notch between digital rays in foot

Knee

Stubby tail

Actual size 23.0 mm

FIG. 2-24

A, Lateral view of an embryo at Carnegie stage 21, about 52 days. **B,** Drawing indicating the structures shown in *A.* The fingers are separated and the toes are beginning to separate. Note that the feet are fan-shaped and that the tail is very short. The scalp vascular plexus now forms a characteristic band across the head. The nose is stubby and the eye is heavily pigmented. (From Nishimura H, et al: *Prenatal development of the human with special reference to craniofacial structures: an atlas,* Washington, DC, 1977, National Institutes of Health.)

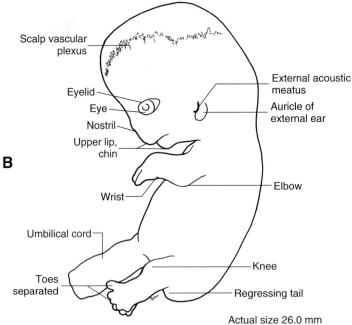

Scalp vascular plexus

Eyelid

Eye

Nostril

Upper lip, chin

Wrist

Umbilical cord

Toes separated

External acoustic meatus

Auricle of external ear

Elbow

Knee

Regressing tail

Actual size 26.0 mm

FIG. 2-25

A, Lateral view of an embryo at Carnegie stage 22, about 54 days. **B,** Drawing indicating the structures shown in *A*. The toes are separate but short. The eyelids and auricle are well developed. The chin and jaw are distinctive but underdeveloped because of the absence of teeth. The tail has almost disappeared. (From Nishimura H, et al: *Prenatal development of the human with special reference to craniofacial structures: an atlas,* Washington, DC, 1977, National Institutes of Health.)

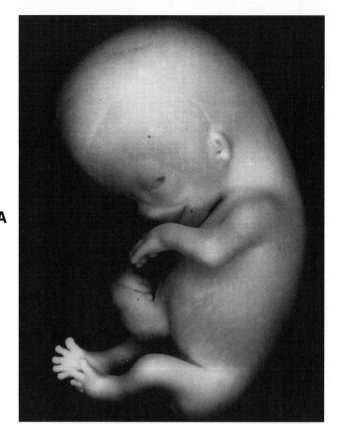

A

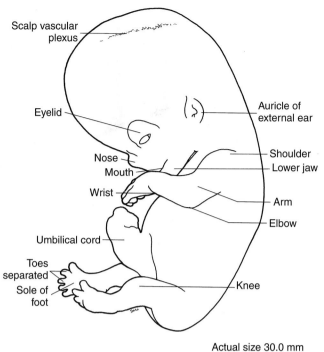

Scalp vascular
plexus

Eyelid

Nose

Mouth

Wrist

Umbilical cord

Toes
separated

Sole of
foot

Auricle of
external ear

Shoulder

Lower jaw

Arm

Elbow

Knee

B

Actual size 30.0 mm

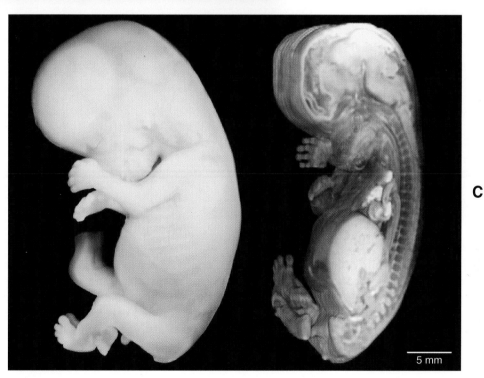

C

5 mm

FIG. 2-26

A, Lateral view of an embryo at Carnegie stage 23, about 56 days (see also Fig. 2-27). **B,** Drawing indicating the structures shown in *A.* The eyelids are closer to each other (compare with Fig. 2-25). The scalp vascular plexus is reduced and the tail has disappeared. The embryo now has a distinct human appearance. **C,** A Carnegie stage 23 human embryo, about 56 days postovulation, imaged with optical microscopy *(left)* and magnetic resonance microscopy (MRM) *(right).* The three-dimensional data set from MRM has been edited to reveal anatomical detail from a midsagittal plane. (**A** and **B,** From Nishimura H, et al: *Prenatal development of the human with special reference to craniofacial structures: an atlas,* Washington, DC, 1977, National Institutes of Health. **C,** Courtesy of Dr. Bradley R. Smith, Center for In Vivo Microscopy, Duke University Medical Center, Durham, North Carolina.)

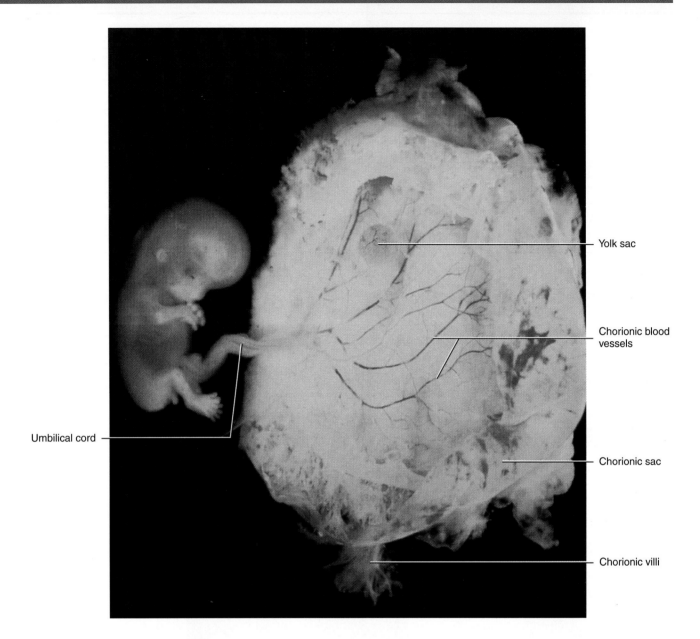

Yolk sac

Chorionic blood vessels

Chorionic sac

Chorionic villi

Umbilical cord

FIG. 2-27

Photograph of an embryo at Carnegie stage 23, about 56 days. The embryo has been removed from its chorionic sac. The yolk sac is very small at this stage and will soon disappear (compare with Fig. 4-3, *A*). Note the large size of the head in comparison to the rest of the body. Although the phallus is large, sex cannot be determined externally at this stage because the primordial genital organ is similar in both sexes at this age (see Chapter 10).

sured for 8-week-old embryos (Table 2-1). To estimate the age of aborted embryos, the *Carnegie Embryonic Staging System* is used. It is based on morphologic developmental landmarks of the embryo. The size of an embryo in a pregnant woman can be estimated using ultrasound measurements (see Chapter 4). *Transvaginal sonographs* permit an earlier and more accurate measurement of CRL in early pregnancy. Current data indicate that there are no confirmed biological effects of ultrasound on embryos or fetuses from the use of diagnostic ultrasound evaluation.

TABLE 2-1

Criteria for Estimating Developmental Stages in Human Embryos

Age (Days)	Figure Reference	Carnegie Stage	No. of Somites	Length (mm)*	Main External Characteristics†
19-21	2-6A₁	9	1-3	1.5-3.0	*Flat embryonic disc. Deep neural groove and prominent neural folds. One to three pairs of somites present.* Head fold evident.
22-23	2-8A 2-9A	10	4-12	2.0-3.5	*Embryo straight or slightly curved.* Neural tube forming or formed opposite somites, but widely open at rostral and caudal neuropores. First and second pairs of branchial arches visible.
24-25	2-10A	11	13-20	2.5-4.5	*Embryo curved opening to head and tail folds.* Rostral neuropore closing. Otic placodes present. Optic vesicles formed.
26-27	2-11A	12	21-29	3.0-5.0	*Upper limb buds appear.* Rostral neuropore closed. Caudal neuropore closing. Three pairs of branchial arches visible. Heart prominence distinct. Otic pits present.
28-30	2-12A 2-13B 2-13C 2-13I 2-13J	13	30-35	4.0-6.0	*Embryo has C-shaped curve.* Caudal neuropore closed. Upper limb buds flipperlike. Four pairs of branchial arches visible. Lower limb buds appear. *Otic vesicles* present. Lens placodes distinct. Attenuated *tail* present.
31-32	2-16A	14	‡	5.0-7.0	*Upper limbs paddle-shaped.* Lens pits and nasal pits visible. Optic cups present.
33-36	2-17A	15		7.0-9.0	*Hand plates formed; digital rays present.* Lens vesicles present. Nasal pits prominent. *Lower limbs paddle-shaped.* Cervical sinuses visible.
37-40	2-18A 2-18C	16		8.0-11.0	*Foot plates formed.* Pigment visible in retina. Auricular hillocks developing.
41-43	2-20A	17		11.0-14.0	*Digital rays clearly visible in hand plates.* Auricle hillocks outline future auricle of external ear. Trunk beginning to straighten. Cerebral vesicles prominent.
44-46	2-21A	18		13.0-17.0	*Digital rays clearly visible in foot plates.* Elbow region visible. Eyelids forming. Notches between the digital rays in the hands. Nipples visible.
47-48	2-22A	19		16.0-18.0	*Limbs extend ventrally.* Trunk elongating and straightening. Midgut herniation prominent.
49-51	2-23A 2-23C	20		18.0-22.0	*Upper limbs longer and bent at elbows. Fingers distinct but webbed.* Notches between the digital rays in the feet. Scalp vascular plexus appears.
52-53	2-24A	21		22.0-24.0	*Hands and feet approach each other. Fingers free and longer. Toes distinct but webbed.* Stubby tail present.
54-55	2-25A	22		23.0-28.0	*Toes free and longer.* Eyelids and auricles or external ears more developed.
56	2-26A 2-26C 2-27	23		27.0-31.0	*Head more rounded and shows human characteristics.* External genitalia still have sexless appearance. Distinct bulge still present in umbilical cord, caused by herniation of intestines. *Tail has disappeared.*

*The embryonic lengths indicate the usual range. In stages 9 and 10, the measurement is greatest length *(GL)*; in subsequent stages crown-rump *(CR)* measurements are given.

†Based on Nishimura, et al (1974), O'Rahilly and Müller (1987), and Shiota (1991).

‡At this and subsequent stages, the number of somites is difficult to determine and so is not a useful criterion.

3

The Ninth to Thirty-Eighth Weeks of Human Development

Development during the **fetal period** (ninth to thirty-eighth weeks) is primarily concerned with rapid growth of the body and differentiation of tissues and organs that started to develop during the embryonic period (see Chapter 2). A notable change occurring during the fetal period is the relative slowdown in the growth of the head compared with the rest of the body. The rate of body growth during the fetal period is rapid, especially between the ninth and sixteenth weeks (Fig. 3-1), and fetal weight gain is phenomenal during the terminal weeks. Periods of normal continuous growth alternate with prolonged intervals of absent growth.

ESTIMATION OF FETAL AGE

If doubt arises about the age of a fetus, ultrasound measurements are taken to determine its size and probable age, and to provide a reliable prediction of the *expected date of confinement* (EDC) for delivery of the fetus. The intrauterine period may be divided into days, weeks, or months, but confusion arises if it is not stated whether the age is calculated from: (1) the onset of the last normal menstrual period (LNMP), or (2) the estimated day of fertilization (see Fig. 1-3). Most uncertainty arises when months are used, particularly when it is not stated whether calendar months (28 to 31 days) or lunar months (28 days) are meant. Fetal age in this atlas is calculated from the estimated time of fertilization, and months refer to calendar months. It is best to express fetal age in weeks and to state whether the beginning or end of a week is meant because statements such as in the tenth week are nonspecific.

Various measurements and external characteristics are useful for estimating fetal age (Table 3-1). *Crown rump length* (CRL) is usually the most reliable measurement, but the length of fetuses, like that of infants, varies considerably for a given

The Fetal Period

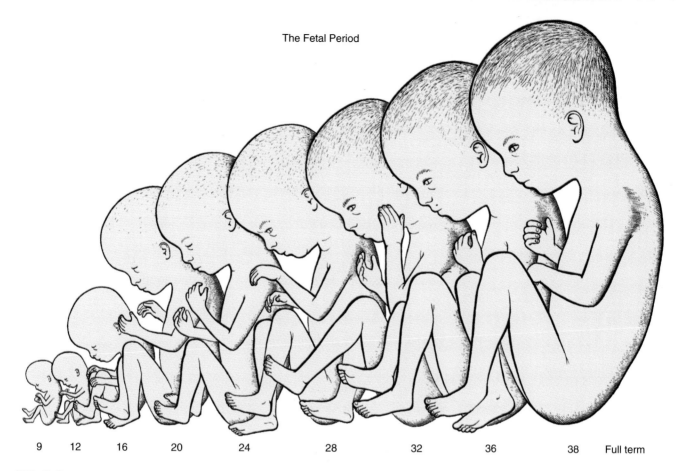

| 9 | 12 | 16 | 20 | 24 | 28 | 32 | 36 | 38 | Full term |

FIG. 3-1

The fetal period, extending from the ninth week to birth, is characterized by growth and elaboration of tissues and organs. Sex is clearly distinguishable by 12 weeks. Fetuses become viable at 22 weeks, but their chances of survival are not good until they are several weeks older. In this drawing, 9- to 38-week fetuses are shown at about half their actual size. Note that head hair begins to appear at 20 weeks, and that eyebrows and eyelashes are recognizable by 24 weeks. Observe that the eyelids are fused at 9 weeks and open at 26 weeks.

age. Foot length correlates well with CRL and is particularly useful for estimating the age of incomplete or macerated fetuses. *Fetal weight* is often a useful criterion for estimating age, but there may be a discrepancy between the fertilization age and the weight of a fetus, particularly when the mother has had metabolic disturbances during pregnancy, for example, diabetes mellitus. In these cases, fetal weight often exceeds values considered normal for CRL.

Fetal dimensions obtained from ultrasound measurements of fetuses closely approximate CRL measurements obtained from aborted fetuses. *Ultrasound CRL measurements* are now predictive of fetal age with an accuracy ± one to two days (Fig. 3-2). In addition, the biparietal diameter of the head and the dimension of the trunk may be obtained. At 9 weeks, the head is still slightly larger than the trunk. Assessment of fetal size and age is enhanced when head and trunk dimensions are considered along with CRL measurements. Recently, cheek-to-cheek and transverse cerebellar measurements have been used for the assessment of fetal growth and gestational age, respectively. Determination of the size of a fetus, especially of its head, is of great value to the obstetrician for the management of patients, for example, women with small pelves and/or those fetuses with intrauterine growth retardation (IUGR) and/or congenital anomalies.

TABLE 3-1

Criteria for Estimating Fertilization Age During the Fetal Period

Age (weeks)	CR Length (mm)*	Foot Length (mm)*	Fetal Weight (gm)†	Main External Characteristics
PREVIABLE FETUSES				
9	50	7	8	*Eye closing or closed.* Head large and more rounded. External genitalia still not distinguishable as male or female. Intestines in proximal part of umbilical cord. Ears low-set.
10	61	9	14	*Intestines in the abdomen.* Early fingernail development.
12	87	14	45	*Sex distinguishable externally.* Well-defined neck.
14	120	20	110	*Head erect.* Eyes face anteriorly. Ears closed to their definitive position. Lower limbs well-developed. Early toenail development.
16	140	27	200	*External ears stand out* from head.
18	160	33	320	*Vernix caseosa covers skin.* Quickening (signs of life) felt by mother.
20	190	39	460	*Head and body hair (lanugo) visible.*
VIABLE FETUSES‡				
22	210	45	630	*Skin wrinkled,* translucent, and pink to red.
24	230	50	820	*Fingernails present.* Lean body.
26	250	55	1000	*Eyes partially open.* Eyelashes present.
28	270	59	1300	*Eyes wide open.* Good head of hair often present. Skin slightly wrinkled.
30	280	63	1700	*Toenails present.* Body filling out. Testes descending.
32	300	68	2100	*Fingernails reach finger tips.* Skin pink and smooth.
36	340	79	2900	*Body usually plump.* Lanugo hairs almost absent. Toenails reach toe tips. Flexed limbs; firm grasp.
38	360	83	3400	*Prominent chest;* breasts protrude. Testes in scrotum or palpable in inguinal canals. Fingernails extend beyond finger tips.

CR, Crown rump.

*These measurements are averages and may not apply to specific cases; dimensional variations increase with age.

†These weights refer to fetuses that have been fixed for about 2 weeks in 10% formalin. Fresh specimens usually weigh about 5% less.

‡There is no sharp limit of development, age, or weight at which a fetus automatically becomes viable or beyond which survival is assured, but experience has shown that it is rare for a baby whose weight is less than 500 gm or whose fertilization age is less than 22 weeks to survive. Even fetuses born between 26 and 28 weeks have difficulty surviving, mainly because the respiratory system and the central nervous system are not completely differentiated. The term *abortion* refers to all pregnancies that terminate before the period of viability.

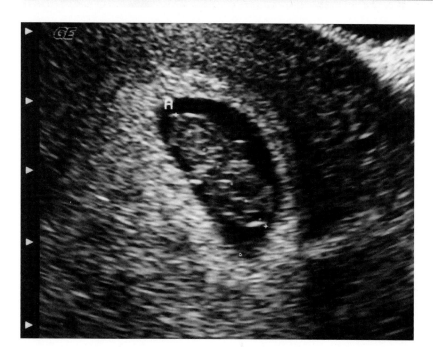

FIG. 3-2

Ultrasound scan of an 8.5-week-old fetus (long axis), showing its relationship to the amniotic and chorionic cavities. (Courtesy of Dr. E.A. Lyons, Department of Radiology, University of Manitoba, Health Sciences Centre, Winnipeg, Manitoba, Canada.)

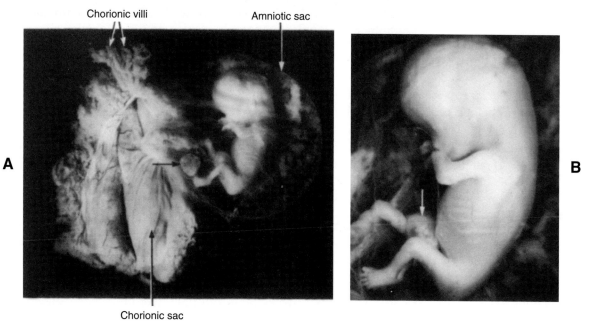

A

B

Chorionic villi

Amniotic sac

Chorionic sac

FIG. 3-3

Photographs of a 9-week fetus in the amniotic sac exposed by removal from its chorionic sac. **A,** Actual size. The remnant of the yolk sac is indicated by an arrow. **B,** Enlarged photograph of the fetus (×2). Note the following features: large head, cartilaginous ribs, intestines in the umbilical cord *(arrow).* (Courtesy of Professor Jean Hay [retired], Department of Human Anatomy and Cell Science, University of Manitoba, Winnipeg, Manitoba, Canada.)

NINE TO TWELVE WEEKS

At the beginning of the ninth week, the head constitutes one half the CRL of the fetus (Fig. 3-3). Subsequently, growth in body length accelerates rapidly so that, by the end of 12 weeks, the CRL has more than doubled. Although growth of the head slows down considerably, it is still disproportionately large compared with the rest of the body. At 9 weeks the face is broad, the eyes widely separated, the ears low-set, and, by the end of the

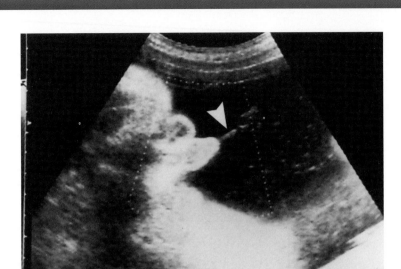

FIG. 3-4

Routine ultrasound examination at 32 weeks of gestation revealed a male fetus. Both conventional gray-scale sonography and Doppler sonography demonstrated fetal micturition. (From Devesa R, Torrents M: *N Engl J Med* 338:170, 1998.)

ninth week, *the eyelids are fused.* The external genitalia of males and females appear similar until the end of the ninth week. Their mature fetal form is not established until the twelfth week. *Urine formation* begins between the ninth and twelfth weeks, and urine is discharged into the amniotic fluid (Fig. 3-4). The fetus reabsorbs some of this fluid after swallowing it. Fetal waste products are transferred to the maternal circulation by passing across the placental membrane (see Chapter 4). Primary ossification centers appear in the skeleton by the end of 12 weeks, especially in the skull and long bones.

THIRTEEN TO SIXTEEN WEEKS

Growth is very rapid during this period (Figs. 3-1, 3-5, and 3-6). By 16 weeks, the head is relatively small compared with that of the 12-week fetus and the lower limbs have lengthened. Limb movements, which first occur at the end of the embryonic period (8 weeks), become coordinated by the fourteenth week but are too slight to be felt by the mother. *Ossification of the skeleton* is active during this period (see Fig. 12-5), and the bones are clearly visible on radiographs of the mother's abdomen by the beginning of the sixteenth week.

Ultrasonography has revealed that slow *eye movements occur at 14 weeks* (16 weeks after LNMP). Scalp hair patterning is also determined during this period. By 16 weeks, the ovaries are differentiated and contain primordial follicles enclosing oogonia. At this time, the appearance of the fetus is even more human because its eyes face anteriorly rather than anterolaterally. In addition, the external ears are close to their definitive position on the sides of the head.

SEVENTEEN TO TWENTY WEEKS

Growth slows down during this period (Fig. 3-1), but the fetus still increases its CRL by about 50 mm. The lower limbs reach their final relative proportions and fetal movements known as **quickening** are commonly felt by the mother. The mean time that intervenes

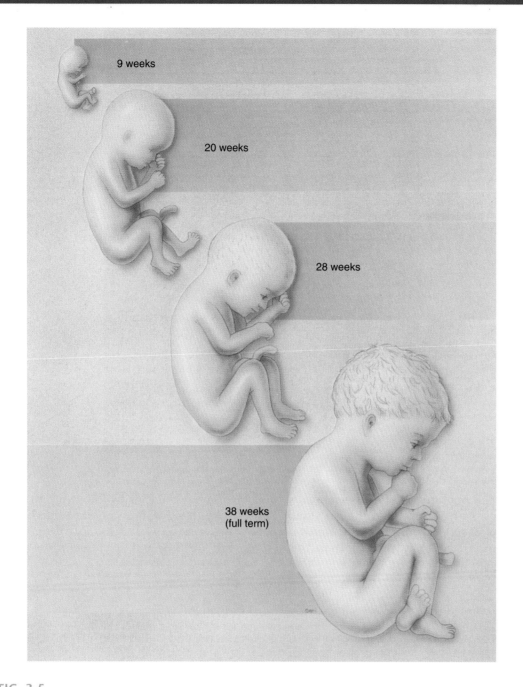

FIG. 3-5

Drawing of fetuses at 9, 20, 28, and 38 weeks, respectively. Note that the eyelids are fused in 9- and 20-week fetuses. They are usually open at 26 weeks. During the last two months, the fetus obtains well-rounded contours resulting from the deposition of subcutaneous fat.

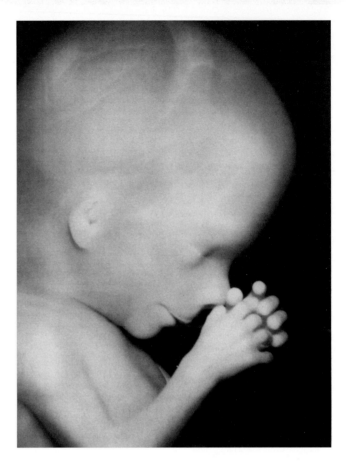

FIG. 3-6

Enlarged photograph of a 13-week fetus. The crown rump length is 84 mm. Note that the eyelids are fused and that the ear stands out from the head. A fetus at this stage has no chance of survival outside of the uterus because of the immaturity of the lungs. (Courtesy of Professor Jean C. Hay [retired], Department of Human Anatomy and Cell Science, University of Manitoba, Winnipeg, Canada.)

between a mother's first detection of fetal movements and delivery is 147 days, with a standard deviation of 15 days.

The skin at 17 weeks is thin because there is very little subcutaneous fat (Fig. 3-7). By 18 weeks, the skin is covered with a greasy, cheeselike material known as *vernix caseosa*. It consists of a mixture of dead epidermal cells and a fatty secretion from the fetal sebaceous glands of the skin. The vernix caseosa protects the delicate fetal skin from abrasions, chapping, and hardening that could result from its exposure to amniotic fluid. The bodies of 20-week fetuses are usually completely covered with fine downy hair called *lanugo;* this hair helps to hold the vernix caseosa on the skin. Eyebrows and head hair are also visible at 20 weeks (Fig. 3-5).

Brown fat forms during the seventeenth through twentieth weeks and is the site of heat production, particularly in the neonate. This specialized adipose tissue produces heat by oxidizing fatty acids. Brown fat is chiefly found at the root of the neck, posterior to the sternum, and in the perirenal area. Brown fat has a high content of mitochondria, giving it a definite brown hue.

By 18 weeks, the uterus is formed and canalization of the vagina has begun. By 20 weeks, the *testes* have begun to descend but are still located on the posterior abdominal

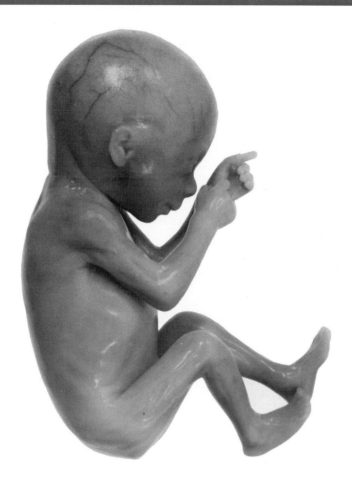

FIG. 3-7

A fetus at 17 weeks. Observe the blood vessels in the scalp. They are visible because the skin is thin at this stage and very little subcutaneous fat is present. Although it appears mature, a fetus at this stage is unable to survive if it aborts spontaneously, as in this case.

wall, as are the *ovaries* in female fetuses. By this time many *primordial ovarian follicles* containing oogonia have formed.

TWENTY-ONE TO TWENTY-FIVE WEEKS

There is a *substantial weight gain* during this period. Although still somewhat lean, the fetus is better proportioned (Fig. 3-8). The skin is usually wrinkled, particularly during the early part of this period, and is more translucent. The skin is pink to red in fresh specimens because blood is visible in the capillaries. At 21 weeks rapid eye movements begin, and *blink-startle responses* have been reported at 22 to 23 weeks following application of a vibroacoustic noise source to the mother's abdomen.

By 24 weeks, the secretory epithelial cells (type II pneumocytes) in the interalveolar walls of the lung have begun to secrete *surfactant*, a surface-active lipid that maintains the patency of the developing alveoli of the lungs (see Chapter 8). *Fingernails* are also present by 24 weeks. Although a 22- to 25-week fetus born prematurely may survive if given intensive care, it may die during early infancy because its respiratory system is still immature.

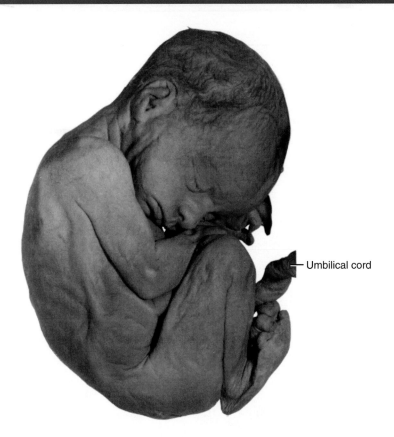

Umbilical cord

FIG. 3-8

Photograph of a 25-week fetus in the fetal position. Note that its fingernails are present and that the skin is wrinkled and the body lean as a result of the scarcity of subcutaneous fat. A fetus born prematurely at this age may survive. Observe that its eyelids are just beginning to separate. They are usually wide open at 26 weeks. Most infants born at 25 weeks or less, and with birth weights less than 500 grams, are unlikely to survive in spite of intensive care.

TWENTY-SIX TO TWENTY-NINE WEEKS

During this period, a prematurely born fetus often survives if given intensive care because its *lungs are now capable of breathing air.* The lungs and pulmonary vasculature have developed sufficiently to provide adequate gas exchange (Fig. 3-9). In addition, the central nervous system has matured to the stage where it can direct rhythmic breathing movements and control body temperature. The greatest neonatal losses occur in infants of low (2500 gm or less) and very low (1500 gm or less) birth weight.

The eyes reopen at 26 weeks, and lanugo and head hair are well developed (Fig. 3-8). Toenails become visible, and considerable subcutaneous fat is now present under the skin, smoothing out many of the wrinkles. During this period, the quantity of white fat increases to about 3.5% of body weight. *The fetal liver and spleen are now important sites of hematopoiesis.* Erythropoiesis in the spleen ends by 28 weeks, by which time bone marrow has become the major site of formation of erythrocytes.

THIRTY TO THIRTY-FOUR WEEKS

The *pupillary light reflex* of the eyes can be elicited by 30 weeks. Usually by the end of this period, the skin is pink and smooth, and the upper and lower limbs have a chubby ap-

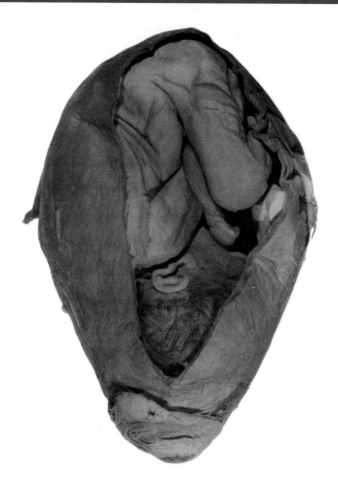

FIG. 3-9

Photograph of a 29-week fetus in the cephalic presentation in utero. A portion of the anterior wall of the uterus and its membranes (amnion and chorion) have been cut away to expose the fetus. At this age the breech (caudal end of fetus) is commonly in the fundus of the uterus and the head is adjacent to the cervix. Fetuses born at this age usually survive because their lungs are capable of breathing air. This fetus and its mother died as a result of injuries sustained in an automobile accident.

pearance. At this stage the quantity of white fat is about 8% of body weight. Fetuses 32 weeks and older usually survive if born prematurely. If a normal-weight fetus is born during this period, it is premature by date as opposed to being premature by weight.

THIRTY-FIVE TO THIRTY-EIGHT WEEKS

Fetuses at 35 weeks have a firm grasp and exhibit a spontaneous orientation to light. As term approaches, the nervous system is sufficiently mature to carry out some integrative functions. Most fetuses during this finishing period are plump (Fig. 3-10). By 36 weeks, the circumferences of the head and abdomen are approximately equal. After this, the circumference of the abdomen may be greater than that of the head. There is a *slowing of growth* as the time of birth approaches. Normal fetuses usually reach a CRL of 360 mm and weigh about 3400 gm. By full term the amount of white fat is about 16% of body weight. A fetus adds about 14 gm of fat a day during these last weeks of gestation. In general, male fetuses are longer and weigh more at birth than female fetuses.

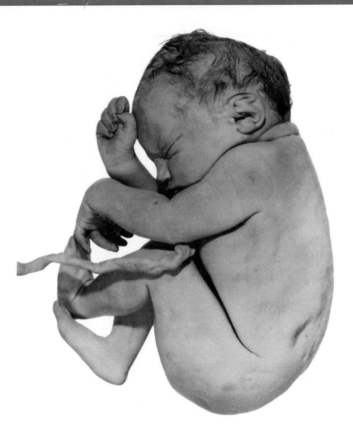

FIG. 3-10

This near-term fetus (36 weeks) is plump as a result of the deposition of subcutaneous fat. Note that its fingernails have reached its fingertips. A fetus born at this age has an excellent chance of survival.

By full term (38 weeks after fertilization; 40 weeks after LNMP), the skin is normally bluish-pink. The chest is prominent, and the breasts protrude slightly in both sexes. The testes are usually in the scrotum in full-term male infants; their descent begins at 28 to 32 weeks. Thus premature male infants commonly have undescended testes (cryptorchism). Although the head at full term is smaller in relation to the rest of the body than it was earlier in fetal life, it still is one of the largest regions of the fetus. This is an important consideration related to its passage through the birth canal (Fig. 3-16; also see Fig. 4-9).

TIME OF BIRTH

The expected time of birth is 266 days or 38 weeks after fertilization, that is, 280 days or 40 weeks after LNMP. However, about 12% of babies are born 1 to 2 weeks after the expected date of confinement (EDC). Prolongation of pregnancy for 3 or more weeks beyond the EDC occurs in 5% to 6% of women. Some infants in prolonged pregnancies develop the *postmaturity syndrome.* They are thin and have dry, parchmentlike skin, but they are often overweight and characterized by absence of lanugo hair, decreased or absent vernix caseosa, long nails, and increased alertness. When delivery is delayed 3 weeks or more beyond term, there is a significant increase in mortality. Because of this, labor is often induced.

The common clinical method of determining EDC is to count back three calendar months from the first day of the LNMP and then add a year and seven days *(Nägeles rule).* In women with regular menstrual cycles, this method gives a reasonably accurate EDC. If the woman's cycles are irregular, however, miscalculations of 2 to 3 weeks may occur. In addition, *implantation bleeding* occurs in some pregnant women at the time of the first missed period (about 2 weeks after fertilization [see Fig. 1-7]). Should the woman interpret this bleeding as a normal menstruation, the estimated time of birth could be miscalculated by 2 or more weeks. Ultrasonographic examinations of the fetus, in particular CRL measurements between 9 and 12 weeks of gestation (7 to 10 weeks after fertilization), are now commonly used for obtaining a more reliable prediction of the EDC (Fig. 3-2).

PERINATOLOGY

This branch of medicine is concerned with the well being of the fetus and neonate, generally covering the period from about 26 weeks after fertilization to 4 weeks after birth. The subspecialty of *perinatal medicine* combines certain aspects of obstetrics and pediatrics. A physician can now determine whether or not a fetus has a particular disease or a congenital anomaly by using various diagnostic techniques. *Prenatal diagnosis* can be made early enough to allow early termination of the pregnancy if elected, for example, when serious anomalies incompatible with postnatal life are diagnosed (e.g., trisomy 13; see Fig. 5-8). In selected cases various treatments can be given to the fetus, for example, the administration of drugs to correct cardiac arrhythmia. Surgical correction of some congenital anomalies in utero is also possible, for example, ureterostomies on fetuses that have ureters that do not open into the bladder.

Chorionic Villus Sampling

Biopsies of chorionic villi may be obtained by inserting a needle, guided by ultrasonography, through the mother's abdominal and uterine walls into the uterine cavity (Fig. 3-11, *A*). Chorionic Villus Sampling (CVS) can be performed by transabdomen approach or transcervically using real-time ultrasound guidance. Biopsies of chorionic villi are used for detecting chromosomal abnormalities, inborn errors of metabolism, and X-linked disorders. CVS can be performed as early as the ninth week of gestation (7 weeks after fertilization). The rate of fetal loss is between 2% and 3%, slightly more than the risk from amniocentesis. The major advantage of CVS over amniocentesis is that it allows the results of chromosomal analysis to be available several weeks earlier. Reports regarding an increased risk of limb defects after CVS are conflicting.

Diagnostic Amniocentesis

This is the most common invasive prenatal diagnostic procedure (Fig. 3-11, *B*). Amniocentesis is usually performed during the fourteenth to sixteenth weeks of gestation (12 to 14 weeks after fertilization). There is an increased risk of spontaneous fetal loss after early amniocentesis. The procedure is relatively devoid of risk, especially when it is performed by an experienced physician who is guided by ultrasonography for outlining the position of the fetus and placenta.

Alpha-Fetoprotein Assay

Alpha-fetoprotein (AFP) assay escapes from the circulation into the amniotic fluid from fetuses with *open neural tube defects* (NTDs), such as spina bifida with myeloschisis or meroanencephaly (see Chapter 13). Measuring the levels of AFP in amniotic fluid was first carried out for the antenatal diagnosis of NTDs (Ross and Elias, 1997). The term *open* refers to lesions that are not covered with skin. AFP also enters the amniotic fluid from open ventral wall defects (VWDs), such as gastroschisis and omphalocele (see Chapter 9).

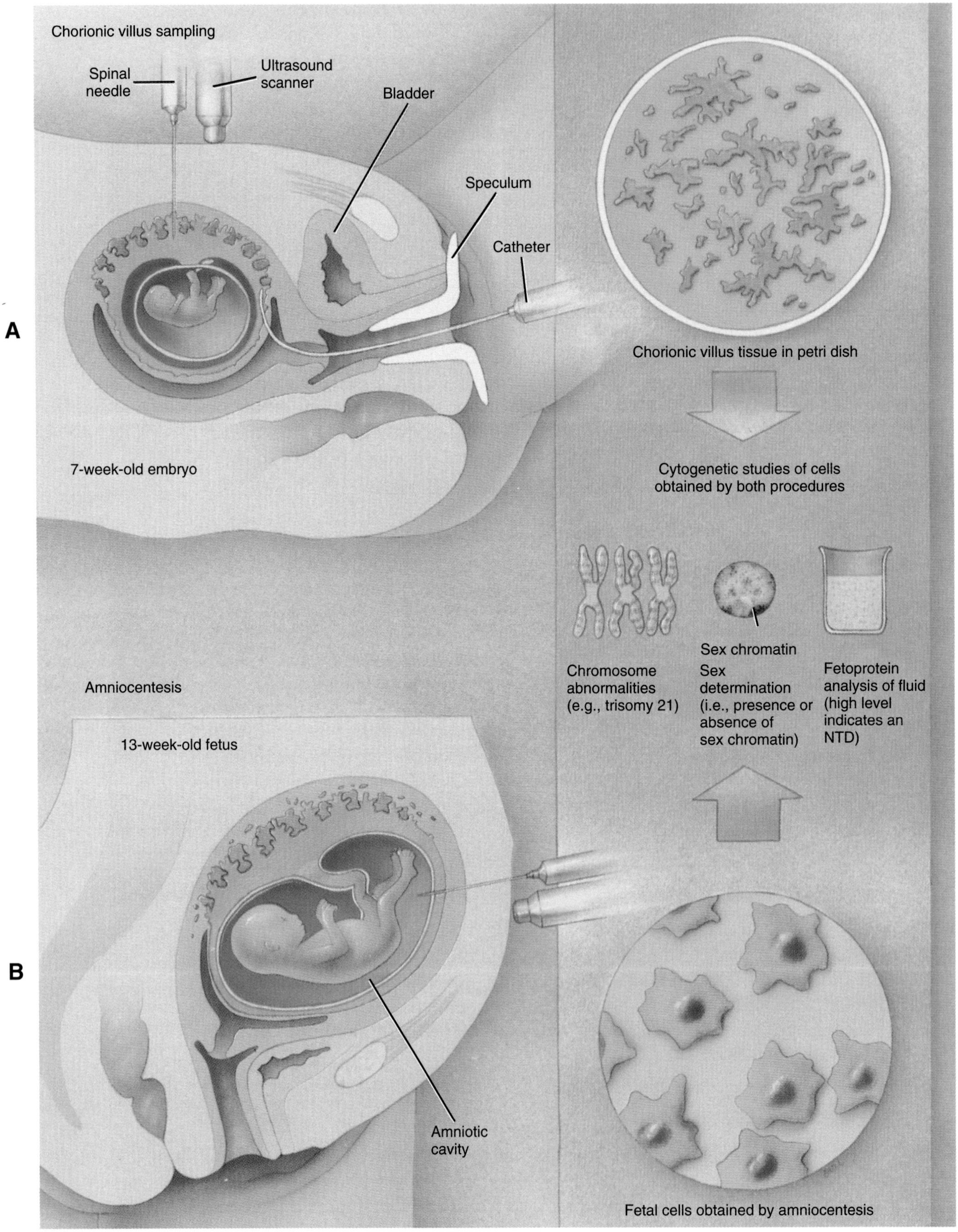

Chorionic villus sampling

Spinal needle

Ultrasound scanner

Bladder

Speculum

Catheter

Chorionic villus tissue in petri dish

A

7-week-old embryo

Cytogenetic studies of cells obtained by both procedures

Sex chromatin

Chromosome abnormalities (e.g., trisomy 21)

Sex determination (i.e., presence or absence of sex chromatin)

Fetoprotein analysis of fluid (high level indicates an NTD)

Amniocentesis

13-week-old fetus

B

Amniotic cavity

Fetal cells obtained by amniocentesis

FIG. 3-11

For legend see opposite page.

FIG. 3-11

A, Drawing illustrating chorionic villus sampling (CVS). Two sampling approaches are illustrated: (1) through the maternal anterior abdominal wall with a spinal needle, and (2) by way of the vagina and cervical canal using a malleable cannula. Success and safety in this approach depend on use of a ultrasound scanner. CVS can be performed as early as the ninth week of gestation (7 weeks after fertilization). **B,** Drawing illustrating amniocentesis. A needle is inserted through the abdominal and uterine walls into the amniotic cavity. A syringe is attached and amniotic fluid is withdrawn for diagnostic purposes (e.g., for cell cultures). Before the procedure is carried out, the placenta is located by ultrasonography so it can be avoided when the needle is inserted. The technique is usually performed at 14 to 16 weeks of gestation (12 to 14 weeks after fertilization). Before this stage of development, there is relatively little amniotic fluid and the difficulties in obtaining it without endangering the mother or fetus are consequently greater.

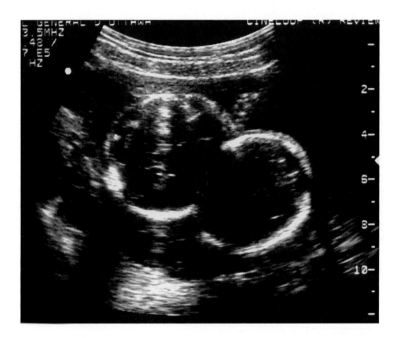

FIG. 3-12

Early second trimester diagnosis of dicephalus conjoined twins. (From Fung Kee Fung KA: *J Soc Obstet Gynaecol Can* 20:641, 1998.)

Percutaneous Umbilical Cord Blood Sampling (PUBS)

Fetal blood samples may be obtained from the umbilical vessels for chromosome analysis. Ultrasonographic scanning facilitates the procedure by outlining the location of the vessels. PUBS is often used about 20 weeks after LNMP for chromosome analysis when ultrasonographic or other examinations have shown a fetal anomaly.

Ultrasonography

The chorionic (gestational) sac and its contents may be visualized during the embryonic and fetal periods by using ultrasound techniques (Fig. 3-2). Placental and fetal sizes, multiple gestation (Fig. 3-12), and abnormal presentations can also be deter-

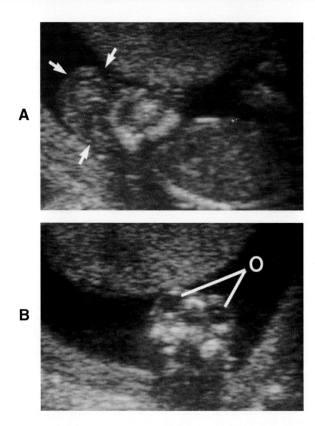

FIG. 3-13

Early second trimester pregnancy showing a fetus with meroanencephaly or anencephaly (partial absence of the brain [see also Fig. 13-16]). **A,** Sagittal sonogram demonstrating a large mass of angiomatous tissue *(arrows)* cephalad to the skull base. **B,** Coronal image of the face demonstrating the absence of the calvaria superior to the orbits *(O)*. (From Filly RA: Ultrasound evaluation of the fetal neural axis. In Callen PW [editor]: *Ultrasonography in obstetrics and gynecology,* ed 3, Philadelphia, 1994, Saunders.)

mined. *Sonograms* give accurate measurements of the biparietal diameter of the fetal skull from which close estimates of fetal age and length can be made. *Neural tube defects,* such as meroanencephaly (anencephaly) and myelomeningocele (Figs. 3-13 and 3-14), as well as many other fetal anomalies, can easily be detected with high-resolution ultrasonography. It is now possible to visualize many parts of the fetus *in utero* (Fig. 3-15).

Computed Tomography and Magnetic Resonance Imaging

When planning fetal treatment, computed tomography (CT) and magnetic resonance imaging (MRI) (Figs. 3-16 and 3-17) may be used to provide more information about an abnormality that has been detected in a sonogram. The major application of CT is in performing *pelvimetry* (measurement of the diameters of the pelvis). The uses of MRI are in the assessment of the cervix, uterus, and placenta, and in the investigation of certain fetal anomalies.

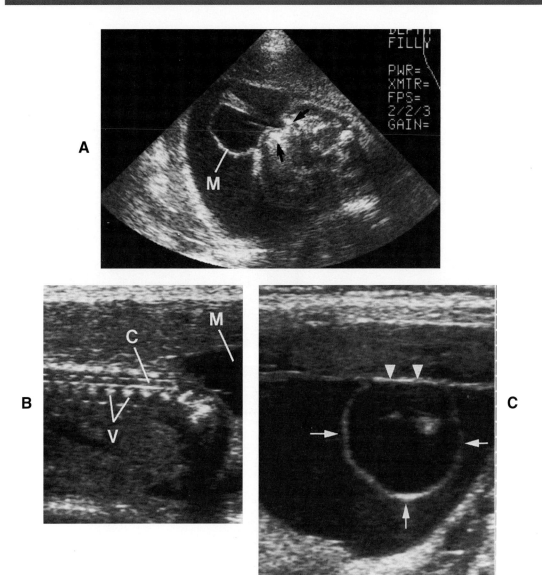

FIG. 3-14

A, Transverse sonogram of the sacrum in a fetus with a myelomeningocele *(M)*. Abnormal posterior ossification centers are seen *(arrows)*. **B,** Longitudinal sonogram demonstrating the myelomeningocele *(M)* extending from the vertebral column. The spinal cord *(C)* ends at an abnormally low level (tethered cord); *V,* vertebral bodies. **C,** Scan oriented through the sac of the myelomeningocele. The sac margin is easily seen where it contacts the amniotic fluid *(arrows)* but virtually disappears where the sac contacts the placental surface *(arrowheads)*. (From Filly RA: Ultrasound evaluation of the fetal neural axis. In Callen PW [editor]: *Ultrasonography in obstetrics and gynecology,* ed 3, Philadelphia, 1994, Saunders.)

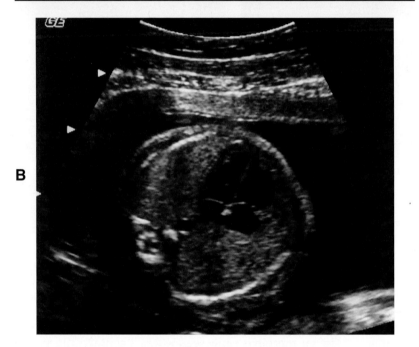

FIG. 3-15

Sonogram (axial scan) of a 22-week fetus. **A,** Profile of the face of the fetus. Observe the nose, lips, and mandible. **B,** This section, through the thorax of the fetus, shows the four chambers of the heart, the descending aorta, and dorsally the spine. (Courtesy of Dr. E.A. Lyons, Department of Radiology, University of Manitoba, Health Sciences Centre, Winnipeg, Manitoba, Canada.)

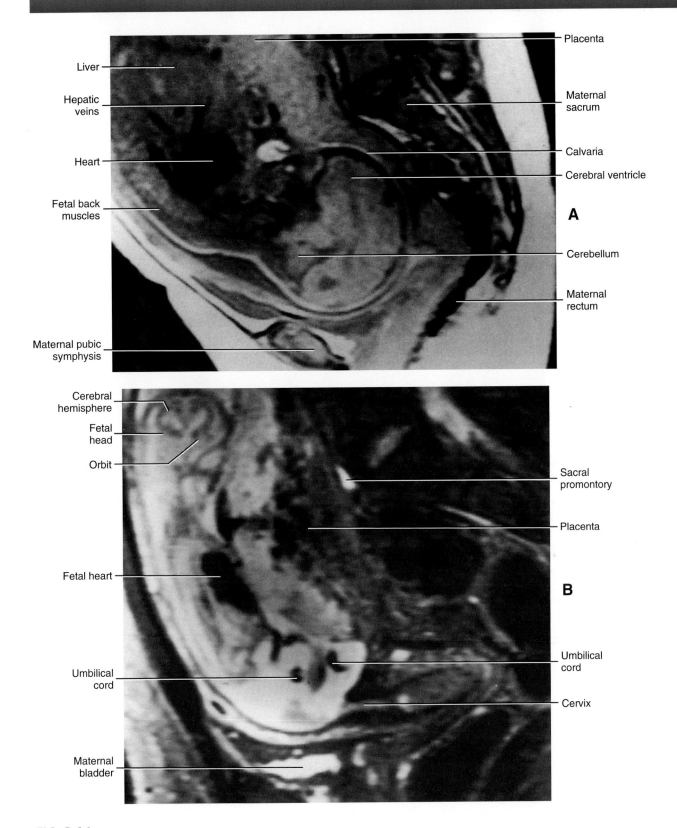

FIG. 3-16

Sagittal magnetic resonance images (MRIs) of the pelves of pregnant women. **A,** The fetus is in the cephalic presentation. The brain, heart, liver, and hepatic veins are well shown, as is the placenta. **B,** The fetus, placenta, and umbilical cord are visible. Note the ventricles of the cerebrum. (Courtesy of Dr. Shirley McCarthy, Director of MRI, Department of Diagnostic Radiology, Yale University School of Medicine, New Haven, Connecticut.)

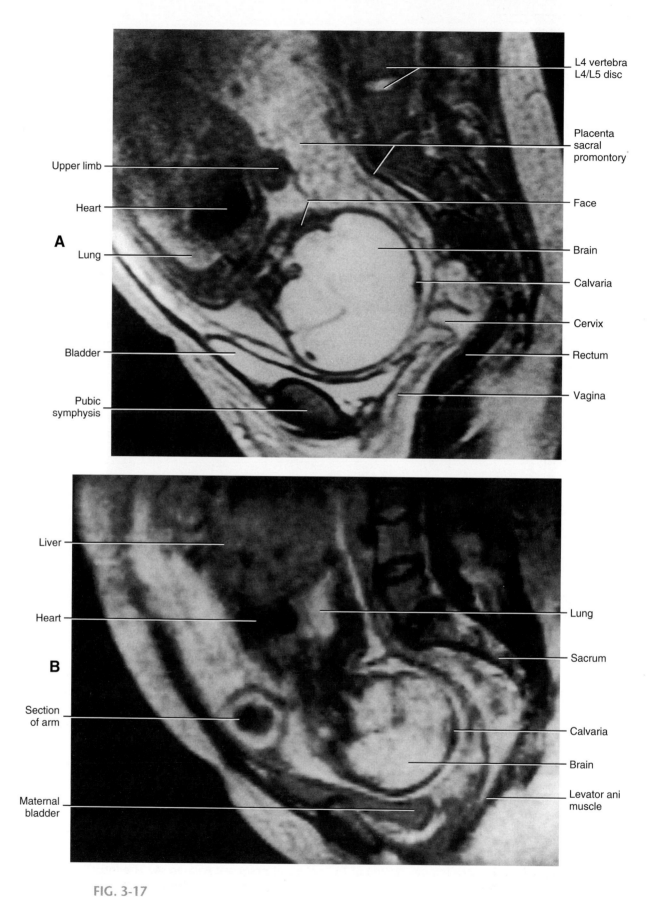

L4 vertebra
L4/L5 disc

Placenta
sacral
promontory

Upper limb

Heart

Face

A

Lung

Brain

Calvaria

Cervix

Bladder

Rectum

Pubic
symphysis

Vagina

Liver

Heart

Lung

B

Sacrum

Section
of arm

Calvaria

Brain

Maternal
bladder

Levator ani
muscle

FIG. 3-17

Sagittal magnetic resonance (MR) scans through the pelves of pregnant women. A, The fetal head is juxtaposed to the cervix. B, The fetal head is opposite the maternal sacrum. Note the heart, lung, arm, placenta, and umbilical cord. (Courtesy of Dr. Shirley McCarthy, Director of MRI, Department of Diagnostic Radiology, Yale University School of Medicine, New Haven, Connecticut.)

Placenta and Fetal Membranes

The placenta is a **fetomaternal organ** that has two components: (1) a *fetal portion* that develops from the chorionic sac, and (2) a *maternal portion* that is derived from the endometrium (Fig. 4-1). The placenta and umbilical cord function as a *transport mechanism* between the mother and the fetus. Oxygen and nutrients pass from the maternal blood through the placenta to the fetus for its nourishment, and carbon dioxide and waste materials pass from the fetus to the mother for disposal.

The fetal membranes and placenta perform the following functions and activities: protection, nutrition, respiration, excretion, and hormone production. At birth, the placenta and fetal membranes are expelled from the uterus, which is referred to as the afterbirth by lay persons (see Fig. 4-9, *H*). Evaluation of the fresh placenta and attached membranes may provide valuable information on the condition of the newborn.

The chorion, amnion, yolk sac, and allantois constitute the fetal membranes, which develop from the zygote but do not form parts of the embryo or fetus (except for parts of the yolk sac and allantois). Part of the yolk sac is incorporated into the embryo as the primordium of the primitive gut (see Chapter 9). The allantois forms a fibrous cord that is known as the urachus in the fetus and the median umbilical ligament in the adult (see Fig. 10-22). It extends from the apex of the urinary bladder to the umbilicus.

THE DECIDUA

The term *decidua* (L. *deciduus*, a falling off) is applied to the *gravid endometrium* (the functional layer of the endometrium in a pregnant woman). The name indicates that this part of the endometrium separates (falls away) from the uterus at *parturition* (childbirth).

Three regions of the decidua are named according to their relation to the implantation site (Fig. 4-1): (1) The part deep to the conceptus that forms the maternal

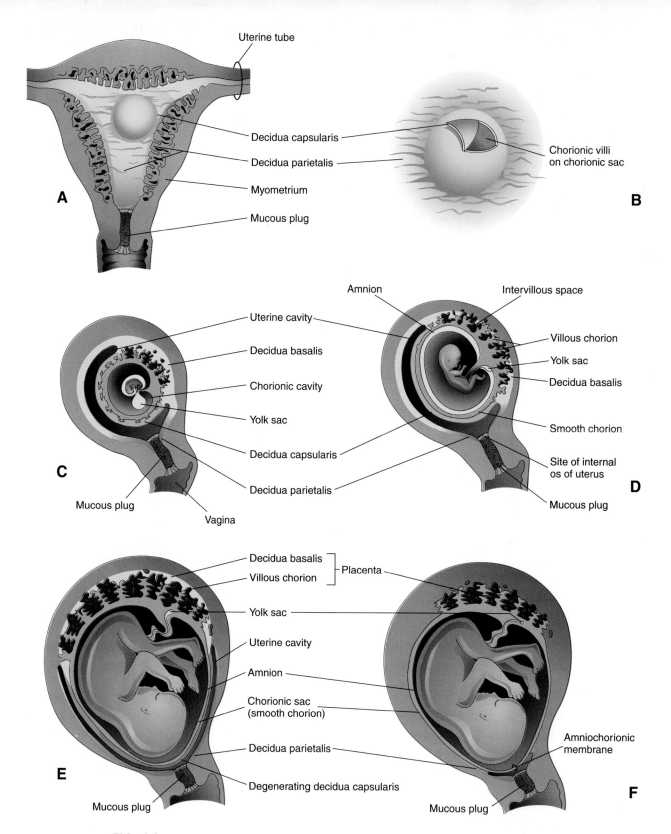

FIG. 4-1

Drawing illustrating development of the placenta and fetal membranes. **A,** Coronal section of the uterus showing elevation of the decidua capsularis by the expanding chorionic sac of a 4-week embryo, implanted in the endometrium on the posterior wall. **B,** Enlarged drawing of the implantation site. The chorionic villi were exposed by cutting an opening in the decidua capsularis. **C** through **F,** Sagittal sections of the gravid uterus from the fifth to twenty-second week, showing the changing relations of the fetal membranes to the decidua. In *F* the amnion and chorion are fused with each other and the decidua parietalis, thereby obliterating the uterine cavity. Note in *D* to *F* that the chorionic villi persist only where the chorion is associated with the decidua basalis.

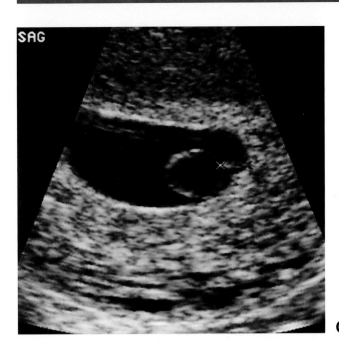

FIG. 4-1, cont'd

G, Sonogram through the uterus and gestational sac at 10 weeks pregnancy. Cardiac activity was detected in the embryo (calipers), which appeared too small for expected dates. The secondary yolk sac adjacent to the embryo is too large (>6 mm), and this is usually associated with an abnormal outcome. (**G,** Courtesy of Dr. E.A. Lyons, Department of Radiology, University of Manitoba, Health Sciences Centre, Winnipeg, Manitoba, Canada.)

G

component of the placenta is called the *decidua basalis;* (2) the superficial portion overlying the conceptus is known as the *decidua capsularis;* and (3) all the remaining endometrium is referred to as the *decidua parietalis* (vera). These decidual regions, clearly recognizable during *ultrasonography,* are important in diagnosing early pregnancy.

Up to the eighth week, chorionic villi cover the entire chorionic sac (Figs. 4-1, *C,* and 4-2). As this sac grows, the villi associated with the decidua capsularis are compressed and the blood supply to them is reduced. These villi soon degenerate, producing a bare area (Figs. 4-1, *D,* and 4-3) known as the *smooth chorion or* chorion laeve (L. *levis,* smooth). As these villi disappear, those associated with the decidua basalis rapidly increase in number, branch profusely, and enlarge.

The bushy part of the chorionic sac is known as the *villous chorion* (Fig. 4-1, *D* through *F*) or chorion frondosum (L. *frondosus,* leafy). The increase in the thickness of the placenta results from the branching of stem villi (Figs. 4-2 to 4-6). As the fetus grows, the uterus and placenta enlarge. Growth in the thickness of the placenta continues until the fetus is about 18 weeks old (20 weeks gestation). The fully developed placenta represents 15% to 30% of the decidua.

The **fetal component of the placenta** is formed by the *villous chorion* (Figs. 4-1, 4-2, 4-4 to 4-6, and 4-8). The villi project into the intervillous space containing maternal blood. The **maternal component of the placenta** is formed by the *decidua basalis.* This is the endometrium that is related to the fetal component of the placenta (Fig. 4-1). By the end of the fourth month the decidua basalis is largely replaced by the fetal component of the placenta.

The Fetomaternal Junction

The fetal portion of the placenta (villous chorion) is attached to the maternal portion of the placenta (decidua basalis) by the *cytotrophoblastic shell* (Fig. 4-5). Stem chorionic villi (anchoring villi) are attached firmly to the decidua basalis through the cytotrophoblastic shell. These villi anchor the placenta and fetal membranes to the decidua basalis. Maternal arteries and veins pass freely through gaps in the cytotrophoblastic shell and open into the intervillous space (Figs. 4-4 and 4-5).

Text continued on p. 77

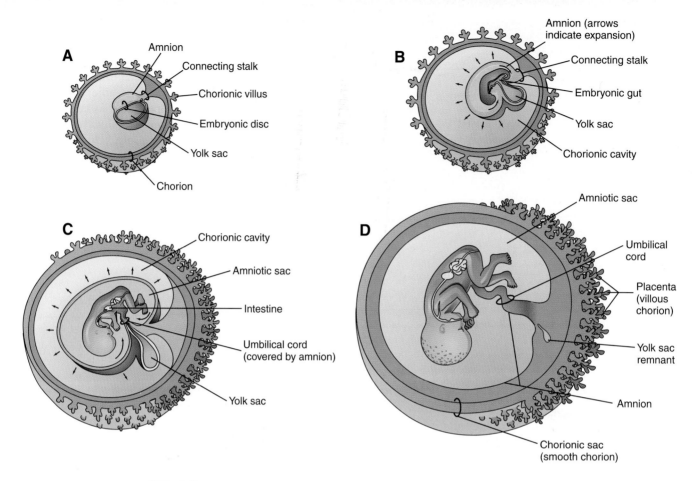

A
Amnion
Connecting stalk
Chorionic villus
Embryonic disc
Yolk sac
Chorion

B
Amnion (arrows indicate expansion)
Connecting stalk
Embryonic gut
Yolk sac
Chorionic cavity

C
Chorionic cavity
Amniotic sac
Intestine
Umbilical cord (covered by amnion)
Yolk sac

D
Amniotic sac
Umbilical cord
Placenta (villous chorion)
Yolk sac remnant
Amnion
Chorionic sac (smooth chorion)

FIG. 4-2

Drawings illustrating how the amnion enlarges, fills the chorionic sac, and envelops the umbilical cord. Observe that part of the yolk sac is incorporated into the embryo as the primitive gut. Formation of the fetal part of the placenta and degeneration of chorionic villi are also shown. **A,** 3 weeks. **B,** 4 weeks. **C,** 10 weeks. **D,** 20 weeks.

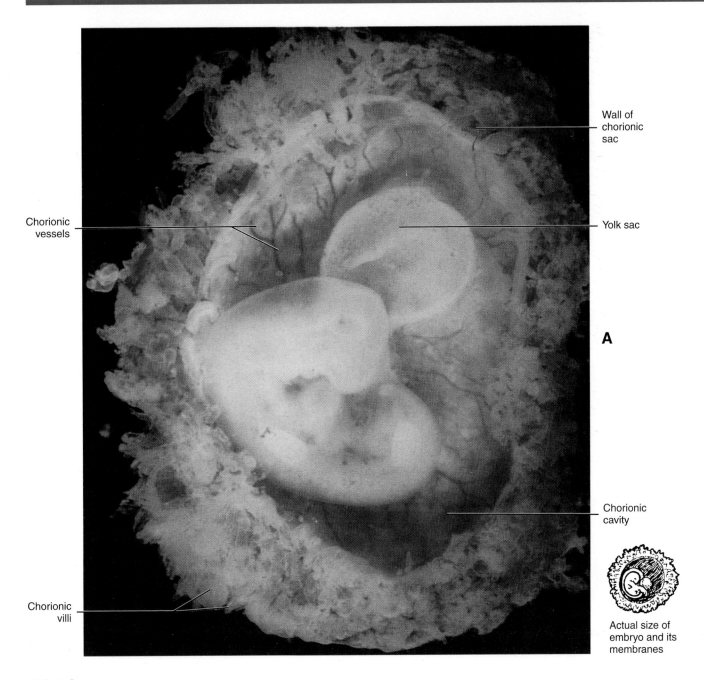

Wall of chorionic sac

Chorionic vessels

Yolk sac

A

Chorionic cavity

Chorionic villi

Actual size of embryo and its membranes

FIG. 4-3

A, Lateral view of an embryo at Carnegie stage 14, about 32 days. The chorionic and amniotic sacs have been opened to show the embryo. Note the large size of the yolk sac at this stage (see Fig. 2-16 for the characteristics of an embryo at this stage). The sketch *(lower right)* is drawn to show the actual size of the embryo and its membranes. (From Nishimura H, et al: *Prenatal development of the human with special reference to craniofacial structures: an atlas,* Washington, DC, 1977, National Institutes of Health.)

Continued

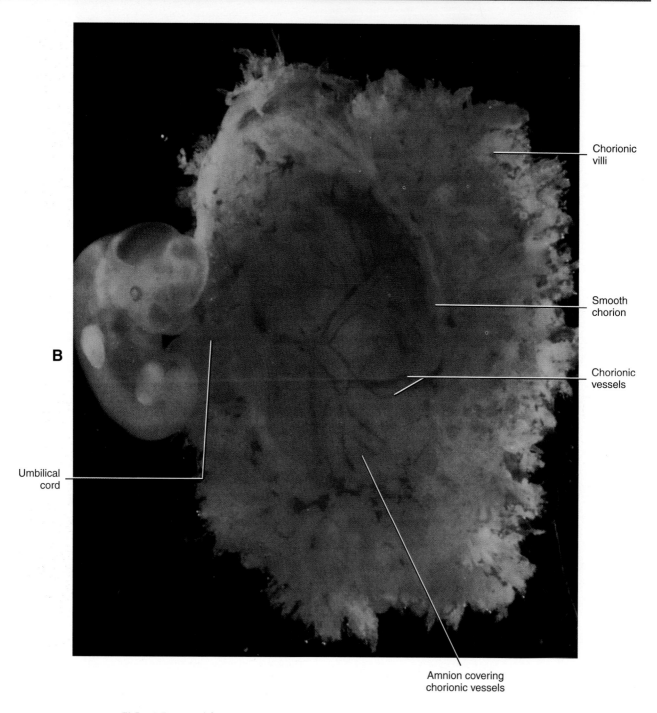

FIG. 4-3, cont'd

B, Lateral view of an embryo at Carnegie stage 15, about 36 days (see Fig. 2-17 for the characteristics of this embryo). Chorionic villi cover the entire chorionic sac at this stage. (From Nishimura H, et al: *Prenatal development of the human with special reference to craniofacial structures: an atlas,* Washington, DC, 1977, National Institutes of Health.)

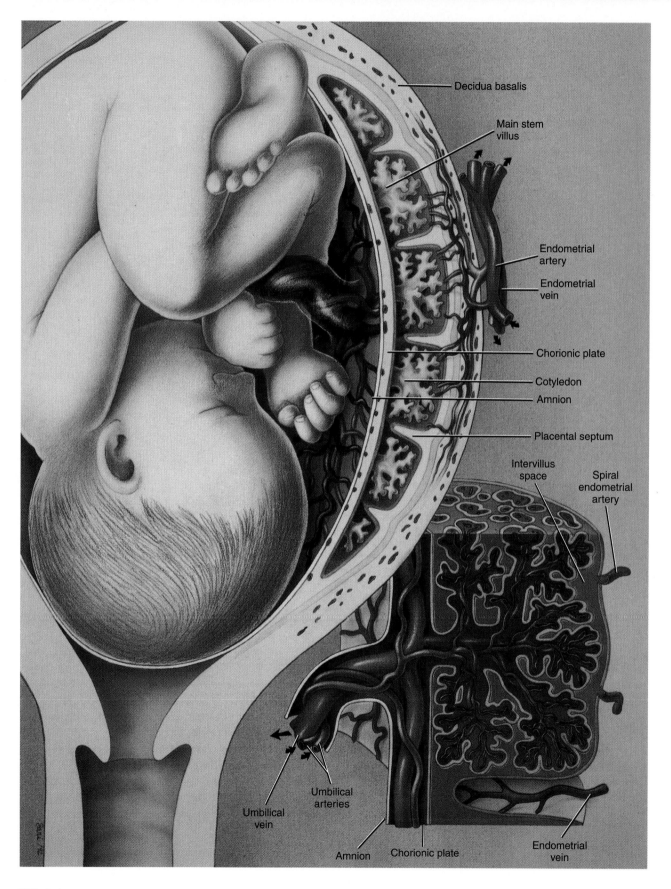

Decidua basalis

Main stem villus

Endometrial artery

Endometrial vein

Chorionic plate

Cotyledon

Amnion

Placental septum

Intervillus space

Spiral endometrial artery

Umbilical vein

Umbilical arteries

Amnion

Chorionic plate

Endometrial vein

FIG 4-4

Drawing of a near-term fetus in the uterus. It is surrounded by the amniotic and chorionic sacs, which have almost obliterated the uterine cavity.

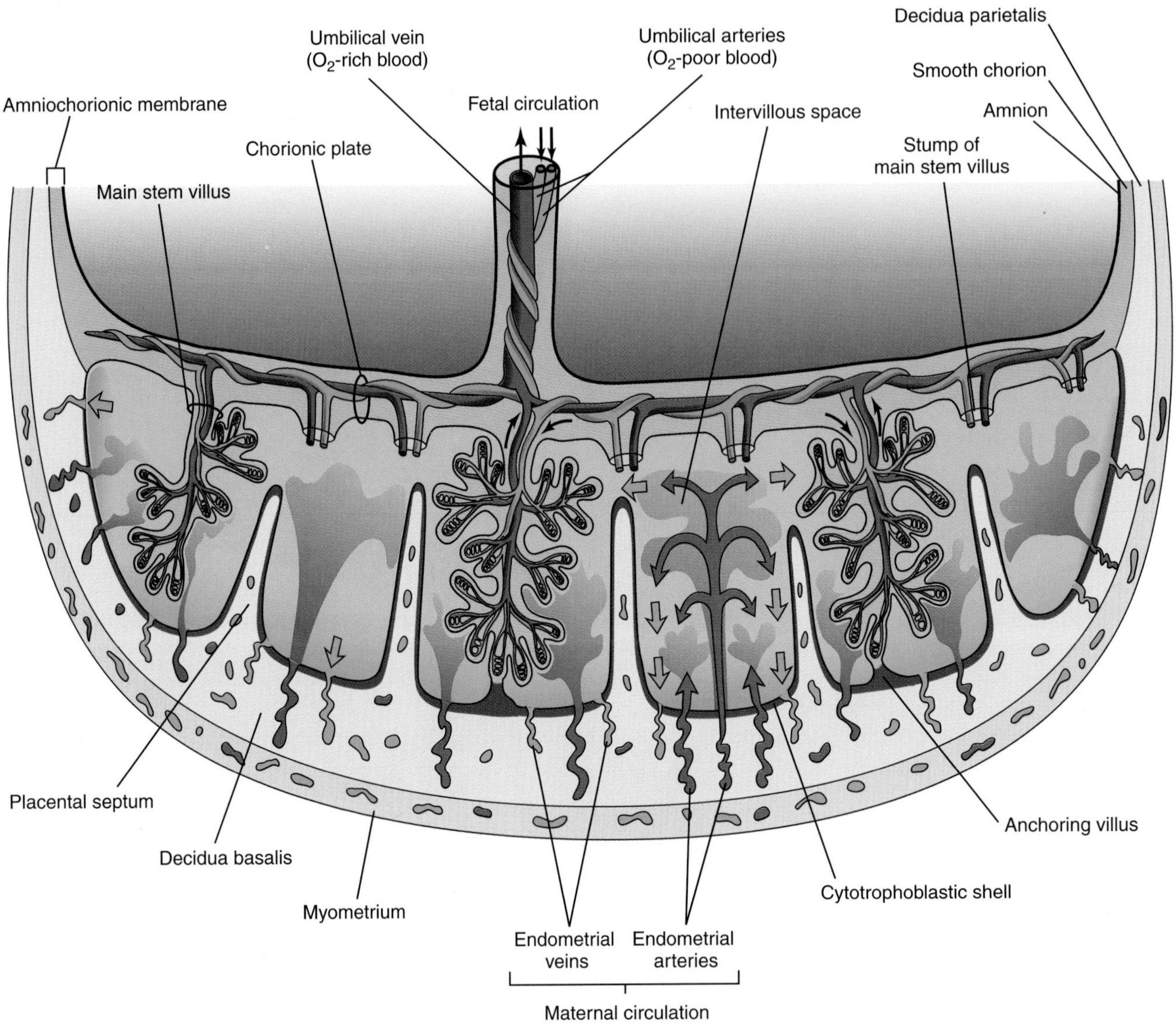

FIG. 4-5

Schematic drawing of a transverse section through a full-term placenta, showing: (1) the relation of the villous chorion (fetal part of placenta) to the decidua basalis (maternal part of placenta), (2) the fetal placental circulation, and (3) the maternal placental circulation. Maternal blood flows into the intervillous spaces in funnel-shaped spurts from the spiral arteries, and exchanges occur with the fetal blood as the maternal blood flows around the branch villi. It is through the branch villi that the main exchange of material between the mother and embryo/fetus occurs. The inflowing arterial blood pushes venous blood out of the intervillous space into the endometrial veins, which are scattered over the entire surface of the decidua basalis. Note that the umbilical arteries carry poorly oxygenated fetal blood (shown in blue) to the placenta and that the umbilical vein carries oxygenated blood (shown in red) to the fetus. Note that the cotyledons are separated from each other by placental septa, projections of the decidua basalis. Each cotyledon consists of two or more main stem villi and their many branches. In this drawing, only one stem villus is shown in each cotyledon, but the stumps of those that have been removed are indicated.

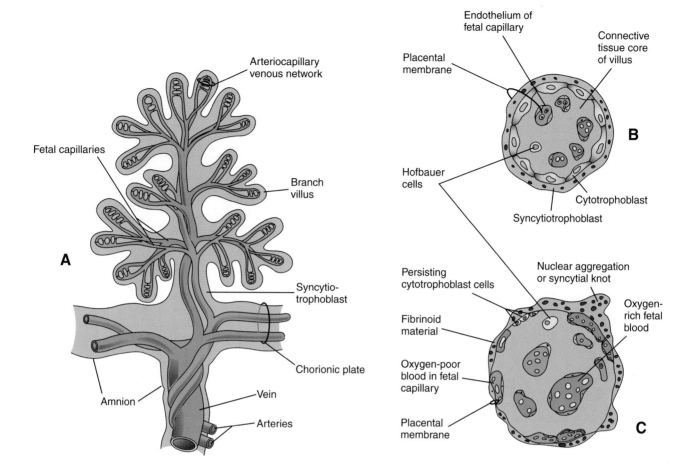

FIG. 4-6

A, Drawing of a stem chorionic villus showing its arteriocapillaryvenous system. The arteries carry poorly oxygenated blood and waste products from the fetus, whereas the vein carries well-oxygenated blood and nutrients to the fetus. **B** and **C,** Drawings of sections through a chorionic villus at 10 weeks and at full term, respectively. The villi are bathed externally in maternal blood. The placental membrane, composed of extrafetal tissues, separates the maternal blood from the fetal blood. Note that this membrane becomes very thin toward the end of pregnancy. Note also that at some sites nuclei in the syncytiotrophoblast form syncytial knots. These aggregations of nuclei break off and enter the maternal circulation. Some of them may lodge in the capillaries of the maternal lungs where they are rapidly destroyed by maternal enzymes. Fibrinoid material consists of fibrin and other substances. Formation of fibrinoid material mainly results from placental aging. (From Moore KL, Persaud TVN: *The developing human,* ed 6, Philadelphia, 1998, Saunders.)

PLACENTAL CIRCULATION

The many branch villi of the placenta provide a large surface area where materials are exchanged across the *placental membrane* (barrier) interposed between the fetal and maternal circulations (Figs. 4-4 to 4-7). It is through the numerous *branch villi,* which arise from the *stem villi,* that the main exchange of material between the mother and fetus takes place. The circulations of the fetus and the mother are separated by the very thin placental membrane consisting of extrafetal tissues (Figs. 4-6 and 4-7).

Fetal Placental Circulation

Poorly oxygenated blood leaves the fetus and passes through the *umbilical arteries* to the placenta. At the site of attachment of the cord to the placenta, these arteries divide into

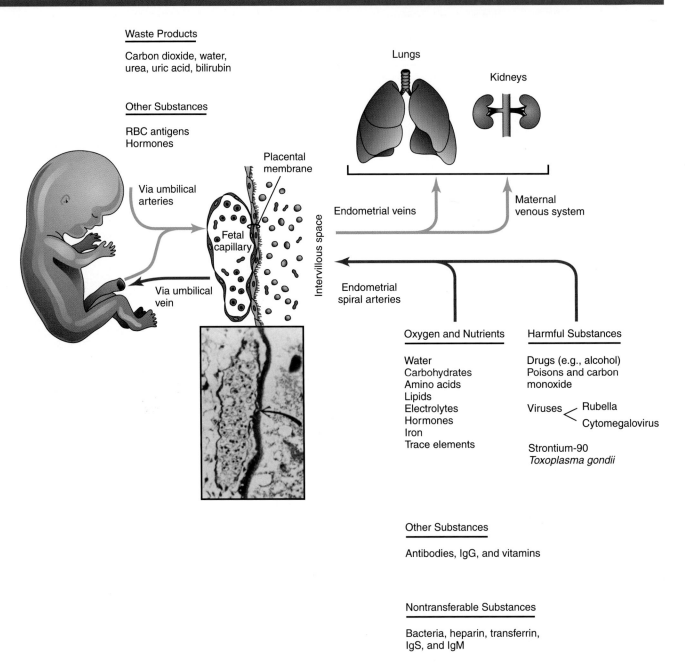

FIG. 4-7

Diagrammatic illustration of transfer across the placental membrane (barrier). The extrafetal tissues, across which transport of substances between the mother and fetus occurs, collectively constitute the placental membrane. (Inset photomicrograph from Javert CT: *Spontaneous and habitual abortion,* **New York, 1957, McGraw-Hill.)**

a number of radially disposed vessels that branch freely in the *chorionic plate* before entering the villi (Figs. 4-4 to 4-6). The blood vessels form an extensive *arteriocapillary-venous system* within the villi, which brings the fetal blood extremely close to the maternal blood (Fig. 4-6). This system provides a very large area for the exchange of metabolic and gaseous products between the maternal and fetal blood streams. There is normally *no intermingling of fetal and maternal blood,* but very small amounts of fetal blood may enter the maternal circulation through minute defects that sometimes develop in the placental membrane. The well-oxygenated fetal blood passes into thin-walled chorionic veins that follow the chorionic arteries to the site of attachment of the umbilical cord, where they converge to form the *umbilical vein*. This large vessel carries the oxygen-rich blood to the fetus (Figs. 4-4 to 4-6). The fetal circulation is illustrated and discussed in Chapter 11.

Maternal Placental Circulation

The blood in the *intervillous space* is temporarily outside the maternal circulatory system (Figs. 4-5 and 4-6). It enters the intervillous space through 80 to 100 *spiral arteries* in the decidua basalis. These vessels discharge oxygen-rich blood into the intervillous space through gaps in the cytotrophoblastic shell. The blood flow from the spiral arteries is pulsatile and is propelled in jetlike fountains by the maternal blood pressure. The entering blood is at a considerably higher pressure than that in the intervillous space; hence it spurts toward the *chorionic plate* forming the roof of the intervillous space. As the pressure dissipates, the blood flows slowly around the branch villi, allowing an exchange of metabolic and gaseous products with the fetal blood. The blood eventually returns to the endometrial veins and the maternal circulation.

The welfare of the embryo and fetus depends more on the adequate bathing of the branch villi with maternal blood than on any other factor. Reductions of uteroplacental circulation (e.g., caused by the effects of nicotine in cigarettes) result in fetal hypoxia and intrauterine growth retardation (IUGR). Severe reductions of uteroplacental circulation can result in fetal death. The intervillous space of the mature placenta contains about 150 ml of blood that is replenished three or four times per minute. The intermittent contractions of the uterus during pregnancy decrease uteroplacental blood flow slightly, but they do not force significant amounts of blood out of the intervillous space. Consequently, oxygen transfer to the fetus is decreased during uterine contractions, but the process does not stop.

Placental Membrane

The placental membrane *consists of the extrafetal tissues* separating the maternal and fetal blood (Figs. 4-6 and 4-7). Until about 20 weeks, it consists of four layers: (1) syncytiotrophoblast, (2) cytotrophoblast, (3) connective tissue in the villus, and (4) endothelium of the fetal capillaries.

Changes occur in the villi that result in the cytotrophoblast in the branch villi becoming attenuated. Eventually it disappears over large areas of the villi leaving only thin patches of syncytiotrophoblast (Fig. 4-6, C). As a result, the placental membrane in near-term placentas consists of three layers only in most places.

Although the **placental membrane** is often called the *placental barrier*, this is an inappropriate term because there are only a few compounds, endogenous or exogenous, that are unable to pass through the placental membrane in detectable amounts. The placental membrane acts as a barrier only when the molecule has a certain size, configuration, and charge (e.g., heparin). Some metabolites, toxins, and hormones, though present in the maternal circulation, do not pass through the placental membrane in sufficient concentrations to affect the embryo/fetus. Most drugs and other substances present in the maternal plasma pass through the placental membrane and are found in the fetal plasma. Syncytial knots of nuclear aggregations are formed during the third trimester. Toward the end of pregnancy, a fibrinoid material, consisting of fibrin and an eosin-staining unidentified substance, forms on the surfaces of the villi. This increases with aging of the placenta and may reduce placental transfer.

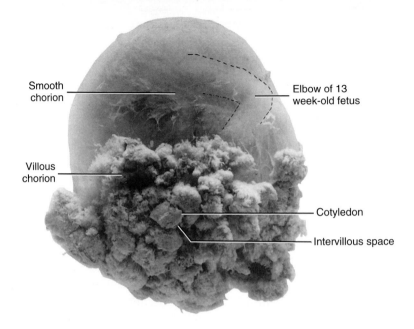

Smooth chorion

Elbow of 13 week-old fetus

Villous chorion

Cotyledon

Intervillous space

FIG. 4-8

Photograph of a human chorionic sac containing a 13-week fetus. The smooth chorion (chorion laeve) forms when the chorionic villi degenerate and disappear from this area of the chorionic sac (see Fig. 4-1). The villous chorion (chorion frondosum) is where chorionic villi persist and form the fetal part of the placenta. In situ the cotyledons were attached to the decidua basalis and the intervillous space was filled with maternal blood (see Figs. 4-4 and 4-5).

PARTURITION

Parturition (L. *parturitio,* childbirth) is the birth process during which the fetus, placenta, and fetal membranes are expelled from the mother's reproductive tract (Fig. 4-9). **Labor** is the sequence of involuntary *uterine contractions* that result in dilation of the cervix and delivery of the fetus and placenta from the uterus. The factors that trigger labor are not completely understood, but several hormones are involved in the initiation and stimulation of uterine contractions.

Stages of Labor

Labor is the process that is involved during the birth of a child that facilitates parturition. There are four stages, discussed in the following (Fig. 4-9).

■ **The first stage of labor** (dilation stage) begins when there is objective evidence of progressive dilation of the cervix. This occurs when the onset of *regular contractions of the uterus occur* less than 10 minutes apart. The first stage ends with complete dilation of the cervix. This stage is by far the most time consuming of the labor process. The average duration is about 12 hours for first pregnancies (nulliparous patients, or *primigravidas*), and about 7 hours for women who have had a child previously (multiparous patients, or *multigravidas*). However, there are wide variations.

■ **The second stage of labor** (expulsion stage) begins when the cervix is fully dilated and ends with delivery of the baby. During this stage the *amniochorionic membrane* (fused amnion and smooth chorion) ruptures and *the fetus descends through the vagina* and is delivered (Fig. 4-9, *E*). As soon as the fetus is outside the mother, it is

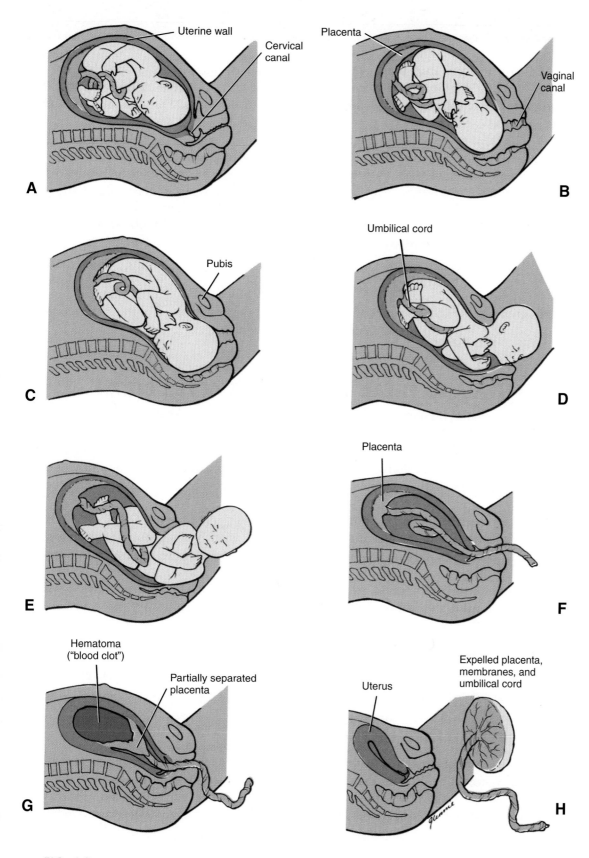

FIG. 4-9

The process of birth or parturition. **A** and **B**, The cervix of the uterus is dilating during the first stage of labor. **C** to **E**, The amniochorionic membrane ruptures and the fetus passes through the cervix and vagina and is delivered during the second stage of labor. **F** and **G**, The uterus contracts during the third stage of labor and the placenta separates from the uterine wall. This results in bleeding and the formation of a large hematoma between the uterine wall and placenta. **H**, As soon as the placenta and membranes are expelled, the recovery or fourth stage of labor begins. The uterus contracts, which constricts the endometrial arteries and prevents excessive bleeding.

called a newborn infant (or neonate). The average duration of this stage for primigravidas is 50 minutes and 20 minutes for multigravidas. Uterine contractions begin again shortly after the baby is born.

■ **The third stage of labor** (placental stage) begins as soon as the baby is born and ends when the placenta and membranes are expelled (Fig. 4-9, *H*). The duration of this stage is 15 minutes in about 90% of pregnancies. *Retraction of the uterus reduces the area of placental attachment;* thus the placenta and fetal membranes separate from the uterine wall and are expelled through the vagina. After delivery of the baby, the uterus continues to contract. A *hematoma* soon forms deep to the placenta and separates it from the uterine wall (Fig. 4-9, *G*).

■ **The fourth stage of labor** (recovery stage) begins as soon as the placenta and fetal membranes are expelled. This stage lasts about two hours. The myometrial contractions constrict the spiral arteries that formerly supplied blood to the intervillous space (Fig. 4-4). This prevents excessive uterine bleeding.

PLACENTA AND FETAL MEMBRANES AFTER BIRTH

A full-term placenta commonly has a discoid shape (Figs. 4-10 to 4-12), with a diameter of 15 to 20 cm and a thickness of 2 to 3 cm. It weighs 500 to 600 gm, usually about one sixth the weight of the fetus. The margins of the placenta are continuous with the ruptured amniotic and chorionic sacs. Careful examination of the placenta and fetal membranes after birth may provide valuable diagnostic information with respect to the mother and the newborn.

As the placenta develops, chorionic villi usually persist only where the villous chorion is in contact with the decidua basalis (Figs. 4-1 and 4-8). This results in the usual discoid placenta (Figs. 4-10 and 4-11). When villi persist elsewhere, several variations in placental shape occur: *accessory placenta* (Fig. 4-13), bidiscoidal placenta, diffuse placenta, and horseshoe placenta. Although there are variations in the size and shape of the placenta, most of them are of little physiologic or clinical significance. However, examination of the placenta may provide information about the causes of (1) placental dysfunction, (2) IUGR, (3) neonatal illness, and (4) infant death. Placental studies can also determine whether the placenta is complete. Retention of a cotyledon or an accessory placenta in the uterus may lead to *uterine hemorrhage*. Occasionally, chorionic villi may become abnormally attached to the underlying myometrium or even penetrate it.

Maternal Surface of the Placenta

The characteristic cobblestone appearance of this surface is produced by the *cotyledons,* which are separated by grooves that were formerly occupied by *placental septa* (Figs. 4-5 and 4-10). The surface of the cotyledons is covered by thin grayish shreds of decidua basalis that separated with the placenta. Most of the decidua is temporarily retained in the uterus and is shed with subsequent uterine bleeding.

Fetal Surface of the Placenta

The umbilical cord usually attaches to the fetal surface and its amniotic covering is continuous with the amnion adherent to the chorionic plate of the placenta (Figs. 4-2, 4-4, 4-5, and 4-11). The chorionic vessels radiating to and from the umbilical cord are clearly visible through the transparent amnion. The *umbilical vessels* branch on the fetal surface to form *chorionic vessels,* which enter the chorionic villi (Figs. 4-4 to 4-6).

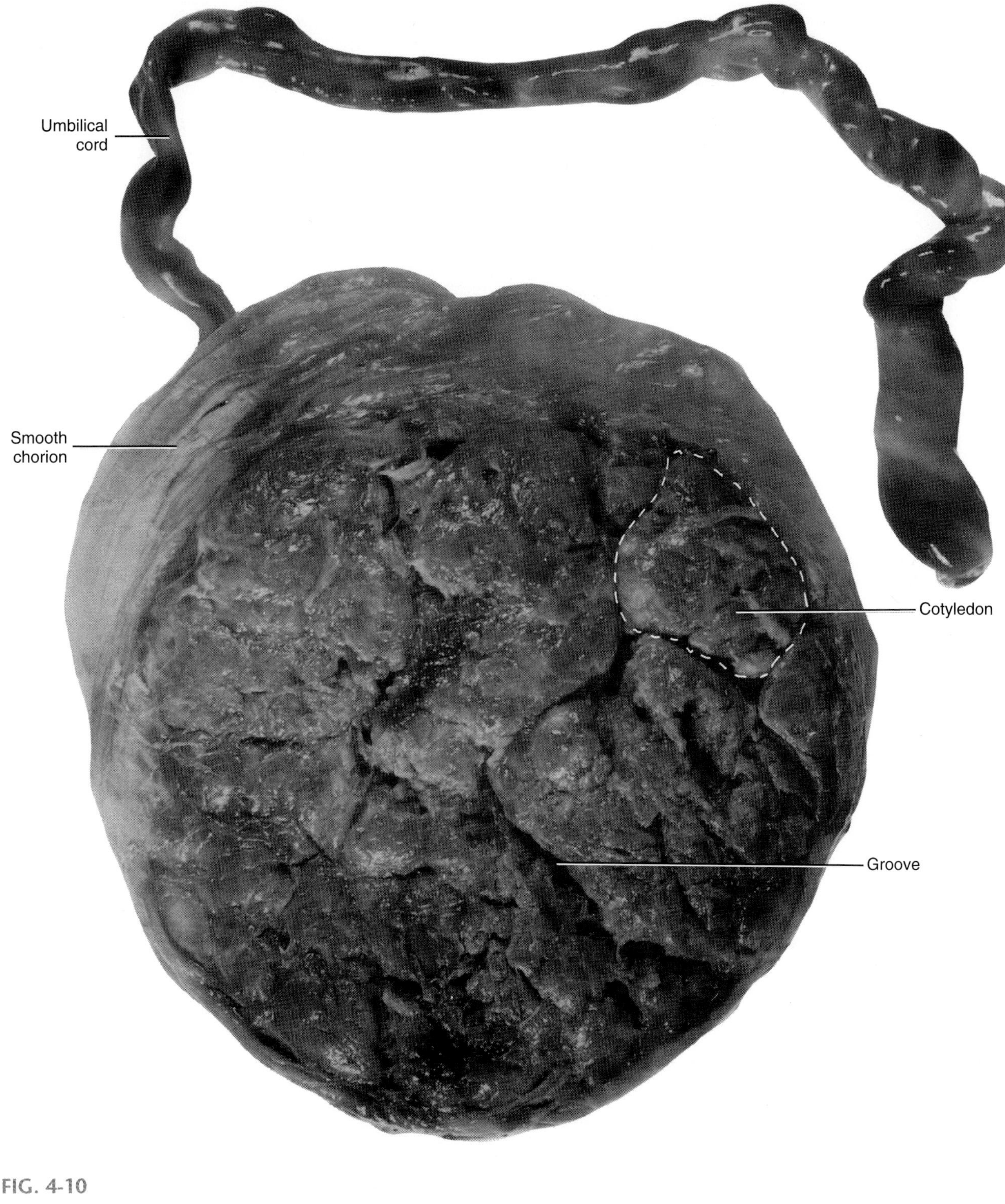

Umbilical cord

Smooth chorion

Cotyledon

Groove

FIG. 4-10

Photograph of the maternal surface of the placenta after birth. Actual size. The characteristic cobblestone appearance of this surface is caused by 15 to 20 cotyledons. Each cotyledon is composed of two or more stem villi and their many branches (see Figs. 4-4 and 4-5). The cotyledons are separated by grooves that in situ were occupied by placental septa. The external surfaces of the cotyledons are covered with remnants of the decidua basalis that separated from the uterus during parturition. The whitish appearance of some of the cotyledons is due to excessive fibrinoid formation (see Fig. 4-6, C) that causes infarction of portions of the villi.

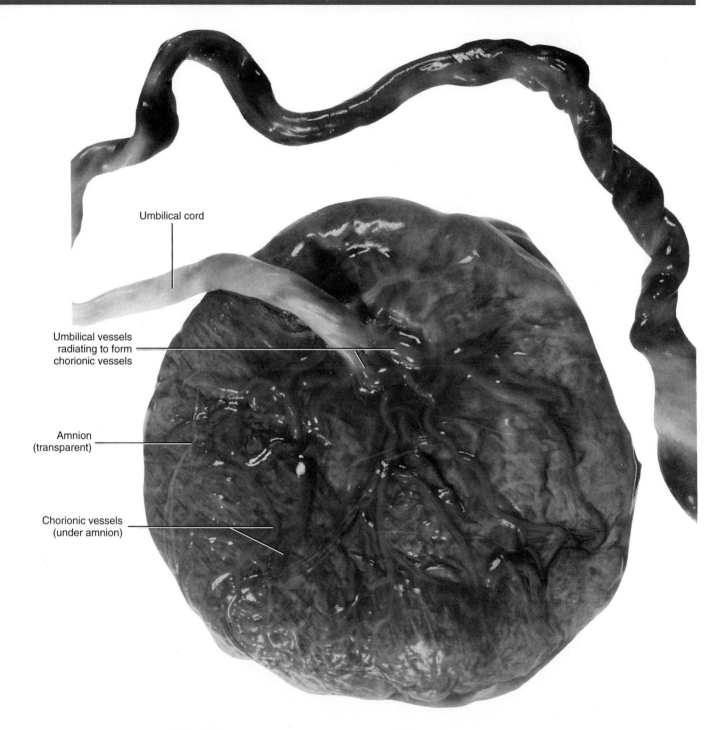

Umbilical cord

Umbilical vessels
radiating to form
chorionic vessels

Amnion
(transparent)

Chorionic vessels
(under amnion)

FIG. 4-11

Photograph of the fetal surface of the placenta after birth. The umbilical cord is attached to this surface. The attachment is usually eccentric as in this specimen. A number of large arteries and veins, the chorionic vessels, may be seen converging toward the umbilical cord, where they form the umbilical vessels. The chorionic vessels are covered by amnion that is continuous with the epithelial covering of the umbilical cord (see Figs. 4-2 and 4-6).

UMBILICAL CORD

The umbilical cord forms from the yolk stalk following folding of the embryo. The attachment of the umbilical cord, which connects the embryo/fetus to the placenta, is usually near the center of the fetal surface of this organ (Fig. 4-11), but it may be found at any point. For example, insertion of it near the placental margin produces a *battledore placenta* (Fig. 4-12) and its attachment to the membranes is called a *velamentous insertion of the cord* (Fig. 4-14). Color flow Doppler ultrasonography may be used for the antenatal detection of the position and structural abnormalities of the umbilical cord and its vessels. As the amniotic cavity enlarges the amnion enfolds the umbilical cord, forming its epithelial covering (Fig. 4-2).

FIG. 4-12

Photograph of the fetal surface of a placenta with the umbilical cord attached near the margin of the placenta. This type of umbilical cord insertion occurs in about 5% of placentas. Usually the cord attaches near the center of the placenta (see Fig. 4-11). A placenta with a marginal attachment of the cord is sometimes called a battledore placenta because of its resemblance to the bat used in the medieval game of battledore and shuttlecock.

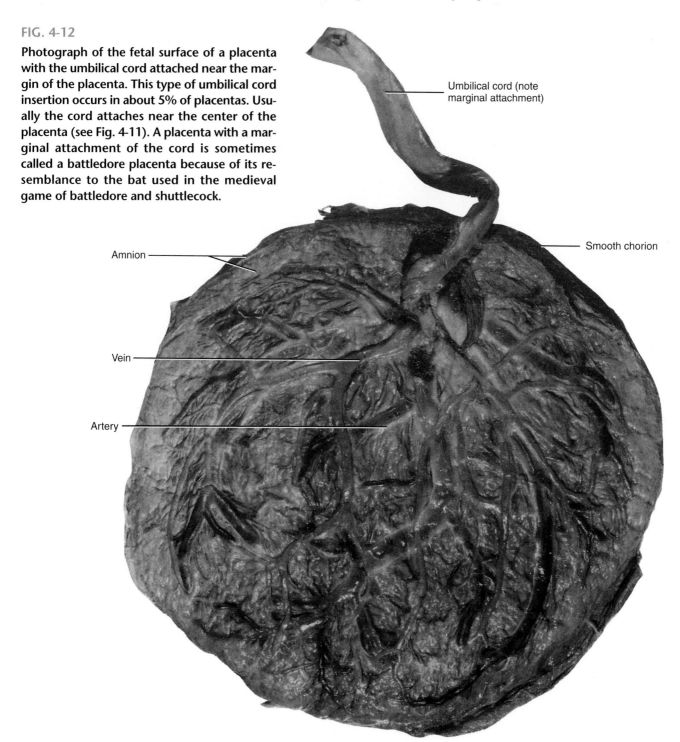

Umbilical cord (note marginal attachment)

Smooth chorion

Amnion

Vein

Artery

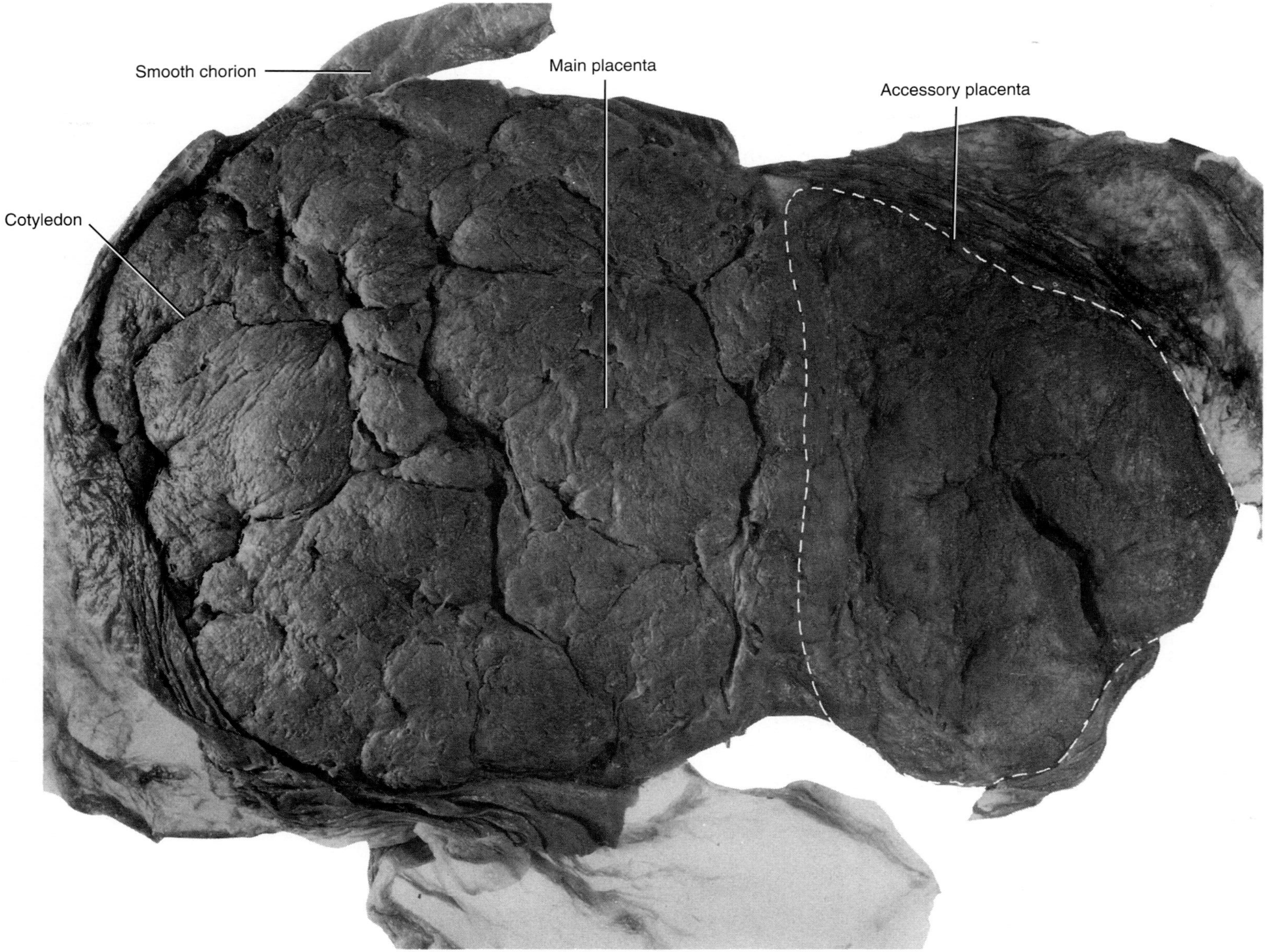

Accessory placenta

Main placenta

Smooth chorion

Cotyledon

FIG. 4-13

Photograph of the maternal surface of an odd-shaped placenta caused by the presence of an accessory placenta. The additional placenta developed from chorionic villi that persisted close to the normal placenta. It resembles the fused placentas of twins except that only one umbilical cord is attached.

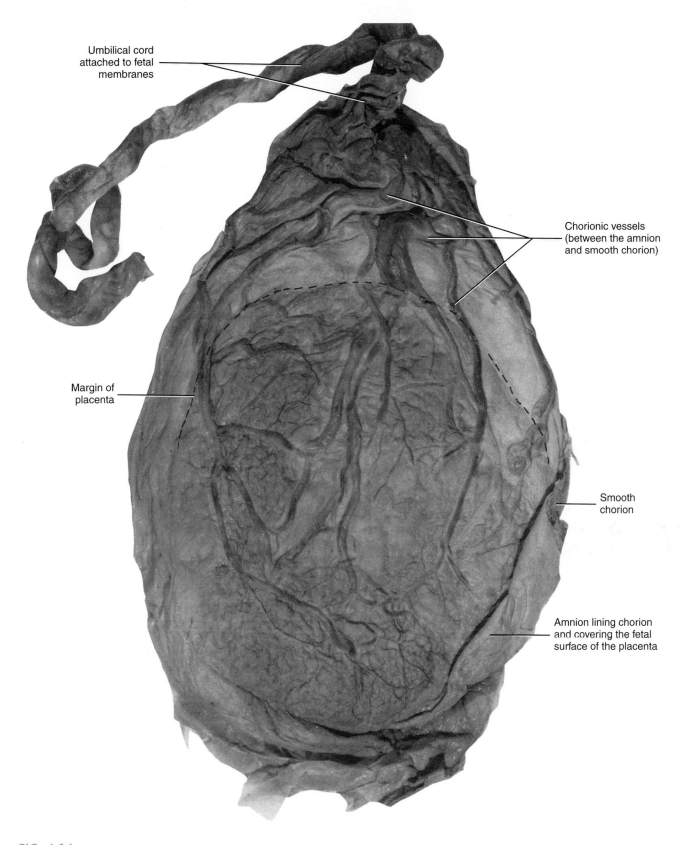

Umbilical cord attached to fetal membranes

Chorionic vessels (between the amnion and smooth chorion)

Margin of placenta

Smooth chorion

Amnion lining chorion and covering the fetal surface of the placenta

FIG. 4-14

Photograph of a placenta with a velamentous insertion of the umbilical cord. The incidence of velamentous umbilical cords is between 1% and 2%. This type of umbilical cord insertion is associated with multiple gestation and developmental abnormalities. In unusual cases, as here, the cord does not attach to the placenta but inserts onto the smooth chorion away from the placenta and chorionic villi. The umbilical vessels leave the umbilical cord and run between the amnion and chorion to reach the placenta and chorionic villi. The blood vessels are easily torn in this location, which results in the loss of fetal blood.

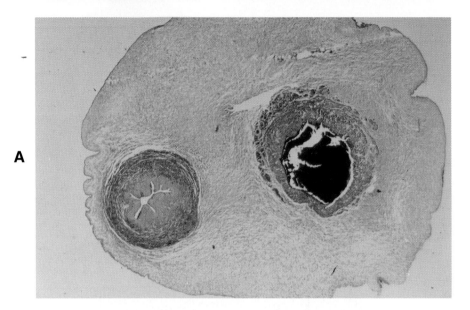

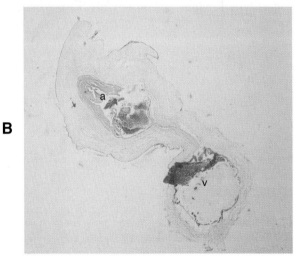

FIG. 4-15

A, Transverse section of umbilical cord from a newborn infant. Observe that the cord is covered by a single-layered epithelium derived from the enveloping amnion. It has a core of mucous connective tissue (Wharton jelly). Observe also that the cord has one umbilical artery and one vein. Usually there are two umbilical arteries. The vein, which carries oxygenated blood from the placenta, is unusual in that its wall, unlike that of most veins, consists principally of a tunica media. **B,** Section of umbilical cord from a fetus at 6 months gestational age. Note the single artery *(a)* and a vein *(v)* in the connective tissue core. The thick wall of the artery appears defective in some areas with hemorrhage within the muscle layer. (**A,** Courtesy of Professor V. Becker, Pathologisches Institut der Universität, Erlangen, Germany. **B,** Courtesy of Dr. E.M. Abdel Meguid and Dr. G.M. Fouad, Departments of Anatomy & Histology, Faculty of Medicine, Alexandria, Egypt.)

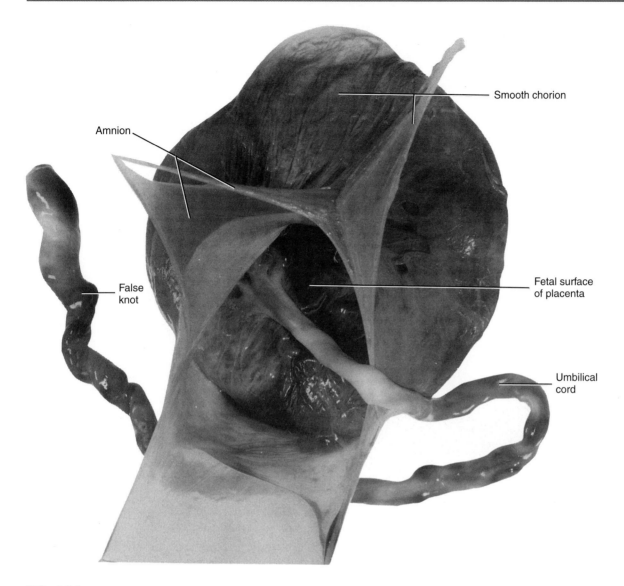

Amnion

Smooth chorion

False
knot

Fetal surface
of placenta

Umbilical
cord

FIG. 4-16

Photograph of the fetal membranes and the fetal surface of the placenta. The amnion and smooth chorion are arranged to show that they are fused and continuous with the margin of the placenta (see also Figs. 4-4 and 4-5). Observe the false knots in the umbilical cord that develop when the umbilical vessels form loops. False knots are common findings and of no clinical significance. A true knot in the cord can cause the death of the fetus if it tightens and obstructs blood flow.

The umbilical cord is usually 1 to 2 cm in diameter and 30 to 90 cm in length (average 55 cm). The normal umbilical cord contains two arteries and one vein. In about 1% of neonates a single umbilical artery is present (Fig. 4-15). This anomaly is often associated with other morphological defects in the infant. Excessively long or short cords are uncommon. Long cords have a tendency to prolapse and/or to coil around the fetus (Figs. 4-16 and 4-17). Prompt recognition of *prolapse of the cord* is important because the cord may be compressed between the presenting body part of the fetus and the mother's bony pelvis. This causes *fetal hypoxia.* If anoxia persists for more than five minutes, the baby's brain may be damaged, producing mental retardation. A very short cord may lead to premature separation of the placenta from the wall of the uterus during delivery.

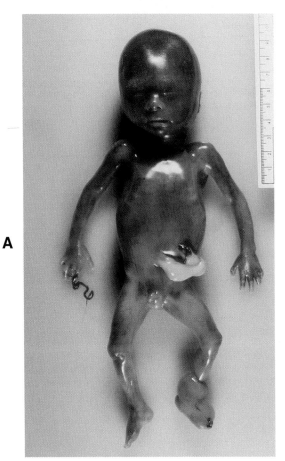 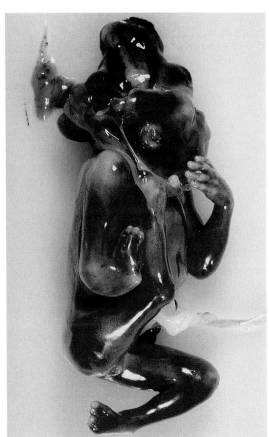

FIG. 4-17

Amniotic rupture sequence with amniotic bands in two fetuses less than 20 weeks of development. **A,** Isolated involvement of extremities with a partial amputation of fingers 2 and 3 on right hand and edema of left ankle and foot resulting from the amniotic band are shown in male fetus of 19 developmental weeks. **B,** Extensive deformations of skull, face, and extremities caused by amniotic bands are illustrated in male fetus of 13.5 developmental weeks. (**A** and **B,** Courtesy of Dr. D.K. Kalousek, Department of Pathology, University of British Columbia, Children's Hospital, Vancouver, B.C., Canada.)

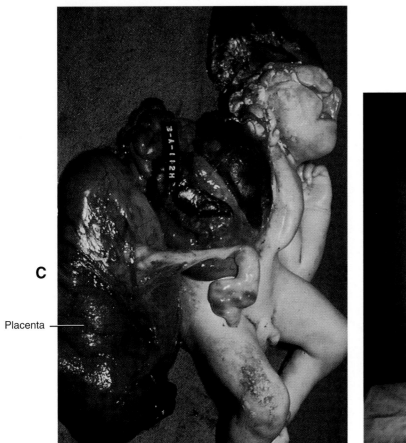

Placenta

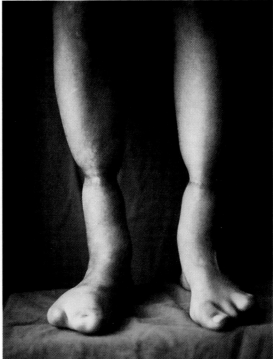

FIG. 4-17, cont'd

C, Photograph of a fetus with the amniotic band syndrome. This stillborn has multiple anomalies including encephalocele, facial clefting, and a lateral abdominal wall defect with exteriorization of the thoracic and abdominal contents resulting from thoracoabdominal schisis (failure of embryonic fusion of the abdominal wall). The right upper limb is rudimentary. Note the short umbilical cord with attachment of the placenta to the intestine. The primary event is believed to be a vascular disruption with secondary adhesion and disruption of the amnion. **D,** Note the circumferential constricting rings involving the lower limbs and deformation of the right foot, caused by aberrant amniotic bands. (**C,** Courtesy of Dr. A.E. Chudley, Department of Pediatrics and Child Health, University of Manitoba, Children's Hospital, Winnipeg, Manitoba, Canada. **D,** Courtesy of Dr. J.C. Fernandes Rodrigues, Servico de Dermatologia, Hospital do Desterro, Lisbon, Portugal.)

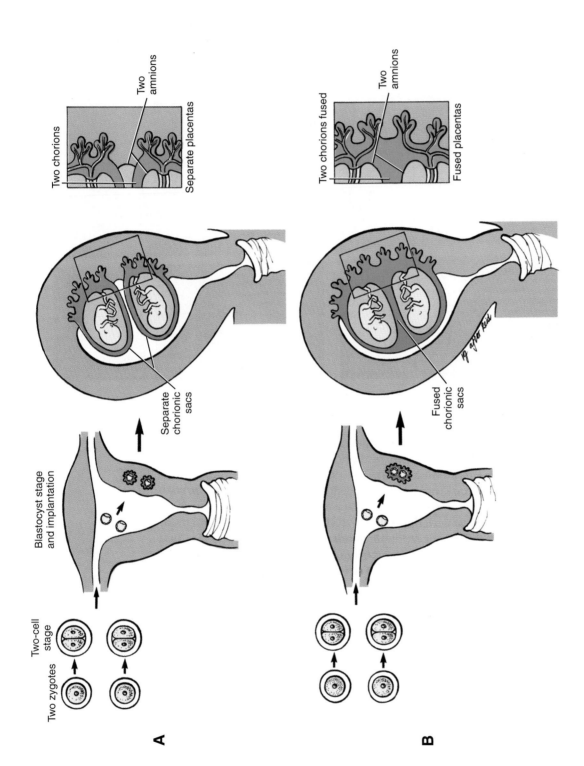

FIG. 4-18

Drawings showing how the most common type of twins, dizygotic (fraternal) twins, develop. They result from the fertilization of two ova by different sperms, which form two zygotes. They always have two amnions and two chorionic sacs and their placentas may be separate or fused. The twins may be of the same sex or different sexes and are no more alike than brothers or sisters born at different times. A, The two blastocysts have implanted separately in the endometrium. B, The blastocysts have implanted close together and their placentas have fused. Similarly the walls of their chorionic sacs have fused. In some cases the blood vessels of the two placentas anastomose (as shown in Fig. 4-19), which results in erythrocyte mosaicism, that is, the twins possess red blood cells of two different types.

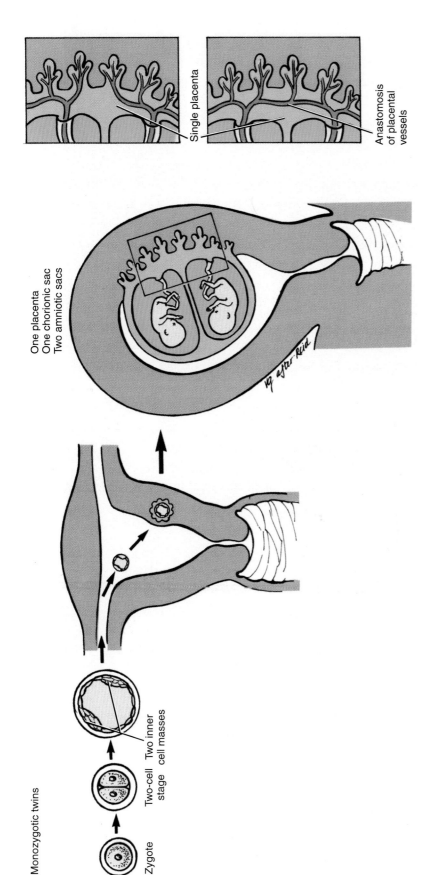

Monozygotic twins

Zygote

Two-cell stage

Two inner cell masses

One placenta
One chorionic sac
Two amniotic sacs

Single placenta

Anastomosis of placental vessels

FIG. 4-19

Drawings showing how monozygotic (identical) twins develop from one zygote. They result from the division of blastomeres at various stages of cleavage (see Figs. 1-3 to 1-5). The separation may occur at the two-cell to morula stage, in which case two blastocysts develop and implant separately. Each embryo has its own placenta and chorionic sac, similar to that which occurs in dizygotic twinning (see Fig. 4-18). In these cases, it is not possible to determine from the membranes alone whether the twins are monozygotic (MZ) or dizygotic (DZ). In most cases, MZ twinning occurs at the early blastocyst stage. The inner cell mass, as shown, splits into two separate groups of embryonic cells. The two embryos that develop have separate amnions but a common chorionic sac and placenta (see also Fig. 4-20, *B*). Often, there is anastomosis of the placental vessels, but this is of no consequence because the flow of blood is similar in both directions. In 15% to 30% of monochorionic diamniotic MZ twins, there is a shunt of arterial blood from one twin through arteriovenous anastomoses into the venous circulation of the other twin. The donor twin is small, pale, and anemic, whereas the recipient twin is large and polycythemic. This condition is known as twin-transfusion syndrome (see Fig. 4-26).

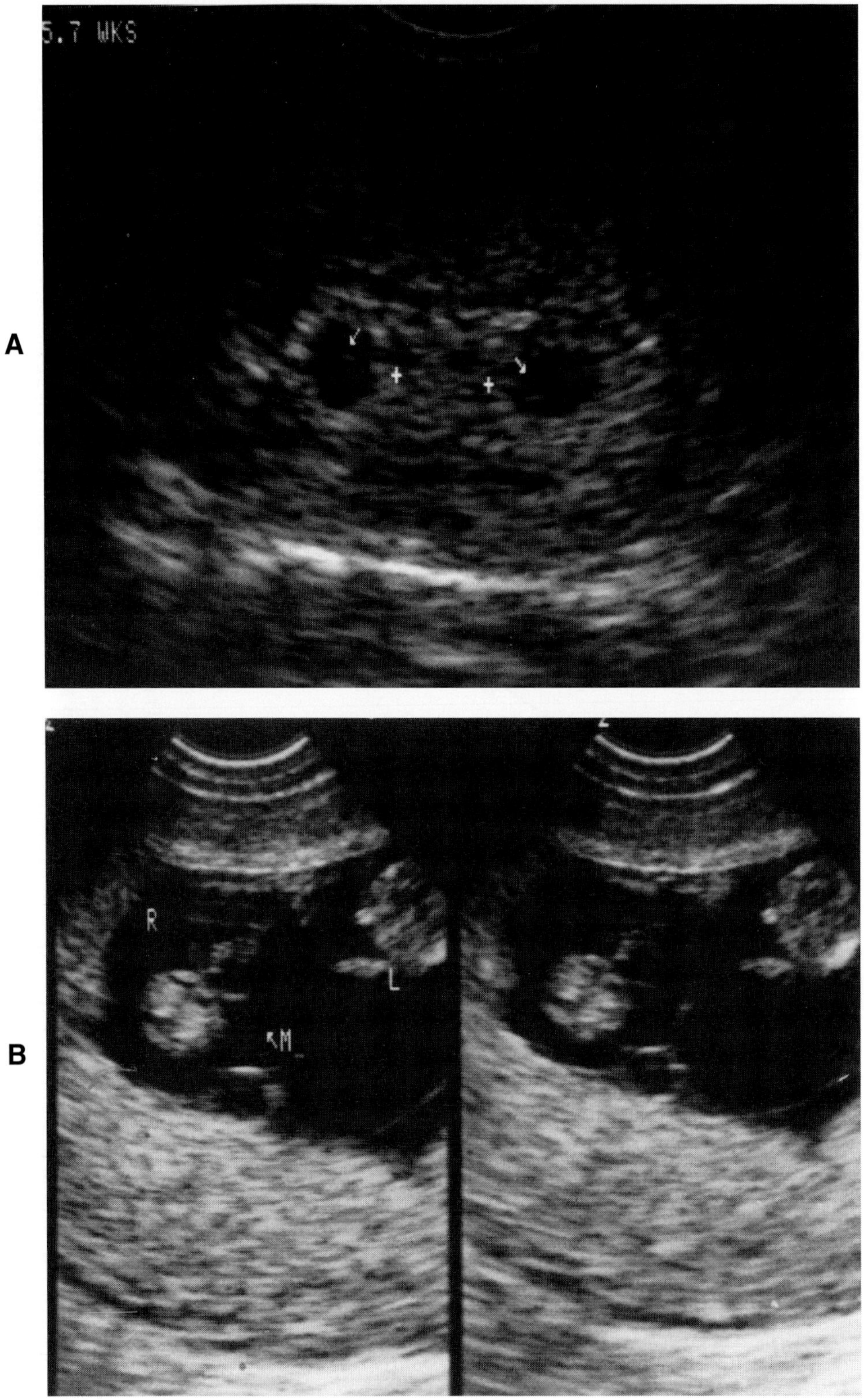

FIG. 4-20

Ultrasound scans of pregnant uteri. **A,** Diamniotic/dichorionic twin gestation at 5.7 weeks. (3.7 weeks after fertilization). The *arrows* indicate the yolk sacs of the dizygotic twins in their chorionic sacs. **B,** Diamniotic/monochorionic twin gestation at 11 weeks (9 weeks after fertilization). The fused amnions *(M)* separate the monozygotic fetuses *(R* and *L).* (Courtesy of Dr. Lyndon M. Hill, Department of Obstetrics and Gynecology, Division of Maternal-Fetal Medicine, University of Pittsburgh, Pittsburgh, Pa.)

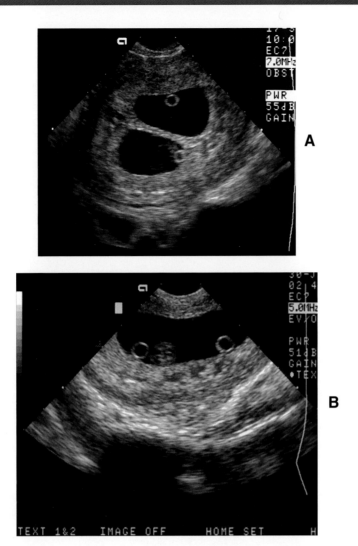

FIG. 4-21

A, Dichorionic, diamniotic twin gestation at 5.5 weeks. Observe the dual yolk sacs with thick interposed chorion. **B,** Monochorionic twin pregnancy at 7.5 weeks of gestation. The two yolk sacs suggest monochorionic, diamniotic twins. A double layer of amnion was detectable one week later. (From Fung Kee Fung KA: *J Soc Obstet Gynaecol Can* 20:641, 1998.)

FIG. 4-22

A, Conjoined twins at 12 weeks of development. Extensive fusion of the chest and abdomen is shown. **B,** In this uncommon case, separation of the embryonic disc occurred early in the third week as the primitive streak was developing. The twins share a placenta and have common chorionic and amniotic sacs. It has been estimated that about once in every 40 monozygotic twin pregnancies, the twinning is incomplete and conjoined twins develop. If the fusion is extensive, as in these cases, it is impossible to separate the infants. (**A,** Courtesy of Dr. D.K. Kalousek, Department of Pathology, University of British Columbia, Children's Hospital, Vancouver, BC, Canada. **B,** Courtesy of Dr. Susan Phillips, Department of Pathology, Health Science Centre, Winnipeg, Manitoba, Canada.)

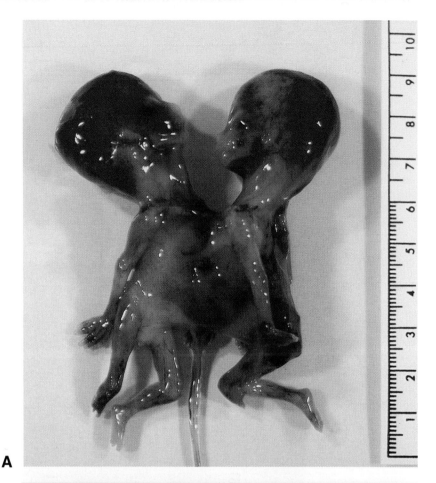

A

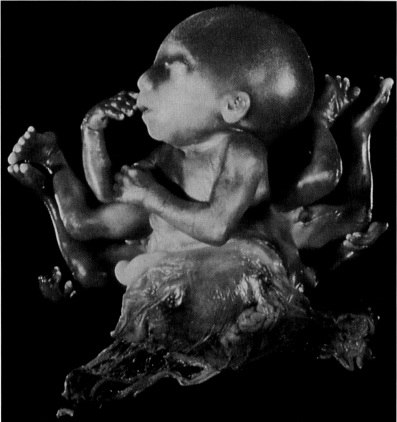

B

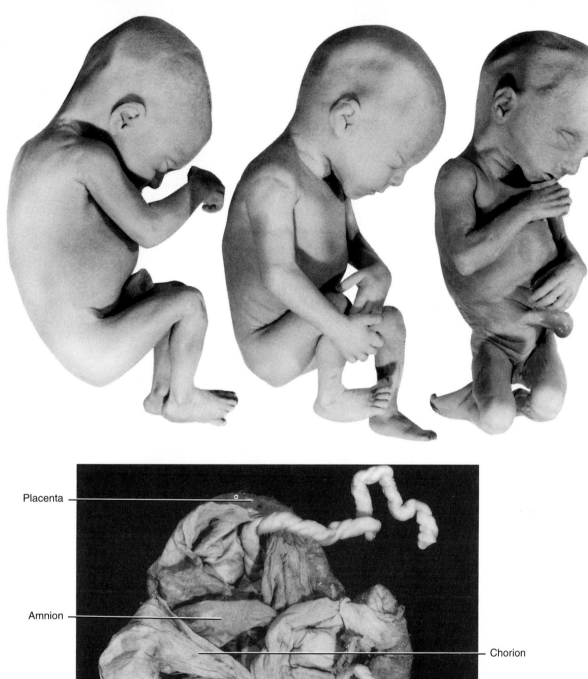

Placenta

Amnion

Chorion

Single placenta

Umbilical cord

FIG. 4-23

Photographs of triplets with their placentas and fetal membranes. Triplets may develop from one, two, or three zygotes. Examination of the placentas and membranes reveals that the two fetuses on the left were identical and the one on the right was a singleton. The diamniotic/monochorionic placenta is on the left and the single placenta is on the right. Thus these three fetuses developed from two zygotes. In recent years multiple births have occurred more frequently in mothers given fertility drugs for ovulatory failure.

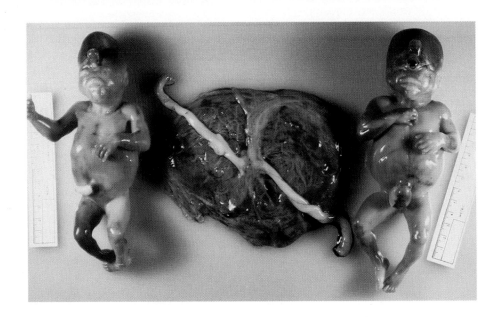

FIG. 4-24

Monozygotic twins with monochorionic and diamniotic placenta showing holoprosencephaly and abnormal facial development as a result of a chromosomal defect (15 to 16 weeks of development). (Courtesy of Dr. D.K. Kalousek, Department of Pathology, University of British Columbia, Children's Hospital, Vancouver, B.C., Canada.)

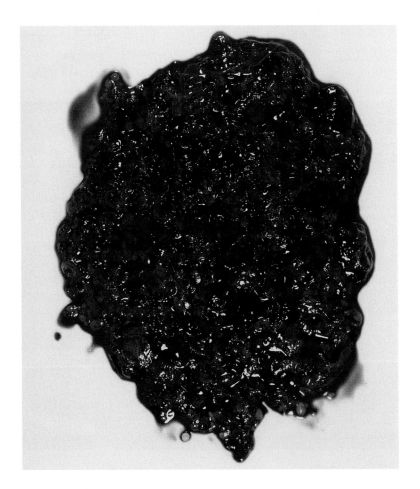

FIG 4-25

Complete hydatidiform mole with a normal diploid karyotype (46,XX) in which both haploid sets of chromosomes (23,X) are of paternal origin. The complete lack of a maternal set of chromosomes causes an abnormal cystic development of the placenta. (Courtesy of Dr. D.K. Kalousek, Department of Pathology, University of British Columbia, Children's Hospital, Vancouver, B.C., Canada.)

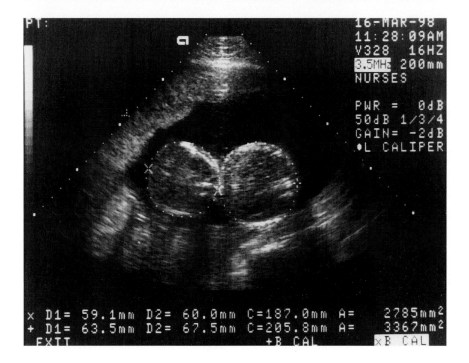

FIG. 4-26

Ultrasound image of discordant twins (24 weeks gestation), twin-twin transfusion syndrome. (Courtesy of Dr. G.J. Reid, Department of Obstetrics, Gynecology and Reproductive Sciences, University of Manitoba, Women's Hospital Winnipeg, Manitoba, Canada.)

Congenital Anomalies or Birth Defects

Congenital anomalies or birth defects may be structural, functional, metabolic, behavioral, or hereditary. More than 20% of infant deaths in North America are attributed to birth defects. Major structural anomalies (e.g., cleft lip and spina bifida cystica) are observed in about 3% of newborn infants. Additional anomalies can be detected after birth; thus the incidence reaches about 6% in 2 year olds and 8% in 5 year olds.

Anomalies may be single or multiple and of major or minor clinical significance. Single *minor anomalies* are present in about 14% of newborns. These defects (e.g., of the external ear) are of no serious medical or cosmetic significance, but they indicate to the clinician the possible presence of associated clinically significant anomalies.

Ninety percent of infants with three or more minor anomalies also have one or more major defects. Of the 3% born with clinically significant congenital anomalies, 0.7% have multiple major anomalies. Most of these infants die during infancy (e.g., those with trisomy 18 [see Fig. 5-7] and trisomy 13 [see Fig. 5-8]). Major developmental defects are much more common in early embryos (10% to 15%), but most of them abort spontaneously. Chromosome abnormalities are present in 50% to 60% of spontaneously aborted early embryos.

The causes of congenital anomalies are often divided into *genetic factors* (e.g., mutant genes and chromosome abnormalities) and *environmental factors,* such as drugs and viruses (Figs. 5-1 and 5-2). However, many common congenital anomalies are caused by multiple genetic and environmental factors acting together. This is called *multifactorial inheritance.* For 50% to 60% of congenital anomalies, it is not possible to identify a single cause (Fig. 5-1).

ANOMALIES CAUSED BY GENETIC FACTORS

Numerically, *genetic factors are the most important causes of congenital anomalies* (Fig. 5-1; Tables 5-1 and 5-2). It has been estimated that they cause about a third of all birth defects and nearly 85% of all those with known causes. Any mechanism as

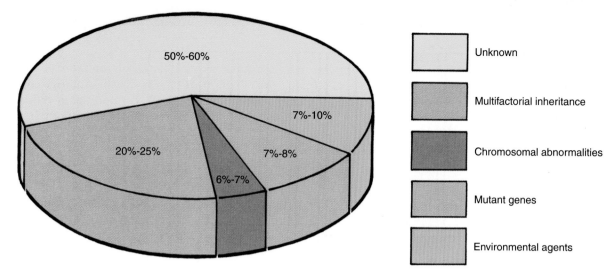

	Unknown
	Multifactorial inheritance
	Chromosomal abnormalities
	Mutant genes
	Environmental agents

FIG. 5-1

Graphic illustration of the causes of human congenital anomalies. Note that the causes of most anomalies are unknown and that 25% of them are caused by a combination of genetic and environmental factors (multifactorial inheritance).

TABLE 5-1

Trisomy of the Autosomes

Chromosomal Aberration/ Syndrome	Incidence	Usual Clinical Manifestations
Trisomy 21 or Down syndrome*	1:800	Mental deficiency; brachycephaly; flat nasal bridge; upward slant to palpebral fissures; protruding tongue; simian crease, clinodactyly of the fifth digit; congenital heart defects.
Trisomy 18 syndrome†	1:8000	Mental deficiency; growth retardation; prominent occiput; short sternum; ventricular septal defect; micrognathia; low-set malformed ears; flexed digits, hypoplastic nails; rocker-bottom feet.
Trisomy 13 syndrome†	1:25,000	Mental deficiency; severe central nervous system malformations; sloping forehead; malformed ears, scalp defects; microphthalmia; bilateral cleft lip and/or palate; polydactyly; posterior prominence of the heels.

*The importance of this disorder in the overall problem of mental retardation is indicated by the fact that persons with Down syndrome represent 10% to 15% of institutionalized mental patients. *The incidence of trisomy 21 at fertilization is greater than at birth;* however, 75% of embryos are spontaneously aborted and at least 20% are stillborn.
†Infants with this syndrome rarely survive beyond 6 months.

TABLE 5-2

Incidence of Down Syndrome in Newborn Infants

Maternal Age (Years)	Incidence	Maternal Age (Years)	Incidence
20-24	1:1400	39	1:140
25-29	1:1100	41	1:85
30-34	1:700	43	1:50
35	1:350	45+	1:25
37	1:225		

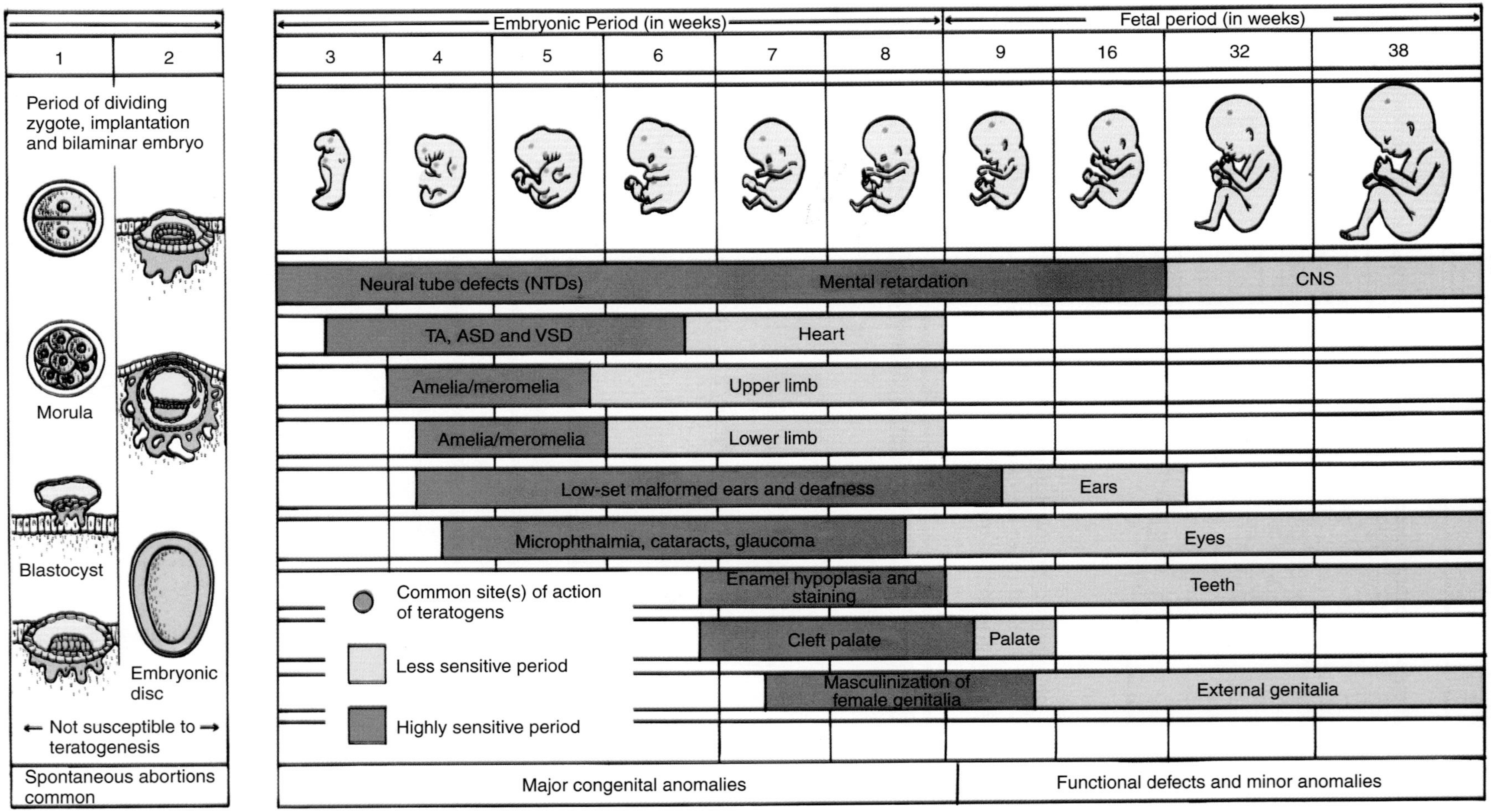

FIG. 5-2

Schematic illustration showing the critical periods of human development. Note that each part or organ of the embryo has a critical period when development may be disrupted, resulting in major congenital anomalies. Thereafter is a period when environmental agents (e.g., drugs and viruses) may cause minor anomalies and functional disturbances (e.g., mental retardation). *TA*, Truncus arteriosus; *ASD*, atrial septal defect; *VSD*, ventricular septal defect; *NTDs*, neural tube defects (e.g., spina bifida).

complex as mitosis or meiosis may occasionally malfunction. Thus *chromosomal aberrations are common* and are present in 6% to 7% of zygotes. Many of these primordial cells never undergo normal cleavage (mitosis) and become blastocysts. *In vitro studies of early embryos* (cleaving human zygotes) less than 5 days old have revealed a high incidence of abnormalities. Many defective zygotes, blastocysts, and early embryos abort spontaneously during the first 3 weeks and the overall frequency of chromosome abnormalities in them is at least 50%.

Two kinds of change occur in chromosome complements: numerical and structural, and they may affect the sex chromosomes and/or the autosomes (Figs. 5-3 to 5-8). In some cases, both kinds of chromosome are affected. People with *numerical chromosome abnormalities* usually have characteristic phenotypes (e.g., the physical characteristics of Down syndrome [Figs. 5-3 and 5-4; Tables 5-1 and 5-2]), and they often look more like other people with the same chromosome abnormality than like their own siblings (brothers or sisters). This characteristic appearance results from genetic imbalance. Structural defects that are present in aneuploid fetuses are commonly diagnosed in utero by ultrasonographic examination.

Text continued on p. 111

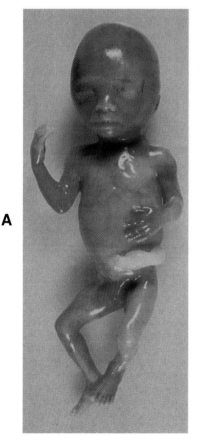
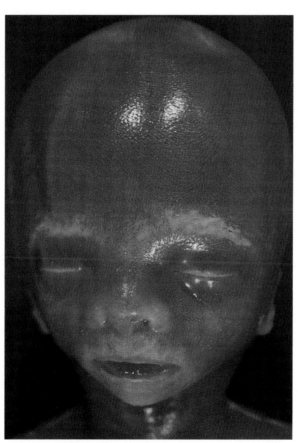

A

B

FIG. 5-3

A, Anterior view of a female fetus (16.5 weeks) with Down syndrome. See Table 5-1 for a list of the usual characteristics associated with this type of trisomy of the autosomes. **B**, Anterior view of the craniofacial region of a fetus with Down syndrome (16 weeks). Note the minimal dysmorphic features. (**A**, Courtesy of Dr. D.K. Kalousek, Department of Pathology, University of British Columbia, Children's Hospital, Vancouver, B.C., Canada. **B**, Courtesy of Dr. A.E. Chudley, Department of Pediatrics and Child Health, University of Manitoba, Children's Hospital, Winnipeg, Manitoba, Canada.) *Continued*

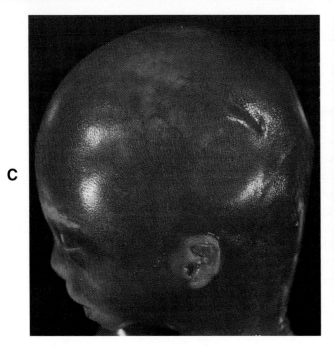

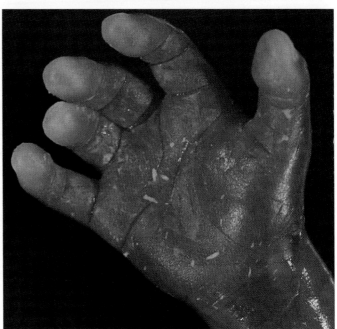

C

D

FIG. 5-3, cont'd

C, Lateral view of the craniofacial region of the fetus. Note the brachycephaly (shortness of the head) and small ears. **D,** Hand of the fetus. Note the single, transverse palmar, flexion (simian) crease and the clinodactyly (incurving) of the fifth digit. Not all persons with Down syndrome have transverse palmar creases. About three quarters of fetuses with Down syndrome (trisomy 21) are lost by spontaneous abortion, usually in the first trimester. The frequency of Down syndrome increases with maternal age (Table 5-2). In most cases the chromosome aberration results from nondisjunction of the number 21 chromosomes during oogenesis rather than spermatogenesis. (**C** and **D,** Courtesy of Dr. A.E. Chudley, Department of Pediatrics and Child Health, University of Manitoba, Children's Hospital, Winnipeg, Manitoba, Canada.)

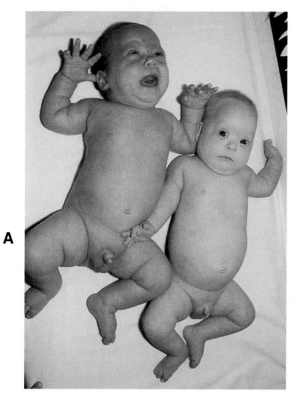

A

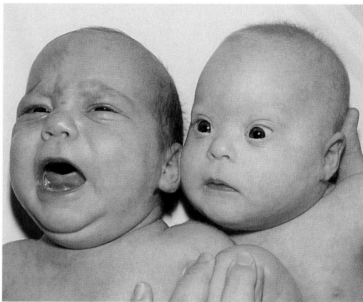

B

FIG. 5-4

Dizygotic (fraternal) male twins that are discordant for Down syndrome (trisomy 21). **A,** Anterior view of the twins. The one on the right is smaller and hypotonic compared with the unaffected twin. The twin on the right developed from a zygote that contained an extra 21 chromosome. **B,** Close-up of their faces. Note the characteristic facial features of Down syndrome in the infant on the right (upslanting palpebral fissures, epicanthal folds and flat nasal bridge). (Courtesy of Dr. A.E. Chudley, Department of Pediatrics and Child Health, University of Manitoba, Children's Hospital, Winnipeg, Manitoba, Canada.)

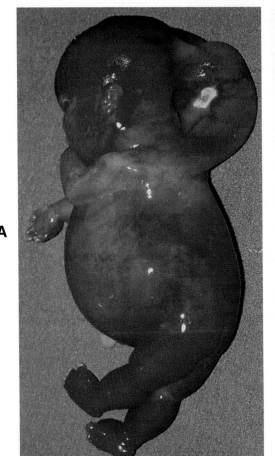
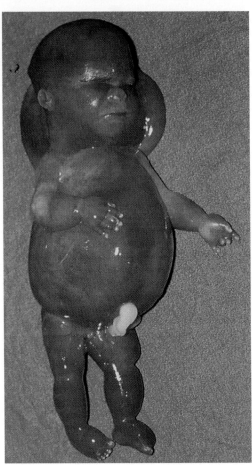

FIG. 5-5
Female fetus (16 weeks) with Turner syndrome and a chromosome constitution of 45,X (sometimes written as 45,XO). She had no second sex chromosome, either X or Y. Note the excessive accumulation of watery fluid (hydrops) and the large cystic hygroma (cystic lymphangioma) in the cervical region. The hygroma causes the loose neck skin and webbing seen postnatally (see Fig. 5-6, *B*). **A**, Lateral view. **B**, Anterolateral view. This chromosomal abnormality is present in 1.5% of all conceptuses and accounts for about 18% of all chromosomally abnormal spontaneous abortions. (Courtesy of Dr. A.E. Chudley, Department of Pediatrics and Child Health, University of Manitoba, Children's Hospital, Winnipeg, Manitoba, Canada.)

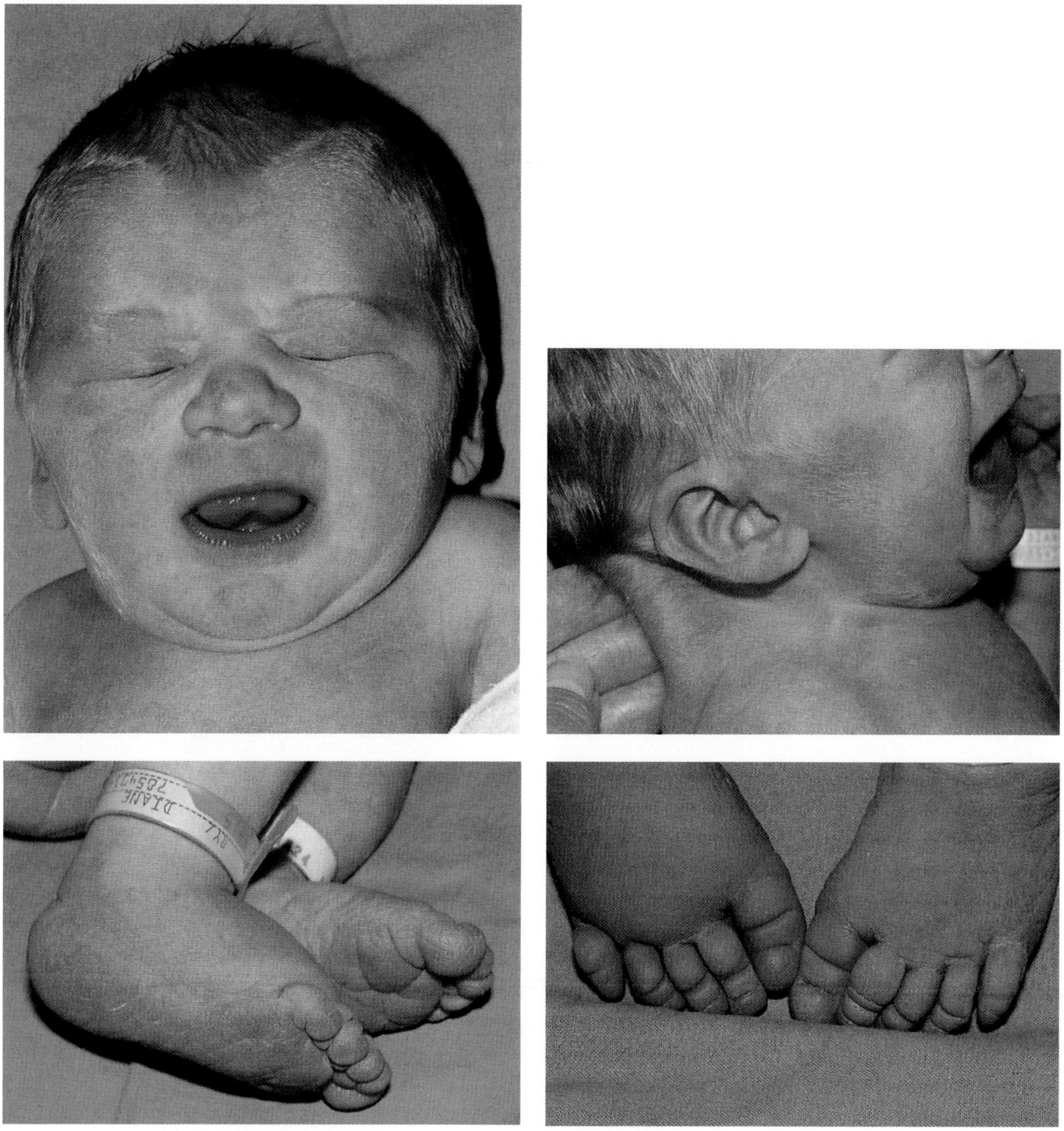

FIG. 5-6

A, Face of a female infant with Turner syndrome (45,X chromosome constitution). Note the short neck. **B,** Lateral view of the infants head and neck, showing the short neck, low-set ears, and redundant skin at the back of the neck. These infants have gonadal dysgenesis (usually streak gonads). **C,** Photograph of the infant's feet showing the characteristic lymphedema, a useful diagnostic sign. **D,** Lymphedema of the toes, a condition that usually leads to nail hypoplasia. In older females with this chromosome abnormality, there is absence of sexual maturation. (Courtesy of Dr. A.E. Chudley, Professor of Pediatrics and Child Health, University of Manitoba, Children's Centre, Winnipeg, Manitoba, Canada.)

FIG. 5-7

Trisomy 18 has an incidence of about 1 in 8000 births. The incidence at fertilization is higher, but about 95% of trisomy 18 fetuses are spontaneously aborted. The features of trisomy 18 always include mental retardation and failure to thrive, and often include a heart anomaly (Table 5-1). Postnatal survival for more than a few months is uncommon. Most affected fetuses and neonates are female. Late maternal age is a causative factor. **A,** Female fetus (15.5 weeks) with trisomy 18. Note the low-set malformed ears and the abnormal position of the hands. **B,** Typical rocker bottom feet in the fetus of 17 developmental weeks with trisomy 18 syndrome. (**A** and **B,** Courtesy of Dr. D.K. Kalousek, Department of Pathology, University of British Columbia, Children's Hospital, Vancouver, B.C., Canada.)

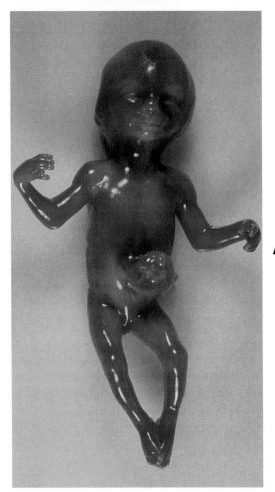

A

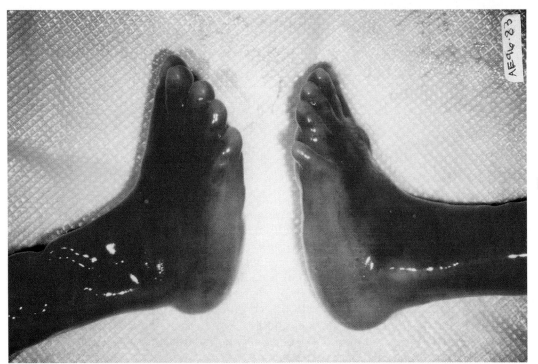

B

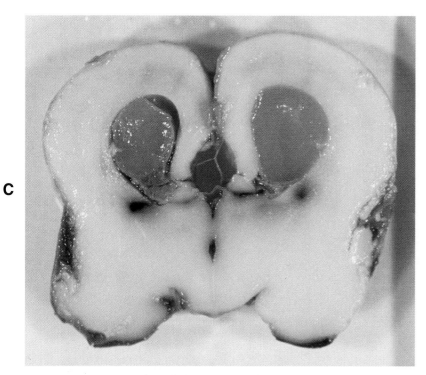

C

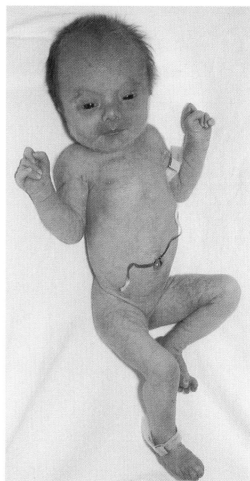

D

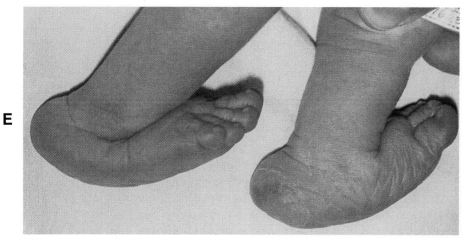

E

FIG. 5-7, cont'd

C, Bilateral choroid plexus cysts in the brain of the female fetus with trisomy 18 syndrome. **D,** Female neonate with trisomy 18. Note the growth retardation, clenched fists with characteristic positioning of the fingers (second and fifth digits overlapping the third and fourth), short sternum, and narrow pelvis. **E,** The feet of another trisomy 18 infant showing the characteristic rocker-bottom appearance as a result of the vertical position of the tali (ankle bones). Also observe the prominent calcanei (heel bones). (**C,** Courtesy of Dr. G. Hendson, Neuropathologist, B.C. Children's Hospital, Canada. **D** and **E,** Courtesy of Dr. A.E. Chudley, Department of Pediatrics and Child Health, University of Manitoba, Children's Hospital, Winnipeg, Manitoba, Canada.)

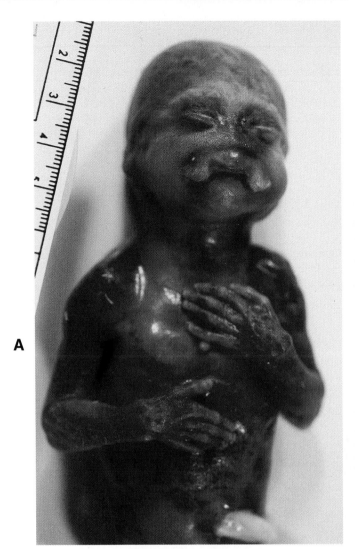

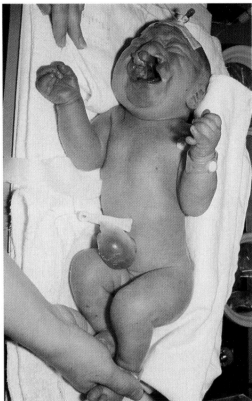

FIG. 5-8
Trisomy 13 is a clinically severe syndrome that occurs in about 1 in 25,000 births. It is lethal in almost all cases by the age of 6 months. Associated with late maternal age, the extra 13 chromosome arises from nondisjunction during the first division of maternal meiosis. **A,** Female fetus (16.5 weeks) with trisomy 13 syndrome, showing a characteristic phenotype with cebocephaly and postaxial polydactyly. Observe the severe cleft lip and low-set ears. **B,** Female neonate with trisomy 13. Note particularly the bilateral cleft lip, low-set malformed ear, and polydactyly (extra digits). A small omphalocele (herniation of viscera into the umbilical cord) is also present. For other defects characteristic of this syndrome, see Table 5-1. (**A,** Courtesy of Dr. D.K. Kalousek, Department of Pathology, University of British Columbia, Children's Hospital, Vancouver, B.C., Canada. **B,** Courtesy of Dr. A.E. Chudley, Department of Pediatrics and Child Health, University of Manitoba, Children's Hospital, Winnipeg, Manitoba, Canada.)

TABLE 5-3

Trisomy of the Sex Chromosomes

Chromosome Complement*	Sex	Incidence†	Usual Characteristics
47, XXX	Female	1:960	Normal in appearance; usually fertile; 15% to 25% are mildly mentally retarded
47,XXY	Male	1:1080	Klinefelter syndrome: small testes, hyalinization of seminiferous tubules; aspermatogenesis; often tall with disproportionately long lower limbs. Intelligence is less than in normal siblings. About 40% of these males have gynecomastia
47,XYY	Male	1:1080	Normal in appearance; usually tall; often exhibit aggressive behavior

*The numbers designate the total number of chromosomes including the sex chromosomes shown after the comma.
†Data from Hook EB, Hamerton JL: The frequency of chromosome abnormalities detected in consecutive newborn studies—Differences between studies—Results by sex and by severity of phenotypic involvement. In Hook EB, Porter IH (eds): *Population cytogenetics: studies in humans*. New York, 1977, Academic Press.

SEX CHROMOSOME TRISOMIES

Trisomy of the sex chromosomes is a common condition (Table 5-3); however, because there are no characteristic physical findings in infants or children, this disorder is not usually detected before puberty. **Sex chromatin studies** were useful in the past in detecting some types of trisomy of the sex chromosomes because two masses of sex chromatin are present in nuclei of XXX females, and nuclei of XXY males contain a mass of sex chromatin. Today, diagnosis is best achieved by chromosome analysis.

Structural chromosome abnormalities result from **chromosome breakage** that is induced by various environmental factors, for example, radiation, drugs, chemicals, and viruses. The type of abnormality that results depends on what happens to the broken pieces of the chromosomes (Fig. 5-9). The only aberrations that are likely to be transmitted from parent to child are structural rearrangements, such as inversion and translocation.

DELETION (FIG. 5-9, A). When a chromosome breaks, a portion of the chromosome may be lost. A partial terminal deletion from the short arm of chromosome number 5 causes the **cri du chat syndrome.** Affected infants have a weak, catlike cry, microcephaly, severe mental retardation, and congenital heart disease. A *ring chromosome* (Fig. 5-9, C) is a type of deletion chromosome from which both ends have been lost, and the broken ends have rejoined to form a ring-shaped chromosome. These abnormal chromosomes have been described in persons with Turner syndrome, trisomy 18, and other abnormalities.

TRANSLOCATION (FIG. 5-9, E). This is the transfer of a piece of one chromosome to a nonhomologous chromosome. Translocation does not necessarily lead to abnormal development (balanced translocation). The offspring of balanced translocation carriers can be phenotypically abnormal.

DUPLICATION (FIG. 5-9, B). This abnormality may be represented as a duplicated portion of a chromosome: (1) within a chromosome, (2) attached to a chromosome, or (3) as a separate fragment. *Duplications are more common than deletions and they are less harmful be-*

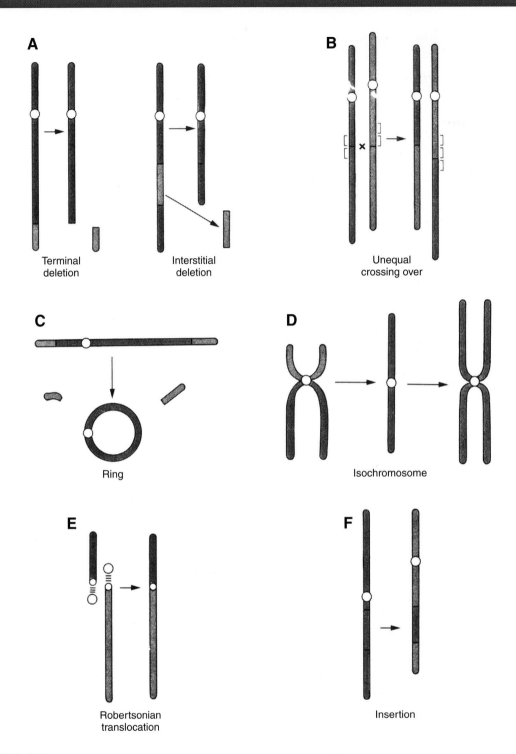

FIG. 5-9

Structural rearrangements of chromosomes. **A,** Terminal and interstitial deletions, each generating an acentric fragment. **B,** Unequal crossing over between segments of homologous chromosomes or between sister chromatids (the duplicated or deleted segment is indicated by brackets). **C,** Ring chromosome with two acentric fragments. **D,** Generation of an isochromosome for the long arm of a chromosome. **E,** Robertsonian translocation between two acrocentric chromosomes. **F,** Insertion of a segment of one chromosome into a nonhomologous chromosome. (From Thompson MW, McInnes RR, Willard HF: *Thompson and Thompson: genetics in medicine,* ed 5, Philadelphia, 1991, Saunders.)

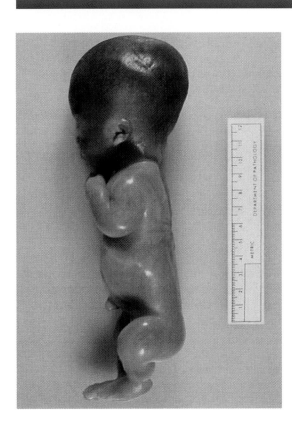

FIG. 5-10

Male fetus (18 weeks) with thanatophoric dwarfism or dysplasia, showing shortening of the limbs, a large head, and depressed nasal bridge. The most likely cause of this condition is a dominant mutation. (Courtesy of Dr. D.K. Kalousek, Department of Pathology, University of British Columbia, Children's Hospital, Vancouver, B.C., Canada.)

cause there is no loss of genetic material. Duplication may involve part of a gene, a whole gene, or a series of genes.

INVERSION. This is a chromosomal aberration in which a segment of a chromosome is reversed.

ISOCHROMOSOME (FIG. 5-9, D). This abnormality results when the centromere divides transversely instead of longitudinally. It appears to be the *most common structural abnormality of the X chromosome.* Patients with this chromosomal abnormality are often short in stature and have other stigmata of the Turner syndrome.

Anomalies Caused by Mutant Genes

Probably 8% of congenital anomalies are caused by mutant genes (see Fig. 5-1). A *mutation* usually involves a loss or a change in the function of a gene. Because a random change is unlikely to lead to an improvement in development, most mutations are deleterious and some are lethal. The mutation rate can be increased by a number of environmental agents, for example, large doses of radiation and some chemicals, especially carcinogenic (cancer-inducing) ones.

Examples of *dominantly inherited congenital anomalies* are **achondroplasia** and some types of polydactyly. Other anomalies are attributed to *autosomal recessive inheritance,* for example, congenital adrenal hyperplasia (see Fig. 10-21) and microcephaly.

Thanatophoric dysplasia or dwarfism (Fig. 5-10) is probably the most frequent lethal congenital skeletal dysplasia. Since the limbs are extremely short, this condition is sometimes misdiagnosed as achondroplasia. The thorax is very narrow in all dimensions and in neonates respiratory distress contributes to early death.

The **human genome** contains an estimated 50,000 to 100,000 structural genes per haploid set, or three billion base pairs. Many disease-causing genes are being identified because of international collaborations and the Human Genome Project. It is expected

TABLE 5-4

Examples of Disorders in Humans Associated With Homeobox Mutations

Name	Clinical Features	Gene
Waardenburg Syndrome (type I)	White forelock, lateral displacement of inner canthus of the eyes, cochlear deafness, heterochromia, tendency to facial clefting, autosomal dominant inheritance.	HuP2 gene in humans, homolog of Pax3 gene of mouse
Synpolydactyly (type II syndactyly)	Webbing and duplication of fingers, supernumerary metacarpal, autosomal dominant inheritance.	HOX D 13 mutation
Holoprosencephaly (one form)	Incomplete separation of lateral cerebral ventricles, anophthalmia or cyclopia, midline facial hypoplasia or clefts, single maxillary central incisors, hypotelorism, autosomal dominant inheritance with widely variable expression.	HPE 3 (Sonic Hedgehog) mutation gene which is homologous to the *Drosophila* segment polarity gene hedgehog
Schizencephaly (type II)	Full-thickness cleft within the cerebral ventricles often leading to seizures, spasticity and mental retardation.	Germline mutation in the EMX2 homeobox gene, homologous to the mouse EMX2

that most genetic diseases will be mapped and all genes sequenced by the early part of the twenty-first century. It is plausible that the majority of infants with congenital anomalies of unknown etiology will be determined to result from gene mutations. Molecular analysis has already confirmed this for many disorders.

Genomic imprinting is an epigenetic process whereby the female and male germline confer a sex-specific mark on a chromosome subregion, so that only the paternal or maternal allele of a gene is active in the offspring. In other words, the sex of the transmitting parent will influence expression or nonexpression of certain genes in the offspring (Table 5-4). This is the reason for Prader-Willi syndrome (PWS) and Angelman syndrome (AS), in which case the phenotype is determined by whether the microdeletion is transmitted by the father (PWS) or by the mother (AS). In a substantial number of cases of PWS and AS, as well as several other genetic disorders, the condition arises from a phenomenon referred to as *uniparental disomy*. In the situation with PWS and AS, both chromosomes 15s originate from only one parent. PWS occurs when both chromosomes 15s are derived from the mother and AS occurs when both are paternally derived. The mechanism for this is believed to begin with a trisomic conceptus, followed by a loss of the extra chromosome in an early postzygotic cell division. This results in a "rescued" cell in which both chromosomes have been derived from one parent.

Homeobox genes are a group of genes found in all vertebrates. They have highly conserved sequences and order. They are involved in early embryonic development and specify identity and spatial arrangements of body segments. Protein products of these genes bind to DNA and form transcriptional factors that regulate gene expression. Disorders associated with homeobox mutations are described in Table 5-4.

ANOMALIES CAUSED BY ENVIRONMENTAL FACTORS

Although the human embryo is well protected in the uterus, certain environmental agents called **teratogens** may cause developmental disturbances following maternal exposure to them (Table 5-5). A teratogen is any agent that can produce a congenital anomaly or raise the incidence of an anomaly in the population. Environmental factors, such as infection and drugs, may simulate genetic conditions; for example, when two or more children of normal parents are affected.

ENVIRONMENTAL FACTORS CAUSE 7% TO 10% OF CONGENITAL ANOMALIES (FIG. 5-1). Because biochemical differentiation precedes morphological differentiation, the period during which structures are sensitive to interference often precedes the stage of their visible development by a few days. Teratogens do not appear to be effective in causing anomalies until cellular differentiation has begun. However, their early actions may cause death of the embryo.

CRITICAL PERIODS IN HUMAN DEVELOPMENT (FIG. 5-2). The organs and parts of an embryo are most sensitive to teratogenic agents during periods of rapid differentiation. The stage of development of an embryo when a teratogenic agent is present determines its susceptibility to a teratogen. The most critical period in development is when cell division, cell differentiation, and morphogenesis are at their peak.

Human Teratogens and Congenital Anomalies

Awareness that certain agents can disrupt embryonic development offers the opportunity to prevent some congenital anomalies (Table 5-5). For example, if women are made aware of the harmful effects of drugs (e.g., alcohol), environmental chemicals (e.g., PCBs), and viruses (e.g., rubella), most of them will not expose their embryos to these teratogenic agents.

Drugs as Teratogens

Drugs vary considerably in their teratogenicity. Some cause severe disturbances in development if administered during the organogenetic period (e.g., thalidomide causes severe limb defects and other anomalies). Other drugs produce mental and growth retardation and other anomalies if used excessively throughout development (e.g., alcohol [Fig. 5-11]).

The use of prescription and nonprescription drugs during pregnancy is surprisingly high. From 40% to 90% of pregnant women consume at least one drug. Several studies have indicated that some pregnant women take an average of four drugs, excluding nutritional supplements, and about half of these women take them during the first trimester of pregnancy. Drug consumption also tends to be higher during the critical period of development among heavy smokers and heavy drinkers.

Infectious Agents as Teratogens

Throughout prenatal life, the embryo and fetus are endangered by a variety of **microorganisms**. In most cases, the assault is resisted; in some cases, a spontaneous abortion or stillbirth occurs; in others, the infants are born with growth retardation, congenital anomalies, or neonatal diseases (Table 5-3). The microorganisms, especially *viruses,* cross the placental membrane and enter the fetal blood stream (see Fig. 4-7). The fetal blood-brain barrier also appears to offer little resistance to microorganisms, because there is a propensity for the central nervous system to be affected. The rubella virus is the prime example of an *infective teratogen.* The risk is about 20% when maternal infection occurs during the first trimester. The usual features of *congenital rubella syndrome* are cataract (Fig. 5-12, *A*), cardiac defects, and deafness. The most common cause of congenital infection is the human cytomegalovirus, which presents serious long-term consequences, including mental retardation, optic atrophy, and neurological disorders. For other teratogenic effects of this and other viruses, see Table 5-3.

TABLE 5-5

Teratogens Known to Cause Human Birth Defects

Agents	Most Common Congenital Anomalies
DRUGS	
Alcohol	*Fetal alcohol syndrome (FAS):* intrauterine growth retardation *(IUGR);* mental retardation, microcephaly; ocular anomalies; joint abnormalities; short palpebral fissures.
Androgens and high doses of progestogens	Varying degrees of masculinization of female fetuses: ambiguous external genitalia resulting in labial fusion and clitoral hypertrophy.
Aminopterin	IUGR; skeletal defects, malformations of the central nervous system (CNS), notably meroanencephaly (most of the brain is absent).
Busulfan	Stunted growth; skeletal abnormalities; corneal opacities; cleft palate; hypoplasia of various organs.
Cocaine	IUGR; microcephaly; cerebral infarction; urogenital anomalies; neurobehavioral disturbances.
Diethystilbesterol	Abnormalities of the uterus and vagina; cervical erosion and ridges.
Isotretinoin (13-cis-retinoic acid)	Craniofacial abnormalities; neural tube defects *(NTDs),* such as spina bifida cystica; cardiovascular defects.
Lithium carbonate	Various anomalies usually involving the heart and great vessels.
Methotrexate	Multiple anomalies, especially skeletal, involving the face, skull, limbs, and vertebral column.
Phenytoin (Dilantin)	*Fetal hydantoin syndrome (FHS):* IUGR; microcephaly; mental retardation; ridged metopic suture; inner epicanthal folds; eyelid ptosis; broad depressed nasal bridge; phalangeal hypoplasia.
Tetracycline	Stained teeth; hypoplasia of enamel.
Thalidomide	Abnormal development of limbs, for example, meromelia (partial absence) and amelia (complete absence); facial anomalies; systemic anomalies, for example, cardiac and kidney defects.
Trimethadione	Developmental delay; V-shaped eyebrows; low-set ears; cleft lip and/or palate.
Valproic acid	Craniofacial anomalies; NTDs; often hydrocephalus; heart and skeletal defects.
Warfarin	Nasal hypoplasia; stippled epiphyses; hypoplastic phalanges; eye anomalies; mental retardation.

TABLE 5-5

Teratogens Known to Cause Human Birth Defects—cont'd

Agents	Most Common Congenital Anomalies
CHEMICALS	
Methylmercury	Cerebral atrophy; spasticity; seizures; mental retardation.
Polychlorinated biphenyls (PCBs)	IUGR; skin discolorization.
INFECTIONS	
Cytomegalovirus	Microcephaly; chorioretinitis; sensorineural loss; delayed psychomotor/mental development; hepatosplenomegaly; hydrocephaly; cerebral palsy; brain (periventricular) calcification.
Herpes simplex virus	Skin vesicles and scarring; chorioretinitis; hepatomegaly; thrombocytopenia; petechiae; hemolytic anemia; hydranencephaly.
Human immunodeficiency virus (HIV)	Growth failure; microcephaly; prominent boxlike forehead; flattened nasal bridge; hypertelorism; triangular philtrum and patulous lips.
Human parvovirus B19	Eye defects; degenerative changes in fetal tissues.
Rubella virus	IUGR; postnatal growth retardation; cardiac and great vessel abnormalities; microcephaly; sensorineural deafness; cataract; microphthalmos; glaucoma; pigmented retinopathy; mental retardation; newborn bleeding; hepatosplenomegaly; osteopathy.
Toxoplasma gondii	Microcephaly; mental retardation; microphthalmia; hydrocephaly; chorioretinitis; cerebral calcifications; hearing loss; neurological disturbances.
Treponema pallidum	Hydrocephalus; congenital deafness; mental retardation; abnormal teeth and bones.
Venezuelan equine encephalitis virus	Microcephaly; microphthalmia; cerebral agenesis; CNS necrosis; hydrocephalus.
Varicella virus	Cutaneous scars (dermatome distribution); neurological anomalies (limb paresis, hydrocephaly, seizures); cataracts; microphthalmia; Horner syndrome; optic atrophy; nystagmus; chorioretinitis; microcephaly; mental retardation; skeletal anomalies (hypoplasia of limbs, fingers, and toes); urogenital anomalies.
HIGH LEVELS OF IONIZING RADIATION	Microcephaly; mental retardation; skeletal anomalies; growth retardation; cataracts.

FIG. 5-11

Neonate with the fetal alcohol syndrome. Note the thin upper lip, short palpebral fissures, flat nasal bridge, short nose, and elongated and poorly formed philtrum. Maternal alcohol abuse is thought to be the most common environmental cause of mental retardation. (Courtesy of Dr. A.E. Chudley, Department of Pediatrics and Child Health, University of Manitoba, Children's Centre, Winnipeg, Manitoba, Canada.)

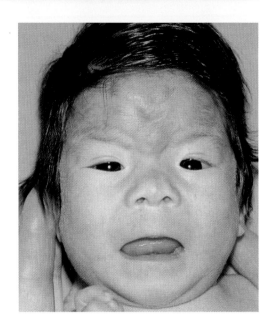

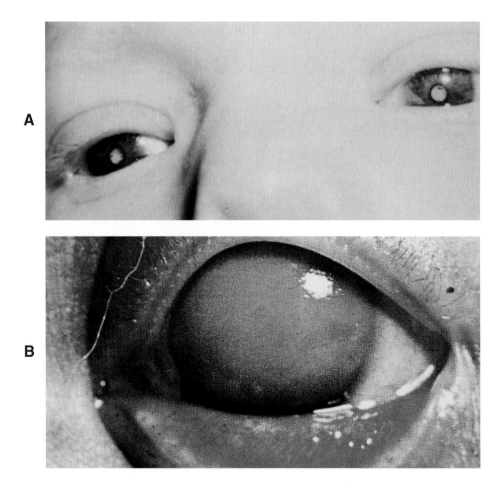

FIG. 5-12

A, Typical bilateral congenital cataracts caused by the teratogenic effects of the rubella virus. Cardiac defects and deafness are other common congenital defects. **B,** Severe congenital glaucoma resulting from rubella. Observe the dense corneal haze, enlarged corneal diameter, and deep anterior chamber. (**A,** Courtesy of Dr. Richard Bargy, Department of Ophthalmology, Cornell-New York Hospital. **B,** Courtesy of Dr. Daniel I. Weiss, Department of Ophthalmology, New York University College of Medicine. From Cooper LA, et al: *Am J Dis Child* 110:416, 1965.)

Radiation as a Teratogen

Exposure to *ionizing radiation* may injure embryonic cells, resulting in cell death, chromosome injury, and retardation of mental development and physical growth. The severity of the embryonic damage is related to the absorbed dose, the dose rate, and the stage of embryonic or fetal development during which the exposure occurs. Data on the group exposed in utero to the atom bomb in Hiroshima and Nagasaki show that severe mental retardation and microcephaly (small head size) occurred after exposures at 8 to 15 weeks of gestational age. In the past, large amounts of ionizing radiation (hundreds to several thousand rads) were given inadvertently to embryos and fetuses of pregnant women who had cancer of the cervix. In all cases, their embryos were severely malformed or killed.

There is no proof that human congenital anomalies have been caused by diagnostic levels of radiation. Scattered radiation from an x-ray examination of a part of the body that is not near the uterus (e.g., the chest, sinuses, teeth) produces a dose of only a few millirads, which is not teratogenic to the embryo.

Ultrasonography is widely used during pregnancy for fetal diagnosis and prenatal care. There are no confirmed biological effects on the fetus from the use of diagnostic ultrasound. Also, there is no evidence of an increased risk of fetal growth retardation and other developmental defects following maternal exposure to low-frequency electromagnetic fields, for example, video display terminals.

ANOMALIES CAUSED BY MULTIFACTORIAL INHERITANCE

Many common congenital anomalies (e.g., cleft lip with or without cleft palate) have familial distribution consistent with multifactorial inheritance (MFI) (Fig. 5-1). Multifactorial inheritance may be represented by a model in which "liability" to a disorder is a continuous variable determined by a combination of genetic and environmental factors, with a developmental threshold dividing individuals with the anomaly from those without it. Multifactorial traits are often single major anomalies, such as cleft lip, isolated cleft palate, neural tube defects (e.g., meroanencephaly and spina bifida cystica), pyloric stenosis, and congenital dislocation of the hip. Some of these anomalies may also occur as part of the phenotype in syndromes determined by single-gene inheritance, chromosome abnormality, or an environmental teratogen. The recurrence risks used for genetic counseling of families having congenital anomalies determined by MFI are empirical risks based on the frequency of the anomaly in the general population and in different categories of relatives. In individual families, such estimates may be inaccurate because they are usually averages for the population rather than precise probabilities for the individual family.

6

Embryonic Body Cavities and the Diaphragm

Early development of the intraembryonic coelom (embryonic body cavity) during the third week is described and illustrated in Chapter 2. By the fourth week, the coelom appears as a horseshoe-shaped cavity in the cardiogenic and lateral mesoderm (Fig. 6-1). The curve or bend in this cavity represents the future *pericardial cavity* and its limbs (or lateral parts) indicate the future *pleural and peritoneal cavities.*

The distal part of each limb of the intraembryonic coelom opens into the *extraembryonic coelom* at the lateral edges of the embryonic disc (Fig. 6-1). This communication is important because most of the midgut normally herniates through this communication into the umbilical cord, where it develops into most of the small intestine and part of the large intestine. During embryonic folding in the horizontal plane, the limbs of the intraembryonic coelom are brought together on the ventral aspect of the embryo (Fig. 6-2). The ventral mesentery degenerates in the region of the future peritoneal cavity, resulting in a large embryonic peritoneal cavity extending from the heart to the pelvic region (Fig. 6-2, *E*).

EMBRYONIC BODY CAVITY

The well-defined intraembryonic coelom gives rise to three well-defined coelomic (body) cavities in the fourth week: (1) a large *pericardial cavity* (Fig. 6-2, *B*), (2) two *pericardioperitoneal canals* connecting the pericardial and peritoneal cavities (Fig. 6-2, *B*), and (3) a large *peritoneal cavity* (Fig. 6-2, *C* to *E*). These cavities have a parietal wall lined by mesothelium (future parietal peritoneum) derived from the somatic mesoderm, and a visceral wall covered by mesothelium derived from the splanchnic mesoderm (Fig. 6-2, *E*). The peritoneal cavity is connected with the extraembryonic coelom but is separated from it during the tenth week as the intestines return to the abdomen from the umbilical cord (see Fig. 9-2).

During formation of the *head fold* during the fifth week, the heart and pericardial cavity are carried ventrocaudally, anterior to the foregut (Fig. 6-2, *A*). As a result, the pericardial cavity opens dorsally into the pericardioperitoneal canals on each

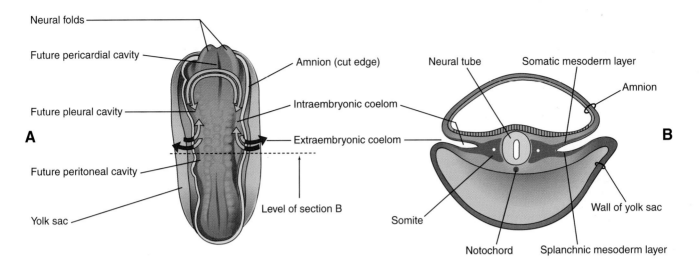

FIG. 6-1

A, Drawing of a dorsal view of a 22-day-old embryo showing the outline of the horseshoe-shaped intraembryonic coelom. The amnion has been removed and the coelom is shown as if the embryo were translucent. The continuity of the intraembryonic coelom, as well as the communication of its right and left limbs with the extraembryonic coelom, is indicated by arrows. **B,** Transverse section through the embryo at the level shown in *A*.

side of the foregut (Fig. 6-2, *B*). After embryonic folding, the caudal part of the foregut, the midgut, and hindgut are suspended in the peritoneal cavity from the posterior abdominal wall by the **dorsal mesentery** (Fig. 6-2, *D*).

A mesentery is a double layer of peritoneum. Transiently, the dorsal and ventral mesenteries divide the peritoneal cavity into right and left halves, but the ventral mesentery soon disappears, except where it is attached to the caudal part of the foregut (primordium of the stomach and the proximal part of the duodenum). The peritoneal cavity then becomes a continuous space (Fig. 6-2, *E*). The arteries supplying the primitive gut (i.e., the celiac [foregut], the superior mesenteric [midgut], and the inferior mesenteric [hindgut]), pass from the dorsal aorta between the layers of the dorsal mesentery.

Division of the Embryonic Body Cavity

Each pericardioperitoneal canal lies lateral to the foregut (future esophagus) and dorsal to the *septum transversum,* which is part of the future diaphragm (Figs. 6-2, *A,* and 6-3). Partitions form concurrently in each pericardioperitoneal canal, which soon separate the pericardial cavity from the pleural cavities and the pleural cavities from the peritoneal cavity. As a result of the *growth of the bronchial buds* (primordia of the lungs) into the pericardioperitoneal canals, a pair of membranous ridges is produced in the lateral wall of each canal. The cranial ridges, called *pleuropericardial membranes,* are located superior to the developing lungs and the caudal ridges, called *pleuroperitoneal membranes,* are located inferior to them.

THE PLEUROPERICARDIAL MEMBRANES (FIG. 6-3, *B*). As these cranial ridges enlarge, they form partitions that separate the pericardial cavity from the pleural cavities. At this stage, the *bronchial buds* are small relative to the heart and pericardial cavity. They grow laterally from the caudal end of the trachea into the corresponding pericardioperitoneal canal (pleural canal), which becomes the *primitive pleural cavity.* As these cavities expand ventrally around the heart, they extend into the body wall and split the mesenchyme into (1) an outer layer that becomes the thoracic wall and (2) an inner layer (the pleuroperi-

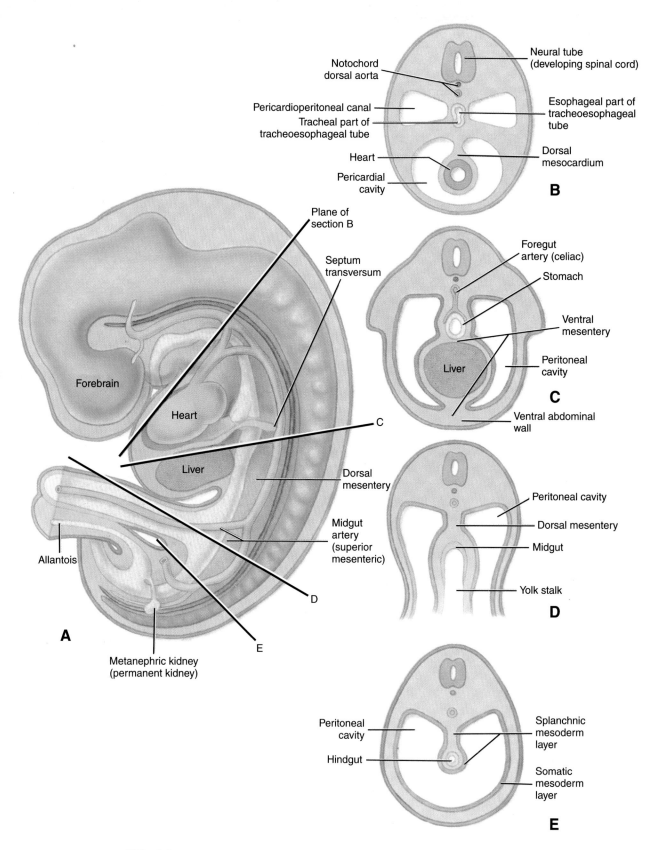

FIG. 6-2

Drawings illustrating the body cavities and mesenteries at the beginning of the fifth week. **A,** Schematic longitudinal section. Note that the dorsal mesentery serves as a pathway for the arteries supplying the developing gut (e.g., midgut artery). Nerves and lymphatics also pass between the layers of this mesentery. **B to E,** Transverse sections through the embryo at the levels indicated in *A.* The ventral mesentery disappears, except in the region of the terminal esophagus, stomach, and the first part of the duodenum. Note that the right and left parts of the peritoneal cavity, which are separate in *C,* are continuous in *E.*

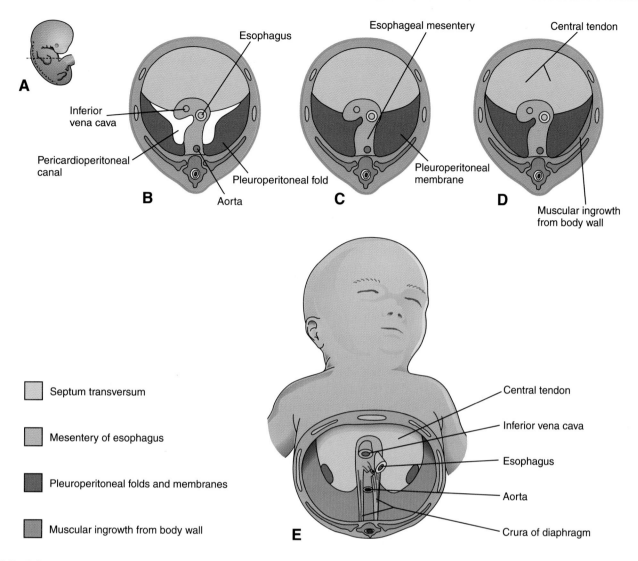

FIG. 6-3

Drawings illustrating development of the diaphragm. **A**, Sketch of a lateral view of an embryo at the end of the fifth week (actual size), indicating the level of sections in *B to D*. **B to E**, The developing diaphragm as viewed inferiorly. **B**, Transverse section showing the unfused pleuroperitoneal membranes. **C**, Similar section at the end of the sixth week after fusion of the pleuroperitoneal membranes with the other two diaphragmatic components. **D**, Transverse section of a 12-week embryo after ingrowth of the fourth diaphragmatic component from the body wall. **E**, View of the diaphragm of a newborn infant, indicating the embryological origin of its components.

cardial membrane) that becomes the *fibrous pericardium,* the outer fibrous layer of the pericardial sac.

THE PLEUROPERITONEAL MEMBRANES. As these caudal partitions in the pericardioperitoneal canals enlarge, they gradually separate the pleural cavities from the peritoneal cavity. This pair of membranes is produced as the developing lungs and pleural cavities expand and invade the body wall. They are attached dorsolaterally to the abdominal wall and their crescentic free edges initially project into the caudal ends of the pericardioperitoneal canals. They become relatively more prominent as the lungs enlarge and the liver expands.

During the sixth week, the pleuroperitoneal membranes extend ventromedially until their free edges fuse with the dorsal mesentery of the esophagus and the septum transversum (Fig. 6-3, C). This separates the pleural cavities from the peritoneal cavity. *Closure of the pleuroperitoneal openings* is assisted by the migration of myoblasts (primitive muscle cells) into the pleuroperitoneal membranes, which form posterolateral parts of the diaphragm (Fig. 6-3, E). The pleuroperitoneal opening on the right side closes slightly before the left one. The reason for this is uncertain, but it may be related to the relatively large right lobe of the liver at this stage of development.

DEVELOPMENT OF THE DIAPHRAGM

This dome-shaped, musculotendinous partition separates the thoracic and abdominal cavities. It has a complex embryonic origin. *The diaphragm develops from four structures:* the septum transversum, the pleuroperitoneal membranes, the dorsal mesentery of the esophagus, and the lateral body walls (Fig. 6-3).

THE SEPTUM TRANSVERSUM. This transverse septum, composed of mesoderm, is the primordium of the *central tendon of the diaphragm* (Fig. 6-3, E). It is located caudal to the pericardial cavity and partially separates it from the developing peritoneal cavity. The septum transversum is first identifiable at the end of the third week as a mass of mesodermal tissue cranial to the pericardial cavity. After the head folds ventrally during the fourth week, the septum transversum forms a thick incomplete partition, or partial diaphragm, between the pericardial and abdominal cavities (Fig. 6-3, B). The septum transversum does not separate the thoracic and abdominal cavities completely. It leaves a large opening, the *pericardioperitoneal canal,* on each side of the esophagus. The septum transversum fuses with the mesenchyme ventral to the esophagus (primordial mediastinum) and with the pleuroperitoneal membranes (Fig. 6-3, C).

THE PLEUROPERITONEAL MEMBRANES (FIG. 6-3, C). These membranes fuse with the dorsal mesentery of the esophagus and the septum transversum. This completes the partition between the thoracic and abdominal cavities and forms the *primitive diaphragm.* Although the pleuroperitoneal membranes form large portions of the embryonic diaphragm, they represent relatively small portions of the infant's diaphragm (Fig. 6-3, E).

THE DORSAL MESENTERY OF THE ESOPHAGUS. As previously described, the septum transversum and pleuroperitoneal membranes fuse with the dorsal mesentery of the esophagus. This mesentery constitutes the median portion of the diaphragm. The *crura of the diaphragm* develop from myoblasts that grow into the dorsal mesentery of the esophagus (Fig. 6-3, E).

THE LATERAL BODY WALLS. During the ninth to twelfth weeks the lungs and pleural cavities enlarge, burrowing into the lateral body walls. During this excavation process the tissue is split into two layers: (1) an outer layer that becomes part of the definitive abdominal wall, and (2) an inner layer that contributes muscle to peripheral portions of the diaphragm, external to the parts derived from the pleuroperitoneal membranes (Fig. 6-3, E).

Congenital Diaphragmatic Defects

Despite the rather complex embryologic development of the diaphragm, congenital anomalies of it are relatively uncommon.

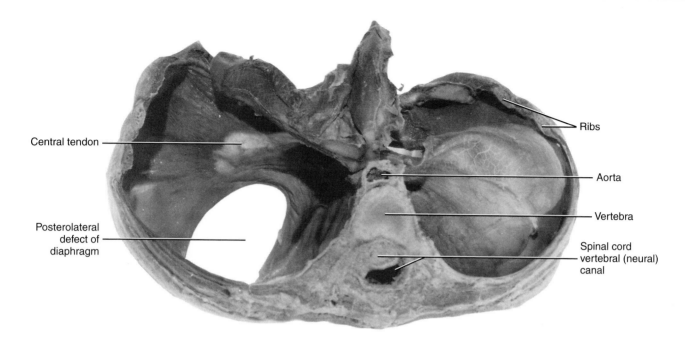

Central tendon

Posterolateral
defect of
diaphragm

Ribs

Aorta

Vertebra

Spinal cord
vertebral (neural)
canal

FIG. 6-4

Photograph of a transverse section through the thoracic region of a stillborn infant, viewed from the thorax. Note the large, left posterolateral defect in the diaphragm, which permitted the abdominal contents to pass into the thorax (CDH), as shown in Fig. 6-5, A.

CONGENITAL DIAPHRAGMATIC HERNIA (CDH). *Posterolateral defect of the diaphragm* is the only relatively common congenital abnormality of the diaphragm (Figs. 6-4 and 6-5). It occurs about once in 2200 newborn infants and is associated with CDH (herniation of abdominal contents into the thoracic cavity) and life-threatening breathing difficulties. *Polyhydramnios* is usually present also. *Prenatal diagnosis of CDH* depends on the sonographic demonstration of abdominal organs in the thorax.

CDH, usually unilateral (97%), results from defective formation and/or fusion of the pleuroperitoneal membrane with the other three parts of the diaphragm (Fig. 6-3). The defect commonly consists of a large opening, sometimes referred to clinically as the foramen of Bochdalek, in the posterolateral region of the diaphragm (Figs. 6-4 and 6-5). The defect usually occurs on the left side (75% to 90%); this preponderance is likely related to the earlier closure of the right pleuroperitoneal opening.

The pleuroperitoneal membranes normally fuse with the other three diaphragmatic components by the end of the sixth week (Fig. 6-3, C). If a pleuroperitoneal membrane is unfused when the intestines return to the abdomen from the umbilical cord in the tenth week, the intestine may pass into the thorax. Often the stomach, spleen, and most of the intestines herniate. Uncommonly, the liver and a kidney also pass into the thoracic cavity and displace the lungs and heart. The viscera usually can move freely through the defect; consequently, they may be in the thoracic cavity when the infant is lying down and in the abdominal cavity when the infant is upright. Most infants born with CDH die not because there is a defect in the diaphragm or viscera in the chest, but because the lungs are hypoplastic as a result of compression during their development (Fig. 6-6).

The lungs in infants with CDH are often hypoplastic and greatly reduced in size. The growth retardation results from lack of room for them to develop normally. The lungs are often aerated and achieve their normal size after reduction (repositioning) of the herniated viscera and repair of the defect in the diaphragm; but the mortality rate is high, approximately 76%. If necessary, CDH can be diagnosed and repaired prenatally between 22 and 28 weeks of gestation (Fig. 6-7), but this intervention carries considerable risk to the fetus and mother.

Congenital diaphragmatic hernia

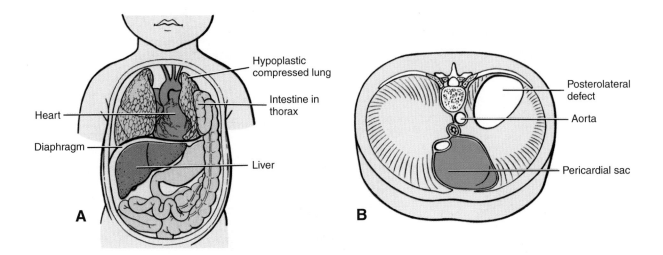

Eventration of the diaphragm

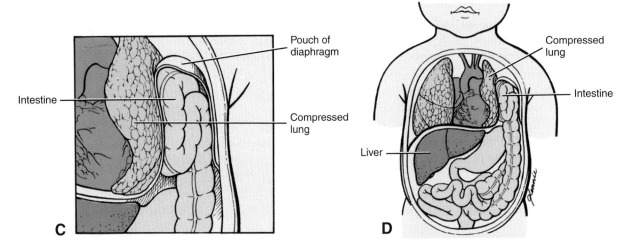

FIG. 6-5

A, Windows have been drawn on the thorax and abdomen to show the herniation of the intestine into the thorax through a posterolateral defect in the left side of the diaphragm similar to that illustrated in Fig. 6-4. Note that the left lung is compressed and hypoplastic. Posterolateral defects of the diaphragm usually occur on the left side (75% to 90%). **B,** Drawing of a diaphragm with a large posterolateral defect on the left side caused by abnormal formation and/or fusion of the pleuroperitoneal membrane on the left side with the mesoesophagus and the septum transversum. **C** and **D,** Eventration of the diaphragm resulting from defective muscular development of the diaphragm. The abdominal viscera are displaced into the thorax within a pouch of diaphragmatic tissue.

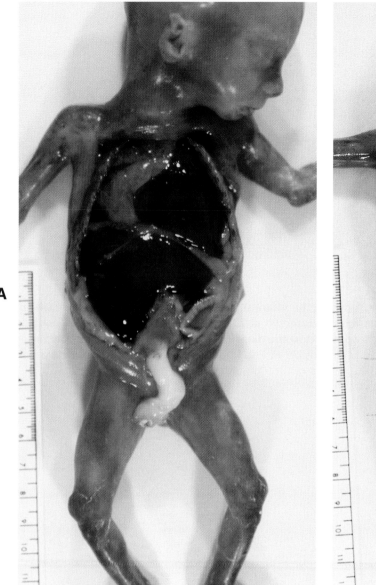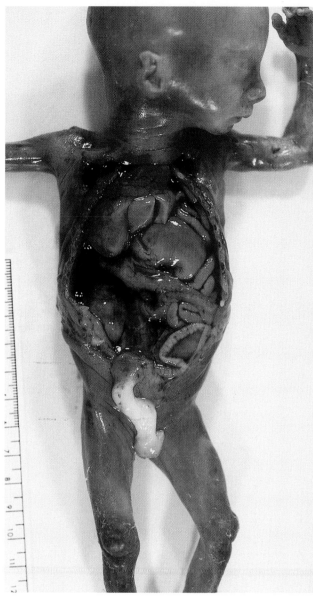

A

B

FIG. 6-6

Diaphragmatic hernia on left side showing herniation of liver (A), stomach and bowel (B) underneath the liver into left chest cavity. Note pulmonary hypoplasia visible after liver removal (female fetus 19 to 20 weeks developmental age). (Courtesy of Dr. D.K. Kalousek, Department of Pathology, University of British Columbia, Children's Hospital, Vancouver, B.C., Canada.)

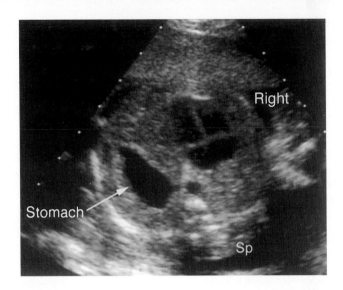

FIG. 6-7

Ultrasound scan of the thorax showing the heart shifted to the right and the stomach on the left. The diaphragmatic hernia was detected at 23.4 weeks' gestation. The stomach has herniated through a posterolateral defect in the diaphragm (CDH). (*Sp,* vertebral column or spine.) (Courtesy of Dr. Wesley Lee, Division of Fetal Imaging, William Beaumont Hospital, Royal Oak, Mich.)

7

The Pharyngeal (Branchial) Apparatus

During the fourth and fifth weeks, the primordial pharynx is bounded laterally by barlike *pharyngeal (branchial) arches* (Figs. 7-1 and 7-2). Each arch consists of a core of mesenchyme covered externally by ectoderm and internally by endoderm. The original mesenchyme in each arch is derived from intraembryonic mesoderm. Later, *neural crest cells* migrate into the arches and are the major source of connective tissue components, including cartilage, bone, and ligaments, in the oral and facial regions. Each arch also contains an artery, a cartilage rod, a nerve, and a muscular component.

Externally, the arches are separated by *pharyngeal (branchial) grooves* (Figs. 7-1 and 7-2). Internally, the arches are separated by evaginations of the pharynx called *pharyngeal pouches*. Where the ectoderm of a groove contacts the endoderm of a pouch, *pharyngeal (branchial) membranes* are formed. The pouches, arches, grooves, and membranes make up the branchial or pharyngeal apparatus. Development of the tongue, face, lips, jaws, palate, pharynx, and neck largely involves transformation of the branchial or pharyngeal apparatus into adult structures (Figs. 7-3 to 7-12). The adult derivatives of the various arch components are summarized in Table 7-1.

The pharyngeal grooves disappear except for the first pair, which persists as the *external acoustic meatus* (see Fig. 7-13). The pharyngeal membranes also disappear except for the first pair, which becomes the *tympanic membranes*. The first pharyngeal pouch gives rise to the *tympanic cavity*, mastoid antrum, and auditory tube. The second pharyngeal pouch is associated with the development of the *palatine tonsil*. The *thymus* is derived from the third pair of pharyngeal pouches, and the *parathyroid glands* are formed from the third and fourth pairs of pharyngeal pouches (Fig. 7-8).

The tongue develops from several mesenchymal proliferations (swellings) in the floor of the primordial pharynx. The anterior two thirds (oral part) of the tongue is formed from the median tongue bud (tuberculum impar) and the distal tongue buds (lateral lingual swellings). The posterior third (pharyngeal part) of the tongue is formed from the copula and hypobranchial eminence. Most of the tongue muscles are derived from myoblasts that migrate during the fifth to the seventh week from the occipital somites (Fig. 7-5). Taste buds develop during weeks 11 to 13.

Text continued on p. 140

TABLE 7-1

Structures Derived from Branchial or Pharyngeal Arch Components*

Arch	Nerve	Muscles	Skeletal Structures	Ligaments
First (mandibular)	Trigeminal† (V)	Muscles of mastication‡ Mylohyoid and anterior belly of digastric Tensor tympani Tensor veli palatini	Malleus Incus	Anterior ligament of malleus Sphenoman-dibular ligament
Second (hyoid)	Facial (VII)	Muscles of facial expressions§ Stapedius Stylohyoid Posterior belly of digastric	Stapes Styloid process Lesser cornu of hyoid bone Upper part of body of the hyoid bone	Stylohyoid ligament
Third	Glossopharyngeal (IX)	Stylopharyngeus	Greater cornu of hyoid bone Lower part of body of the hyoid bone	
Fourth and Sixth‖	Superior laryngeal branch of vagus (X) Recurrent laryngeal branch of vagus (X)	Cricothyroid Levator veli palatini Constrictors of pharynx Intrinsic muscles of larynx Striated muscles of the esophagus	Thyroid cartilage Cricoid cartilage Arytenoid cartilage Corniculate cartilage Cuneiform cartilage	

(Adapted from Moore KL, Persaud TVN: *The developing human,* ed 6, Philadelphia, 1998, Saunders.)

*The aortic arch arteries are described in Chapter 11.

†The ophthalmic division does not supply any pharyngeal arch components.

‡Temporalis, masseter, medial, and lateral pterygoids.

§Buccinator, auricularis, frontalis, platysma, orbicularis oculi.

‖The fifth pharyngeal arch is often absent. When present, it is rudimentary and usually has no recognizable cartilage bar. The cartilaginous components of the fourth and sixth arches fuse to form the cartilages of the larynx.

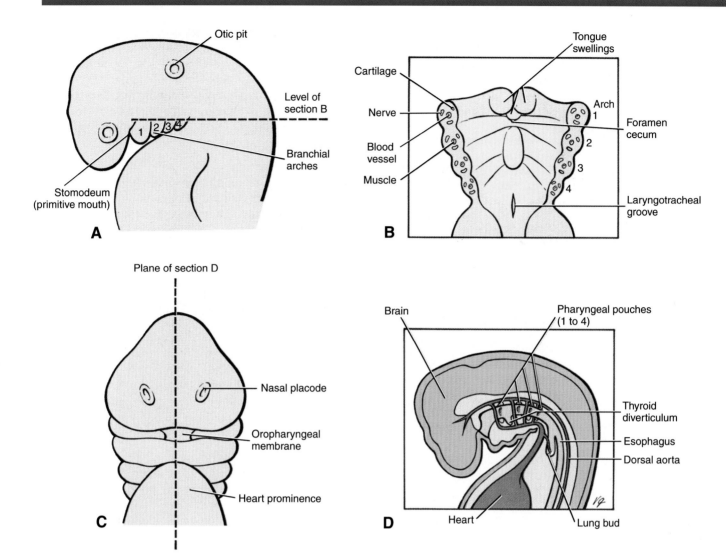

FIG. 7-1

Drawings illustrating the human branchial or pharyngeal apparatus. A, Lateral view of the cranial part of an early embryo. B, Horizontal section through the cranial region of the embryo. C, Ventral or facial view illustrating the relationship of the first arch to the stomodeum. At this stage the oropharyngeal membrane separates the stomodeum from the primitive pharynx. D, Schematic drawing showing the pharyngeal pouches and the related arteries known as aortic arches.

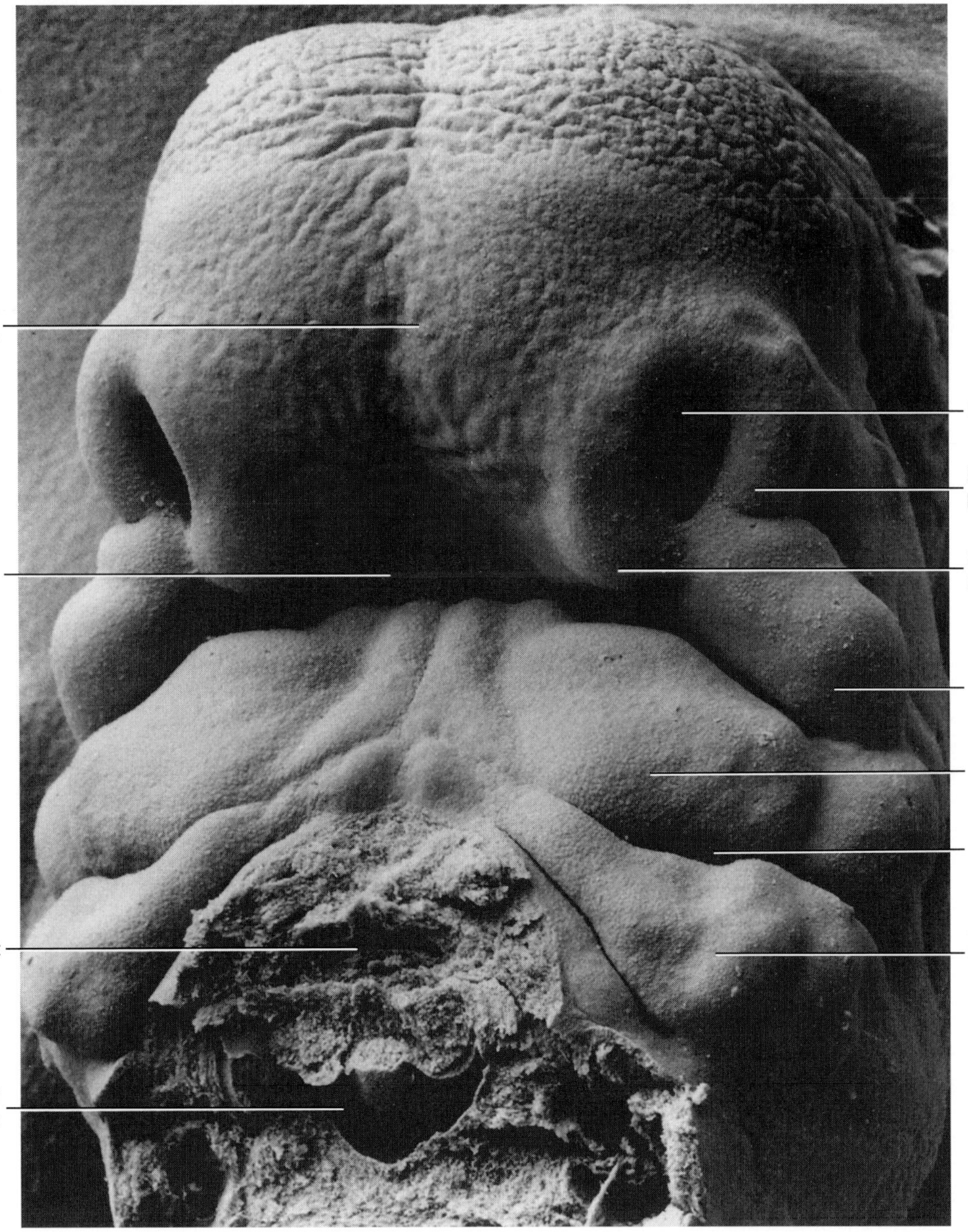

Frontonasal process

Nasal pit

Lateral nasal prominence

Stomodeum (primitive mouth)

Medial nasal prominence

Maxillary prominence

Mandibular prominence

First branchial (pharyngeal) groove

Foregut

Second branchial (hyoid) arch

Cavity of hindbrain

FIG. 7-2

Scanning electron micrograph of the craniofacial region of a human embryo at Carnegie stage 16, about 37 days (CRL 10.5 mm). The wide stomodeum (primordial mouth) is limited caudally by the fused mandibular prominences. The nasal pits are surrounded by the medial and lateral nasal prominences and the maxillary prominences. At this stage, the medial nasal prominences have not merged but the mandibular prominences have fused. (Courtesy of Professor Dr. Klaus Hinrichsen, Ruhr-Universitat, Bochum, Germany.)

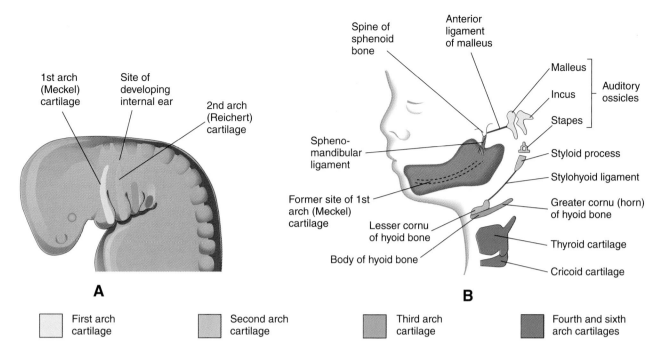

First arch cartilage   Second arch cartilage   Third arch cartilage   Fourth and sixth arch cartilages

FIG. 7-3

A, Schematic lateral view of the head, neck, and thoracic regions of a 4-week embryo, illustrating the location of the cartilages in the pharyngeal arches. **B,** Similar view of a 24-week fetus illustrating the adult derivatives of the arch cartilages. Note that the mandible is formed by membranous ossification of mesenchymal tissue surrounding the first arch (Meckel) cartilage. This cartilage acts as a template for development of the mandible, but does not contribute directly to the formation of it. Occasionally ossification of the second arch cartilage may extend from the styloid process along the stylohyoid ligament. When this occurs, it may cause pain in the region of the palatine tonsil.

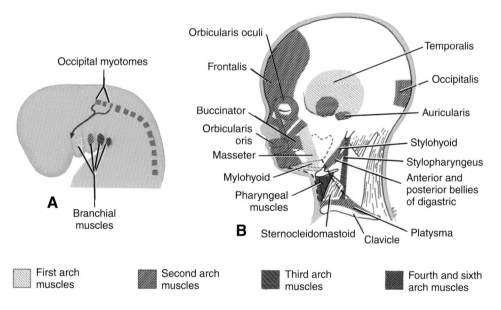

First arch muscles   Second arch muscles   Third arch muscles   Fourth and sixth arch muscles

FIG. 7-4

A, Sketch of lateral view of the head and neck region of a 4-week embryo showing the branchial or pharyngeal muscles. The arrow shows the pathway taken by myoblasts (developing muscle cells) from the occipital myotomes to form the tongue musculature. **B,** Sketch of the head and neck of a 20-week fetus dissected to show the muscles derived from the branchial or pharyngeal arches. Parts of the platysma and sternocleidomastoid muscles have been removed to show the deeper muscles. Note that myoblasts from the second branchial arch migrate from the neck region to the head and give rise to the muscles of facial expression. These muscles are therefore supplied by the facial nerve, the nerve of the second arch.

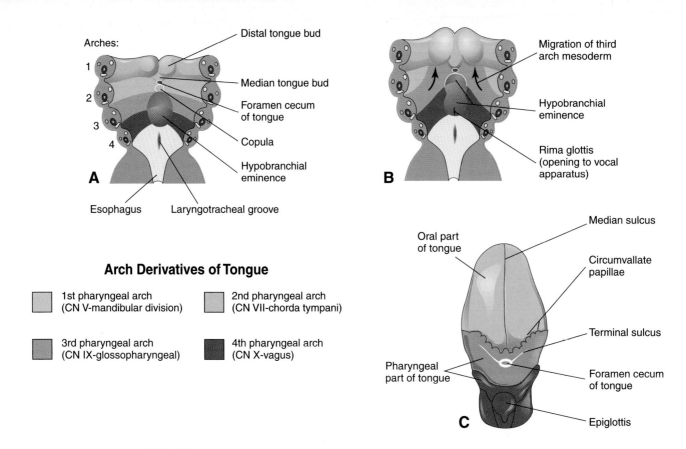

Arch Derivatives of Tongue

- 1st pharyngeal arch (CN V-mandibular division)
- 2nd pharyngeal arch (CN VII-chorda tympani)
- 3rd pharyngeal arch (CN IX-glossopharyngeal)
- 4th pharyngeal arch (CN X-vagus)

FIG. 7-5

A and **B**, Schematic horizontal sections through the pharynx at the level shown in Fig. 7-1, *A*, showing successive stages in the development of the tongue during the fourth and fifth weeks. **C**, Drawing of the adult tongue showing the pharyngeal arch derivation of the nerve supply of its mucosa.

FIG. 7-6

Macroglossia in an infant. An excessively large tongue is uncommon. It results from generalized hypertrophy of the tongue, usually from lymphangioma or muscular hypertrophy. (Courtesy of Dr. A.E. Chudley, Department of Pediatrics and Child Health, University of Manitoba, Children's Hospital, Winnipeg, Manitoba, Canada.)

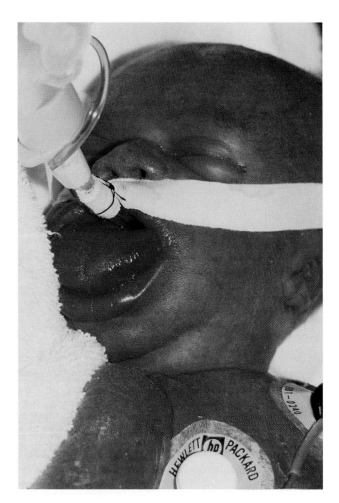

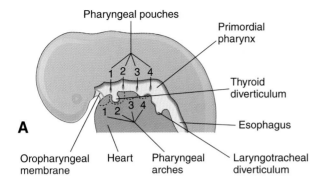

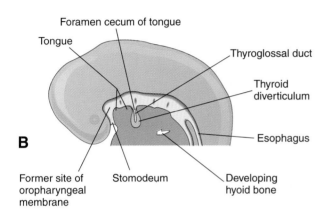

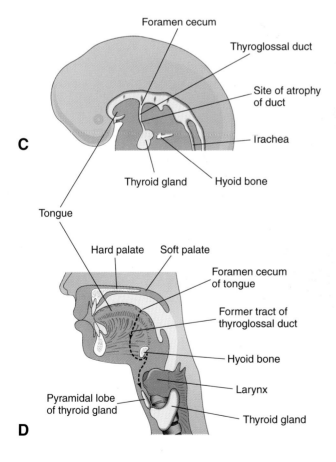

FIG. 7-7

Development of the thyroid gland. A, B, and C, Schematic sagittal sections of the head and neck regions of embryos at 4, 5, and 6 weeks, illustrating successive stages in the development of the thyroid gland. **D,** Similar section of an adult head and neck showing the path taken by the thyroid gland during its embryonic descent (indicated by the former tract of the thyroglossal duct).

FIG. 7-8

Photomicrographs illustrating the histology of the thyroid and parathyroid glands (×60). A, Thyroid and parathyroid glands located lateral to the trachea. The lobes of the developing thymus are located lateral to the esophagus. **B,** The thyroid and parathyroid glands at 21 weeks (×130). Colloid is first visible in the follicles at 11 weeks; thyroxine forms shortly thereafter.

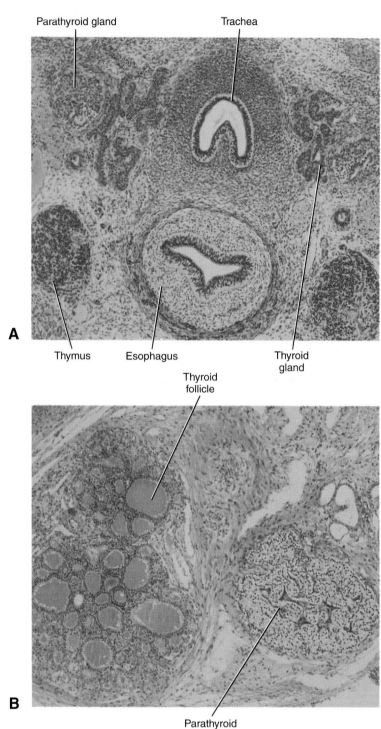

A

B

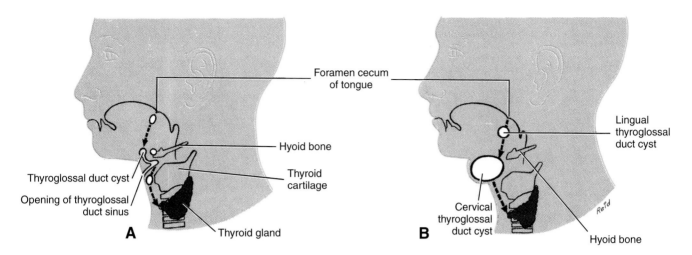

FIG. 7-9

A, Diagrammatic sketch of the head and neck showing the possible locations of thyroglossal duct cysts. A thyroglossal duct sinus is also illustrated. The *broken line* indicates the course taken by the thyroglossal duct during descent of the developing thyroid gland from the foramen cecum in the tongue to its final position in the anterior part of the neck. **B,** Similar sketch illustrating lingual and cervical thyroglossal duct cysts. Most thyroglossal duct cysts are located just inferior to the hyoid bone. (From Moore KL, Persaud TVN: *The developing human,* ed 6, Philadelphia, 1998, Saunders.)

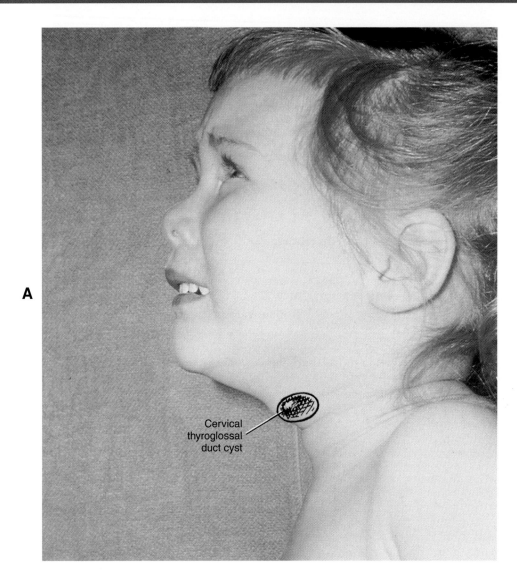

A

Cervical
thyroglossal
duct cyst

FIG. 7-10

Typical thyroglossal duct cyst in a female child **(A).** The round, firm mass (indicated by the sketch) produced a swelling in the median plane of the neck just inferior to the hyoid bone. (From Ueda D, Yoto Y, Sato T: *Pediatr Radiol* 28:126-128, 1998).

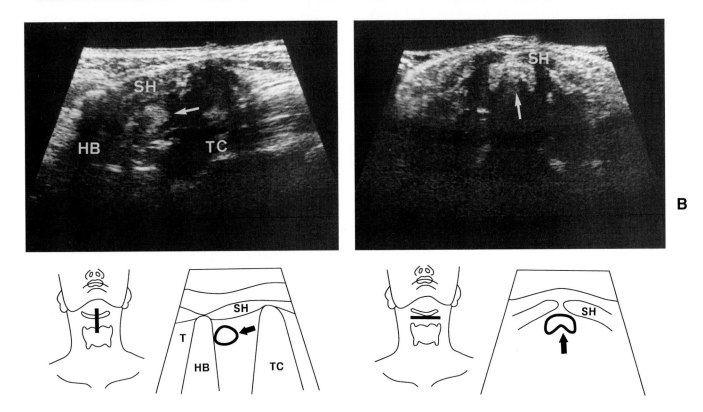

FIG. 7-10, cont'd

B, Representative ultrasound images of the lingual thyroid obtained by a midline sagittal scanning and posterior coronal scanning. An abnormal mass *(arrow)* was delineated on the caudal side of the hyoid bone and deep to the sternohyoid muscle. *SH,* sternohyoid muscle; *T,* tongue; *HB,* acoustic shadow of hyoid bone; *TC,* acoustic shadow of thyroid cartilage.

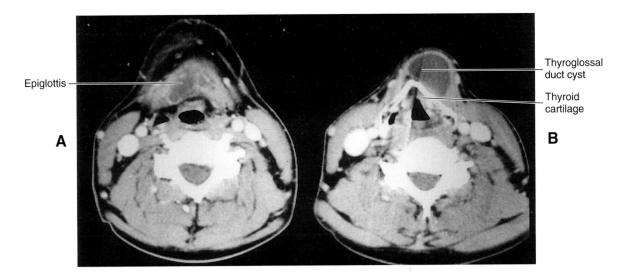

FIG. 7-11

Computed tomography (CT) images. **A,** Level of the thyrohyoid membrane and base of the epiglottis. **B,** Level of thyroid cartilage, which is calcified. The thyroglossal duct cyst extends cranially to the margin of the hyoid bone. (Courtesy of Dr. G.S. Smyser, Altru Health System, Grand Forks, ND.)

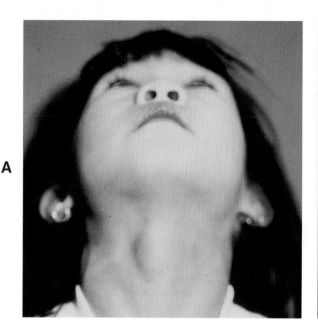

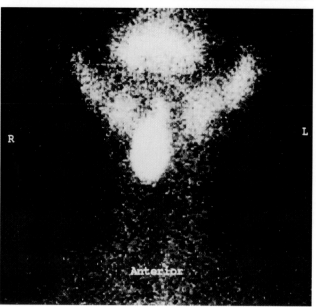

FIG. 7-12

A, Photograph of a sublingual thyroid mass in a 5-year-old girl. **B,** Technetium-99m pertechnetate scan showing a sublingual thyroid without evidence of functioning thyroid tissue in lower neck. (From Leung AKC, Wong AL, Robson WLLM: *Can J Surg* 38:87, 1995.)

Congenital anomalies of the tongue occur infrequently. These include congenital lingual cysts, ankyloglossia (tongue-tie), macroglossia (excessively large tongue, Fig. 7-6), and microglossia (excessively small tongue, usually associated with micrognathia and bifid tongue resulting from incomplete fusion of the distal tongue buds, extremely rare). Fissuring of the tongue and hypertrophy of the lingual papillae are often found in children with Down syndrome.

The **thyroid gland** develops from a downgrowth from the floor of the primordial pharynx in the region where the tongue develops (Figs. 7-7 and 7-8). The parafollicular cells (C cells) in the thyroid gland are derived from the *ultimobranchial bodies,* which are derived mainly from the fourth pair of pharyngeal pouches.

The face develops from five primordia: the single frontonasal prominence and the paired maxillary and mandibular prominences (Figs. 7-13 to 7-15). The *palate* develops from two primordia, the primary palate (median palatine process) and the secondary palate (Figs. 7-16 and 7-22). The secondary palate develops from two mesenchymal projections that extend from the internal aspects of the maxillary prominences. These shelflike structures are called lateral palatine processes or palatal shelves. Anteriorly, these processes (shelves) fuse with the primary palate and later with each other.

The nasolacrimal duct develops from a rodlike thickening of ectoderm in the floor of the nasolacrimal groove (Fig. 7-13). This solid epithelial cord of cells separates from the ectoderm and sinks into the mesenchyme. Later, as a result of cell degeneration, it canalizes to form the nasolacrimal duct. Occasionally, part of the nasolacrimal duct fails to canalize, resulting in atresia or obstruction of the nasolacrimal duct at birth.

Most congenital anomalies of the head and neck originate during transformation of the pharyngeal (branchial) apparatus into adult structures. Branchial cysts, sinuses, and fistulas may develop from parts of the second branchial groove, the cervical sinus, or the second pharyngeal pouch that fail to obliterate. An *ectopic thyroid gland* results when the thyroid gland fails to descend completely from its site of origin in the tongue. The thyroglossal duct may persist or remnants of it may give rise to a *thyroglossal duct cyst*

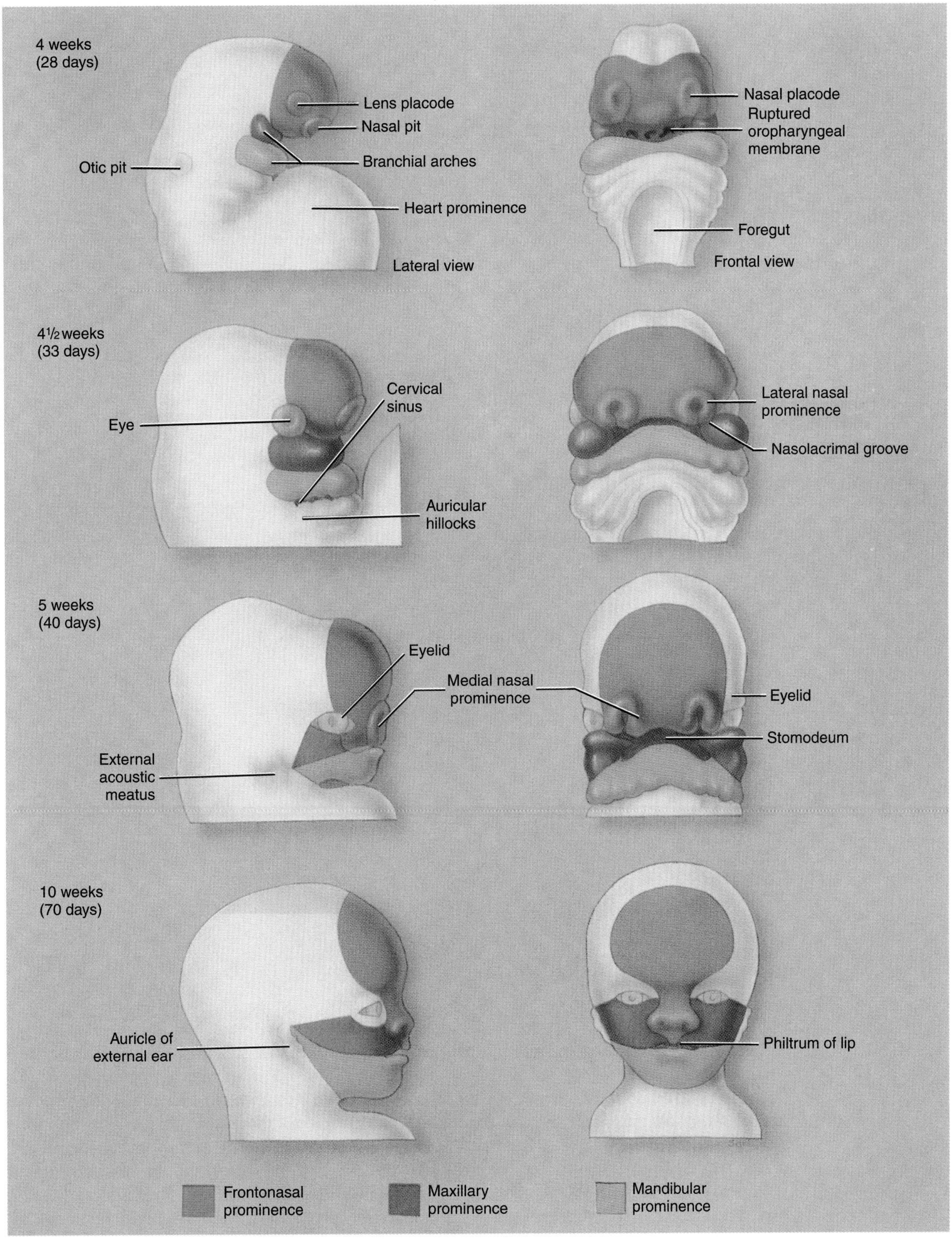

4 weeks (28 days)

Lateral view:
- Lens placode
- Nasal pit
- Branchial arches
- Heart prominence
- Otic pit

Frontal view:
- Nasal placode
- Ruptured oropharyngeal membrane
- Foregut

4½ weeks (33 days)

- Cervical sinus
- Eye
- Auricular hillocks
- Lateral nasal prominence
- Nasolacrimal groove

5 weeks (40 days)

- Eyelid
- Medial nasal prominence
- External acoustic meatus
- Eyelid
- Stomodeum

10 weeks (70 days)

- Auricle of external ear
- Philtrum of lip

Legend:
- Frontonasal prominence
- Maxillary prominence
- Mandibular prominence

FIG. 7-13

Drawings illustrating progressive stages in the development of the face from the fourth to tenth weeks. Observe that the face develops from five primordia that surround the stomodeum (primordium of mouth). The prominences are a single frontonasal prominence and paired maxillary and mandibular prominences.

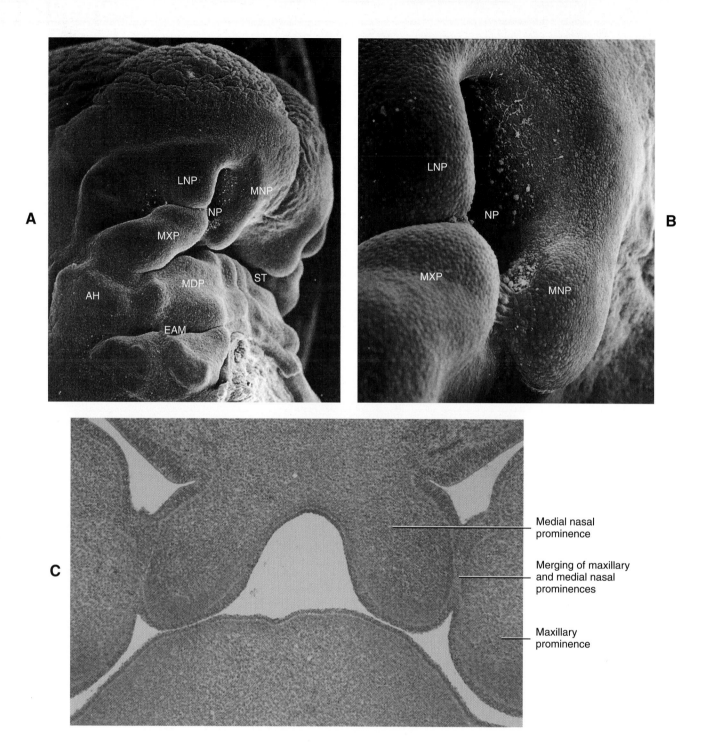

FIG. 7-14

A, Scanning electron micrograph of the craniofacial region of a human embryo at Carnegie stage 16, about 41 days (CRL 10.8 mm), viewed obliquely. The maxillary prominence *(MXP)* appears puffed up laterally and is wedged between the lateral *(LNP)* and medial *(MNP)* nasal prominences surrounding the nasal pit *(NP)*. The auricular hillocks *(AH)* can be seen on both sides of the groove between the first two arches that will form the external acoustic meatus *(EAM)*. **B,** Scanning electron micrograph of the right nasal region of a human embryo of about 41 days showing the maxillary and nasal prominences. Epithelial bridges can be seen between these prominences. Observe the furrow representing the nasolacrimal groove between the maxillary prominence *(MXP)* and the lateral nasal prominence *(LNP)*. Observe the large nasal pit *(NP)*. **C,** Photomicrograph of a coronal section of the face of an embryo at Carnegie stage 18, about 44 days, showing the medial nasal prominences fusing with the maxillary prominences (×25). (**A** and **B,** From Hinrichsen K: The early development of morphology and patterns of the face in the human embryo. In *Advances in anatomy, embryology, and cell biology,* vol 98, New York, 1985, Springer-Verlag.)

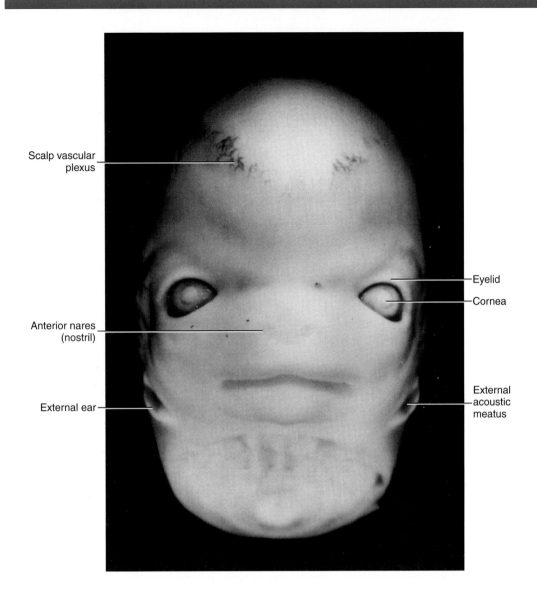

FIG. 7-15

Ventral view of the face of an embryo at Carnegie stage 22, about 54 days (15). Observe that the eyes are widely separated and the ears low-set at this stage. (From Nishimura H, et al: *Prenatal development of the human with special reference to craniofacial structures: an atlas,* Washington, DC, 1977, National Institutes of Health.)

(Figs. 7-7 to 7-12). Infected cysts may perforate the skin and form *thyroglossal duct sinuses* that open anteriorly in the median plane of the neck.

Because of the complex development of the face and palate, congenital anomalies of the face and palate are common. *Anomalies usually result from maldevelopment of neural crest tissue* that gives rise to the skeletal and connective tissue primordia of the face. Neural crest cells may be deficient in number, may not complete their migration to the face, or they may fail in their inductive capacity. Anomalies of the face and palate result from an arrest of development and/or a failure of fusion of the prominences and processes involved.

Cleft lip is a common congenital anomaly (Figs. 7-17 to 7-23). Although it is frequently associated with cleft palate, cleft lip with or without cleft palate, and isolated cleft palate are etiologically distinct anomalies that involve different developmental processes occurring at different times. Cleft lip results from failure of mesenchymal masses in the medial nasal and the maxillary prominences to merge, whereas *cleft palate* results from failure of mesenchymal masses in the palatine processes (palatal shelves) to meet and fuse.

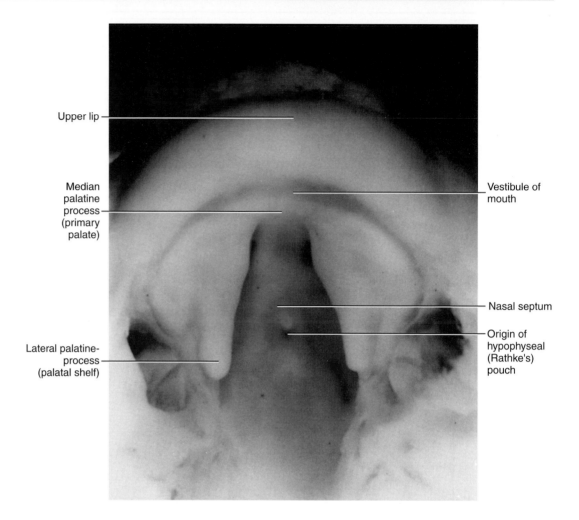

Upper lip

Median palatine process (primary palate)

Lateral palatine process (palatal shelf)

Vestibule of mouth

Nasal septum

Origin of hypophyseal (Rathke's) pouch

FIG. 7-16

Roof of the oral cavity of an embryo at Carnegie stage 22, about 54 days (×20). Note that the lateral palatine processes (palatal shelves) are widely separated at this stage. They fuse in the median plane with each other and the nasal septum at 12 weeks. Failure of these processes to fuse, as shown in Fig. 7-22 results in various types of cleft palate. (From Nishimura H, et al: *Prenatal development of the human with special reference to craniofacial structures: an atlas,* **Washington, DC, 1977, National Institutes of Health.)**

Most cases of cleft lip, with or without cleft palate, are caused by a combination of genetic and environmental factors *(multifactorial inheritance).* These factors interfere with the migration of neural crest cells into the maxillary prominences of the first branchial and pharyngeal arch. If the number of cells is insufficient, clefting of the lip and/or palate may occur. Complex cellular and molecular mechanisms are involved.

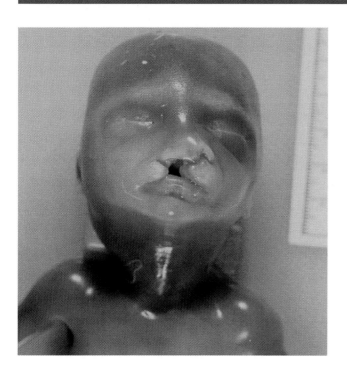

FIG. 7-17

Male fetus (16 weeks) with unilateral cleft lip and palate. The eyelids are normally fused at this age. They open during the twenty-sixth week. (Courtesy of Dr. D.K. Kalousek, Department of Pathology, University of British Columbia, Children's Hospital, Vancouver, B.C., Canada.)

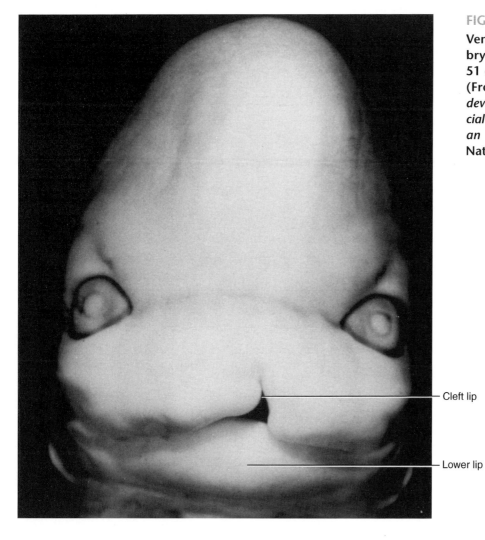

FIG. 7-18

Ventral view of the face of an embryo at Carnegie stage 20 (about 51 days) with a unilateral cleft lip. (From Nishimura H, et al: *Prenatal development of the human with special reference to craniofacial structures: an atlas,* Washington, DC, 1977, National Institutes of Health.)

Cleft lip

Lower lip

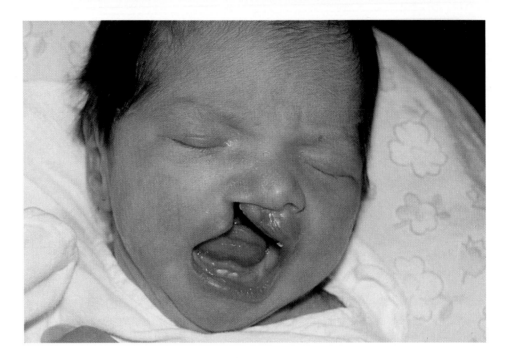

FIG. 7-19

Infant with unilateral cleft lip and palate. Clefts of the lip, with or without cleft palate, occur about once in 1000 births; 60% to 80% of affected infants are males. Unilateral cleft lip results from failure of the maxillary prominence on the affected side to unite with the merged medial nasal prominences (Figs. 7-13 and 7-14). (Courtesy of Dr. A.E. Chudley, Department of Pediatrics and Child Health, University of Manitoba, Children's Hospital, Winnipeg, Manitoba, Canada).

FIG. 7-20

Neonate with bilateral cleft lip and palate. Note the pits in the lower lip, which suggest the autosomal dominant cleft lip-lip pit syndrome of van der Woude. Bilateral cleft lip results from failure of the mesenchymal masses in the maxillary prominences to meet and unite with the merged medial nasal processes. Bilateral cleft palate results from failure of the mesenchymal masses in the lateral palatine processes (palatal shelves) to meet and fuse with the primary palate, with each other, and the nasal septum. (Courtesy of Dr. A.E. Chudley, Department of Pediatrics and Child Health, University of Manitoba, Children's Hospital, Winnipeg, Manitoba, Canada.)

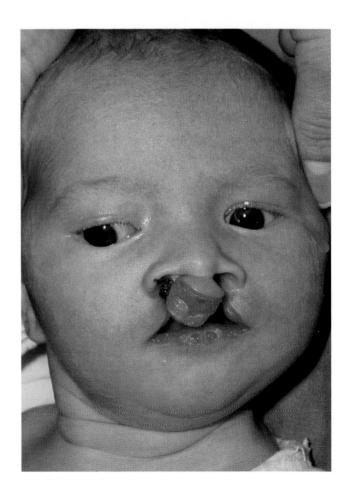

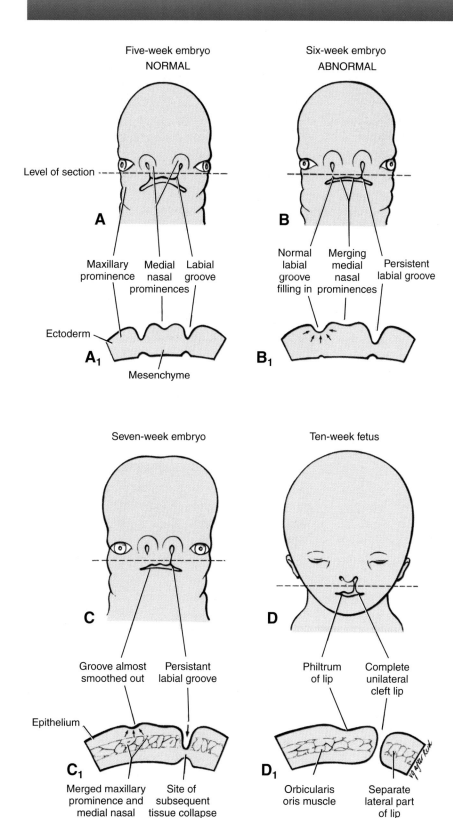

Five-week embryo
NORMAL

Level of section ------

A

Maxillary
prominence

Medial
nasal
prominences

Labial
groove

Ectoderm

A₁

Mesenchyme

Six-week embryo
ABNORMAL

B

Normal
labial
groove
filling in

Merging
medial
nasal
prominences

Persistent
labial groove

B₁

Seven-week embryo

C

Groove almost
smoothed out

Persistant
labial groove

Epithelium

C₁

Merged maxillary
prominence and
medial nasal
prominences

Site of
subsequent
tissue collapse

Ten-week fetus

D

Philtrum
of lip

Complete
unilateral
cleft lip

D₁

Orbicularis
oris muscle

Separate
lateral part
of lip

FIG. 7-21

Drawings illustrating the embryologic basis of complete unilateral cleft lip. A, Five-week embryo. A₁, Horizontal section through the head illustrating the grooves between the maxillary prominences and the merging medial nasal prominences. B, Six-week embryo showing a persistent labial groove on the left side. B₁, Horizontal section through the head showing the groove gradually filling in on the right side following proliferation of mesenchyme (arrows). C, Seven-week embryo. C₁, Horizontal section through the head showing that the epithelium on the right has almost been pushed out of the groove between the maxillary prominence and medial nasal prominence. D, Ten-week fetus with a complete unilateral cleft lip. D₁, Horizontal section through the head after stretching of the epithelium and breakdown of the tissues in the floor of the persistent labial groove on the left side forming a complete unilateral cleft lip.

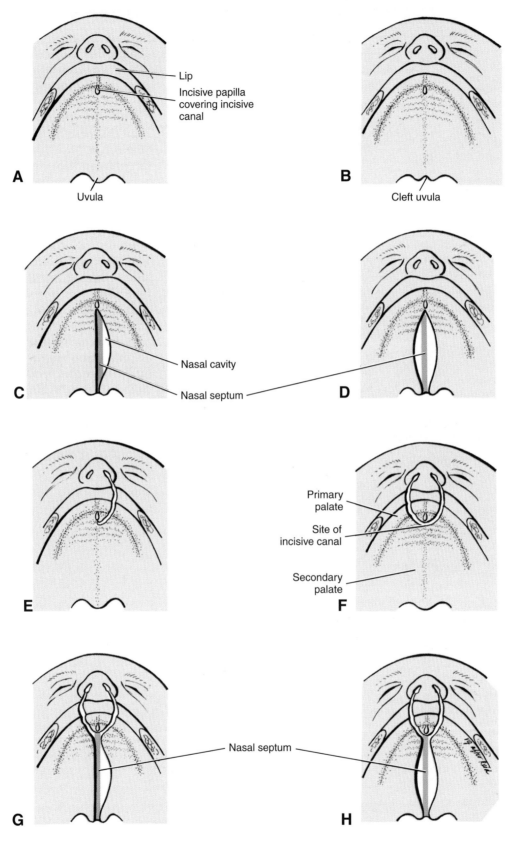

FIG. 7-22

For legend see opposite page.

FIG. 7-22

Drawings illustrating various types of cleft lip and palate. **A,** Normal lip and palate. **B,** Cleft uvula. **C,** Unilateral cleft of the posterior or secondary palate. **D,** Bilateral cleft of the posterior palate. **E,** Complete unilateral cleft of the lip and alveolar process of the maxilla with a unilateral cleft of the anterior or primary palate. **F,** Complete bilateral cleft of the lip and alveolar processes of the maxillae with bilateral cleft of the anterior palate. **G,** Complete bilateral cleft of the lip and alveolar processes of the maxillae with bilateral cleft of the anterior palate and unilateral cleft of the posterior palate. **H,** Complete bilateral cleft of the lip and alveolar processes of the maxillae with complete bilateral cleft of the anterior and posterior palate.

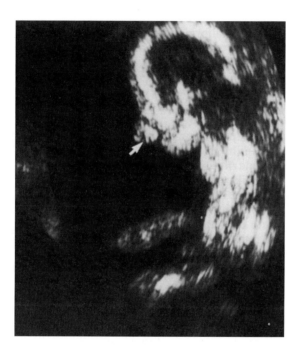

FIG. 7-23

Ultrasound image of the head of an early second-trimester fetus with complete bilateral cleft lip and palate showing anterior displacement of the intermaxillary part of the upper lip *(arrow).* (From Benacerraf BR: Ultrasound evaluation of the fetal face. In Callen PW [editor]: *Ultrasonography in obstetrics and gynecology,* ed 3, Philadelphia, 1994, Saunders.)

8

The Respiratory System

The lower respiratory system begins to develop around the middle of the fourth week from a median *laryngotracheal groove* in the floor of the primordial pharynx (see Fig. 7-1, *B*). This groove deepens to produce a *laryngotracheal diverticulum,* which soon separates from the foregut as tracheoesophageal folds fuse to form the *tracheoesophageal septum* (Figs. 8-1 and 8-2). This results in the formation of the primordial esophagus and the *laryngotracheal tube.* The endoderm of this tube gives rise to the epithelium of the lower respiratory organs and to the *tracheobronchial glands.* The splanchnic mesenchyme surrounding the laryngotracheal tube forms the connective tissue, cartilage, muscle, and blood and lymphatic vessels of these organs (Fig. 8-4).

Pharyngeal arch mesenchyme contributes to formation of the epiglottis and the connective tissue of the larynx. The laryngeal muscles and the skeleton of the larynx are derived from mesenchyme in the caudal pharyngeal arches (Fig. 8-1). The cartilages are derived from neural crest cells. The laryngeal cartilages develop from the cartilaginous bars in the fourth and sixth pairs of branchial or pharyngeal arches (Fig. 8-4; also see Table 7-1).

During the fourth week, the laryngotracheal tube develops a *lung bud* at its distal end, which soon divides into two *bronchial buds* during the early part of the fifth week (Figs. 8-1, *B,* and 8-3). Each bud soon enlarges to form a *primary bronchus,* and then each of these gives rise to two new bronchial buds, which develop into *secondary bronchi.* The right inferior secondary bronchus soon divides into two bronchi. The secondary bronchi supply the lobes of the developing lungs (Fig. 8-1, *C*). Each secondary bronchus undergoes progressive branching to form *segmental bronchi.* Each segmental bronchus with its surrounding mesenchyme is the primordium of a *bronchopulmonary segment.* Branching continues until about 17 orders of branches have formed. Additional airways are formed after birth until about 24 orders of branches are present. Fibroblast growth factor signaling has been implicated as an important regulator of the branching process.

Congenital anomalies of the lower respiratory system are uncommon except for *tracheoesophageal fistula.* Tracheoesophageal fistula is the most common developmental defect of the lower respiratory tract. It occurs about once in 3000 to 4500 live births, more commonly in male infants. The fistula is usually associated with *esophageal atresia* (Figs. 8-5 and 8-6). These anomalies result from faulty partitioning of the foregut into the esophagus and trachea during the fourth and fifth weeks.

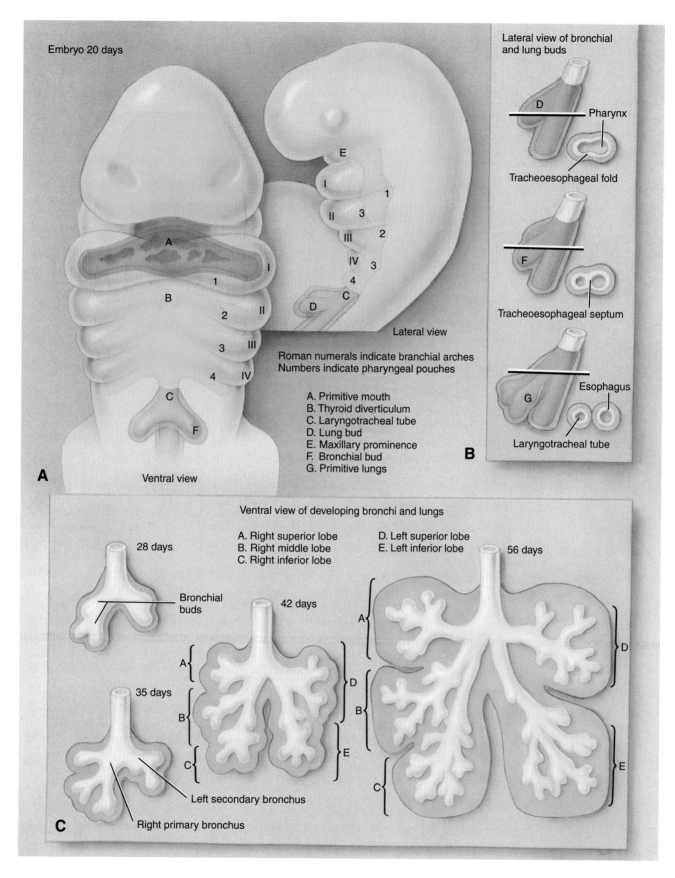

FIG. 8-1

Drawings illustrating various stages in the development of the respiratory system. **A,** The relationship of the branchial (pharyngeal) apparatus to the respiratory system. The laryngotracheal tube *(C)* opens into the primitive pharynx and its caudal end divides into two bronchial buds *(F)*. **B,** Early development of the lung bud into the bronchial buds and primitive lungs. Formation of the laryngotracheal tube and esophagus is also illustrated. **C,** Successive stages in the development of the bronchi and lungs from the fourth to eighth weeks.

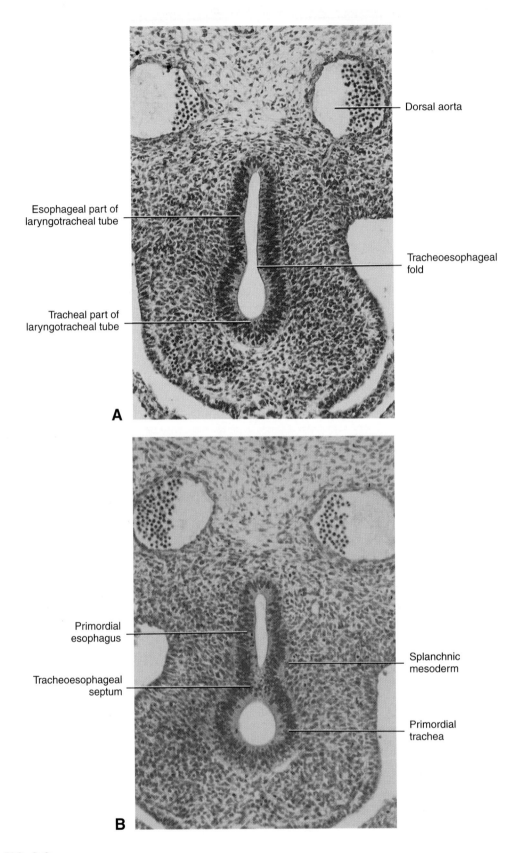

Dorsal aorta

Esophageal part of
laryngotracheal tube

Tracheoesophageal
fold

Tracheal part of
laryngotracheal tube

A

Primordial
esophagus

Splanchnic
mesoderm

Tracheoesophageal
septum

Primordial
trachea

B

FIG. 8-2

Photomicrographs of sections through an embryo (×50) at Carnegie stage 16, about 40 days, showing division of the laryngotracheal tube into the primordia of the esophagus and trachea (see also Fig. 8-1, *B*). The endoderm of the tube gives rise to the tracheal epithelium and glands and the splanchnic mesoderm gives rise to the cartilage, connective tissues and muscles of the trachea (see Fig. 8-4). **A,** Formation of the tracheoesophageal folds. **B,** Fusion of the tracheoesophageal folds to form the primordia of the trachea and esophagus.

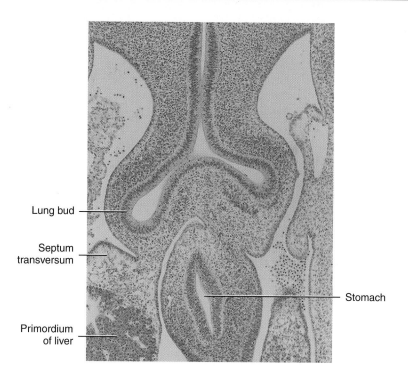

Lung bud

Septum
transversum

Stomach

Primordium
of liver

FIG. 8-3

Photomicrograph of a section of the lung buds of an embryo at Carnegie stage 14. Lung buds with pseudostratified epithelium develop into the pericardioperitoneal cavity from which the future pleural cavity is formed.

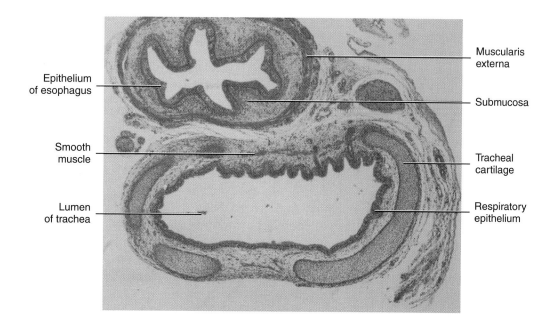

Epithelium
of esophagus

Muscularis
externa

Submucosa

Smooth
muscle

Tracheal
cartilage

Lumen
of trachea

Respiratory
epithelium

FIG. 8-4

Photomicrograph of a transverse section of the developing esophagus and trachea at 14 weeks (×50). The respiratory epithelium is derived from the endoderm of the laryngotracheal tube and the cartilage, connective tissue and smooth muscle differentiate from the splanchnic mesoderm surrounding the laryngotracheal tube.

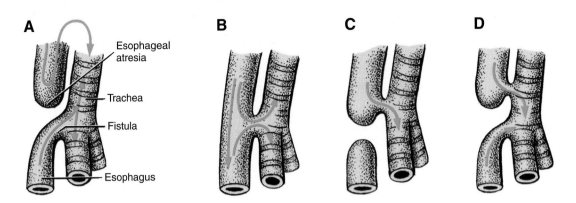

FIG. 8-5

Sketches illustrating the four main varieties of tracheoesophageal fistula. Possible direction(s) of flow of contents is indicated by arrows. Esophageal atresia, as illustrated in *A*, is associated with tracheoesophageal fistula in about 85% of cases. The abdomen rapidly becomes distended as the intestines fill with air. In *C*, air cannot enter the lower esophagus and stomach.

Lung development is divided into four stages (Figs. 8-7 and 8-8). During the *pseudoglandular period* (5 to 17 weeks), the bronchi and terminal bronchioles form. During the *canalicular period* (16 to 25 weeks), the lumina of the bronchi and terminal bronchioles enlarge, the respiratory bronchioles and alveolar ducts develop, and the lung tissue becomes highly vascular. During the *terminal sac period* (24 weeks to birth), the alveolar ducts give rise to terminal sacs (or primitive alveoli). The terminal sacs are initially lined with cuboidal epithelium that begins to attenuate to squamous epithelium at about 26 weeks. By this time, capillary networks have proliferated close to the alveolar epithelium, and the lungs are usually sufficiently well developed to permit survival of the fetus if it is born prematurely. The *alveolar period*, the final stage of lung development, occurs from the late fetal period to about 8 years of age. The number of respiratory bronchioles and primitive alveoli increases.

The respiratory system develops so that it is capable of immediate function at birth. To be capable of respiration, the lungs must acquire an *alveolocapillary membrane* that is sufficiently thin, and an adequate amount of *surfactant* must be present. Pulmonary surfactant is secreted by type II alveolar cells, which develop by **24 weeks.** A deficiency of surfactant appears to be responsible for the failure of primitive alveoli to remain open, resulting in *hyaline membrane disease* (HMD), a major cause of the *respiratory distress syndrome* (RDS). About 2% of live newborn infants are affected by this disease; premature infants are most susceptible. Growth of the lungs after birth results mainly from an increase in the number of respiratory bronchioles and alveoli. New alveoli form for at least 8 years after birth. Characteristic mature alveoli do not form until after birth; about 95% of alveoli develop postnatally.

Agenesis of the lungs results from failure of the bronchial buds to develop. It rarely occurs. Pulmonary sequestration, a small accessory lung, usually located at the base of the left lung, is also uncommon. Lung hypoplasia occurs in infants with congenital diaphragmatic hernia or congenital heart disease. Bronchogenic cysts (filled with fluid or air) are believed to be formed by the dilation of terminal bronchi. Benign lesions are usually located in the mediastinum or at the periphery of the lung and probably result from a disturbance in bronchial development.

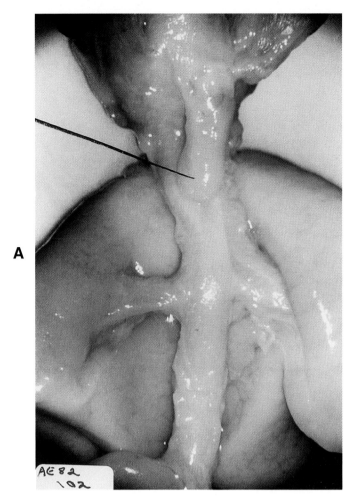

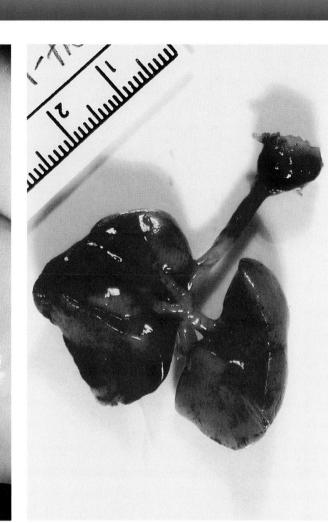

FIG. 8-6

A, Tracheoesophageal fistula in a 17-week male fetus with Trisomy 18 syndrome. The upper esophageal segment ends blindly *(arrow).* **B,** Tracheal agenesis (type II) with a small laryngeal pouch and esophagocarinal fistula in the male fetus, developmental age 15.5 weeks. (**A,** From Kalousek DK, et al: *Pathology of the human embryo and previable fetus,* New York, 1990, Springer Verlag. **B,** Courtesy of Dr. D.K. Kalousek, Department of Pathology, University of British Columbia, Children's Hospital, Vancouver, B.C., Canada.)

STAGES OF LUNG DEVELOPMENT

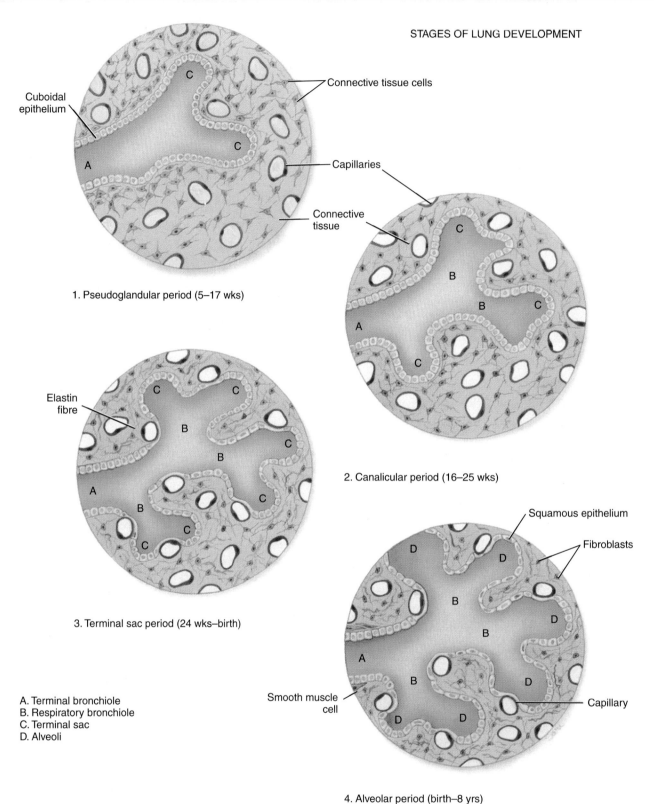

Cuboidal epithelium

Connective tissue cells

Capillaries

Connective tissue

C

A

C

1. Pseudoglandular period (5–17 wks)

C

B

B

A

C

C

2. Canalicular period (16–25 wks)

Elastin fibre

C

C

B

C

B

A

C

B

C

C

3. Terminal sac period (24 wks–birth)

A. Terminal bronchiole
B. Respiratory bronchiole
C. Terminal sac
D. Alveoli

Squamous epithelium

Fibroblasts

D

D

B

D

B

A

B

D

Smooth muscle cell

D

D

Capillary

4. Alveolar period (birth–8 yrs)

FIG. 8-7

Diagrammatic sketches of histologic sections illustrating progressive stages of lung development. 1, Pseudoglandular period (about 8 weeks). 2, Late canalicular period (about 24 weeks). 3, Early terminal sac period (about 26 weeks). 4, Newborn infant. Early alveolar period. Note that the alveolocapillary membrane is thin and that some of the capillaries have begun to bulge into the primordial alveoli.

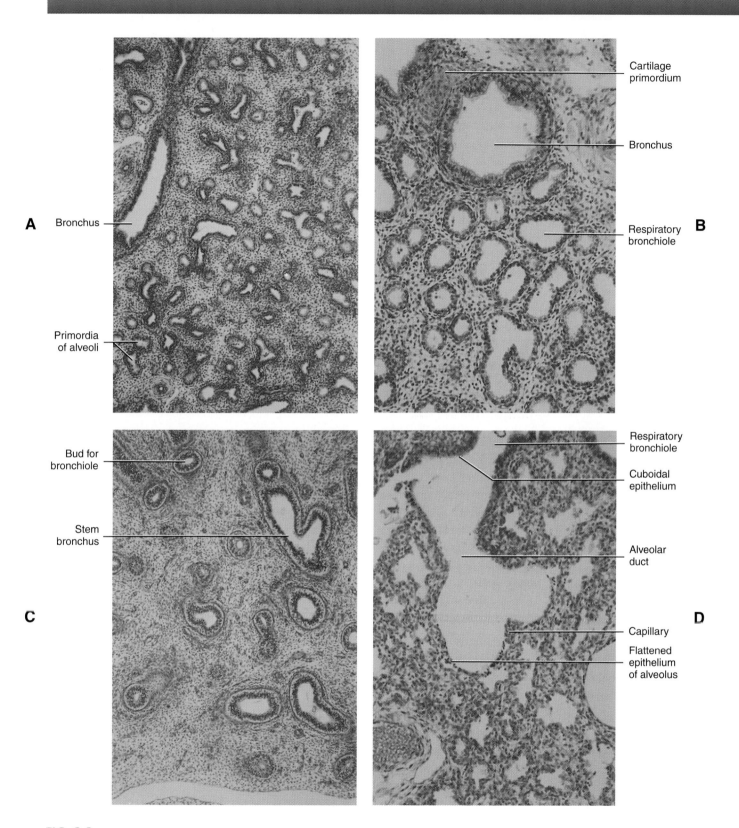

FIG. 8-8

Photomicrographs of sections of developing human lungs. **A,** Pseudoglandular period, 8 weeks. Note the glandular appearance of the lung at this stage. **B,** Canalicular period, 16 weeks. The lumina of the bronchi and terminal bronchioles are enlarging. **C,** Canalicular period, 18 weeks. Note that many blood vessels are developing in the mesenchyme surrounding the sections of bronchi and terminal bronchioles. **D,** Terminal sac period, 24 weeks. Observe the thin-walled terminal sacs (primitive alveoli) that have developed at the ends of the respiratory bronchioles. Also observe that the number of blood vessels has increased and that some of them are closely associated with the terminal sacs or primordial alveoli.

9

The Digestive System

The **primordial gut** (foregut, midgut, and hindgut) forms during the fourth week from the part of the *yolk sac* that is incorporated into the embryo (Fig. 9-1; see also Fig. 6-2). The endoderm of the primordial gut (Fig. 9-2) gives rise to the epithelial lining of most of the digestive tract and biliary passages, together with the parenchyma of its glands including the liver and pancreas. The epithelium at the cranial and caudal extremities of the digestive tract is derived from the ectoderm of the stomodeum and proctodeum, respectively. The muscular and connective tissue components of the digestive tract are derived from the splanchnic mesenchyme surrounding the primordial gut (Fig. 9-3).

The **foregut** gives rise to the pharynx, lower respiratory system, esophagus, stomach, duodenum (proximal to the opening of the bile duct), liver, pancreas, and biliary apparatus (Figs. 9-4 to 9-8). Because the trachea and esophagus have a common origin from the foregut, incomplete partitioning by the tracheoesophageal septum results in stenoses or atresias, with or without fistulas between them (see Figs. 8-5 and 8-6). *Congenital duodenal atresia* results from failure of the vacuolization and recanalization process to occur following the normal solid stage of the duodenal development (Fig. 9-9). Usually these epithelial cells degenerate and the lumen of the duodenum is restored.

The *hepatic diverticulum*, the primordium of the liver, gallbladder, and biliary duct system, is an outgrowth of the endodermal epithelial lining of the foregut. The epithelial liver cords and primordia of the *biliary system* develop from the hepatic diverticulum between the layers of the *ventral mesentery*, which is derived from the septum transversum (see Fig. 6-2, *A*). These primordial cells differentiate into the *parenchyma of the liver* and the lining of the ducts of the biliary system. The fibrous and hemopoietic tissues of the liver are derived from mesenchyme in the septum transversum (Fig. 9-6).

The *pancreas* develops from dorsal and ventral *pancreatic buds* that originate from the endodermal lining of the foregut (Figs. 9-5, *A* to *C*, and 9-8). As the duodenum rotates to the right, the ventral pancreatic bud moves dorsally and fuses with the dorsal pancreatic bud. The *ventral pancreatic bud* forms most of the head of the pancreas, including the uncinate process. The *dorsal pancreatic bud* forms the remainder of the pancreas. In some fetuses the duct systems of the two buds fail to fuse, and an *accessory pancreatic duct* forms.

Neural groove

Ectoderm

Mesoderm

Endoderm

Yolk sac

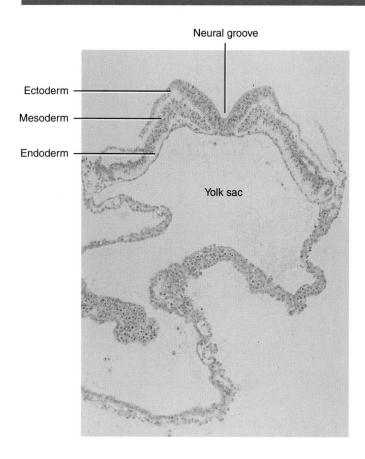

FIG. 9-1

Photomicrograph of a transverse section of an embryo at Carnegie stage 9 illustrating three germ layers and yolk sac.

Somite

Neural tube

Notochord

Foregut

Coelom

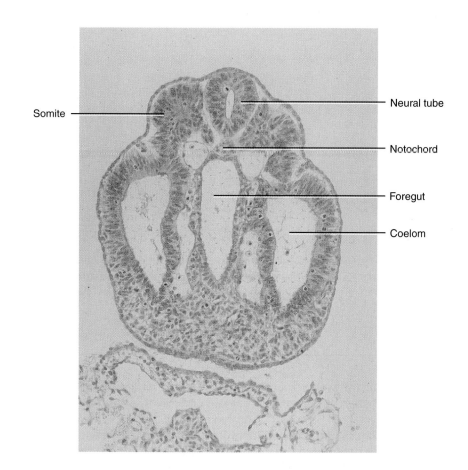

FIG. 9-2

Photomicrograph of a transverse section of an embryo at Carnegie stage 11. The primitive gut has been formed by the endoderm incorporated into the embryonic body. Observe the foregut and bilateral pericardioperitoneal cavities.

The **midgut** gives rise to the duodenum (distal to the bile duct), jejunum, ileum, cecum, vermiform appendix, ascending colon, and the right half to two thirds of the transverse colon. The midgut forms a U-shaped intestinal loop that herniates into the proximal part of the umbilical cord during the sixth week because there is no room for it in the abdomen (Figs. 9-5, *A*, and 9-7). While in the umbilical cord, the *midgut loop* rotates counterclockwise 90 degrees. During the tenth week, the intestines rapidly return to the abdomen, rotating a further 180 degrees during this process (Fig. 9-5, *C*).

Congenital anomalies of the intestine are common; most of them are abnormalities of midgut rotation. *Omphaloceles,* malrotations, and abnormalities of fixation of the intes-

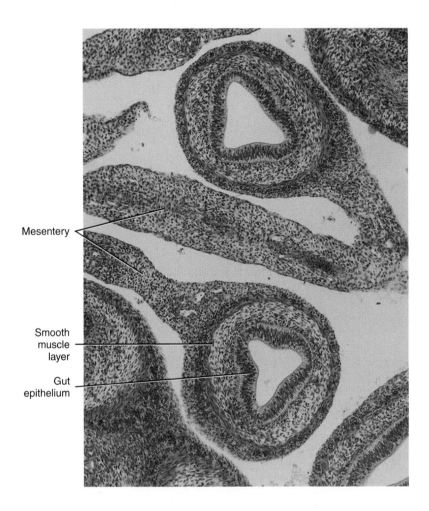

Mesentery

Smooth
muscle
layer

Gut
epithelium

FIG. 9-3

Photomicrograph of a section of the intestinal tube and mesentery in an embryo at Carnegie stage 23. Muscle layers are differentiating in the mesenchymal tissue of the intestinal wall.

FIG. 9-4

The development and rotation of the stomach and formation of the omental bursa (lesser sac) and greater omentum. **A,** Median section of a 28-day-old embryo. **B,** Anterolateral view of a 28-day-old embryo. **C,** Embryo about 35 days. **D,** Embryo about 40 days. **E,** Embryo about 48 days. **F,** Lateral view of the stomach and greater omentum of an embryo at about 52 days. The transverse section shows the omental foramen and omental bursa. **G,** Sagittal section showing the omental bursa and greater omentum.

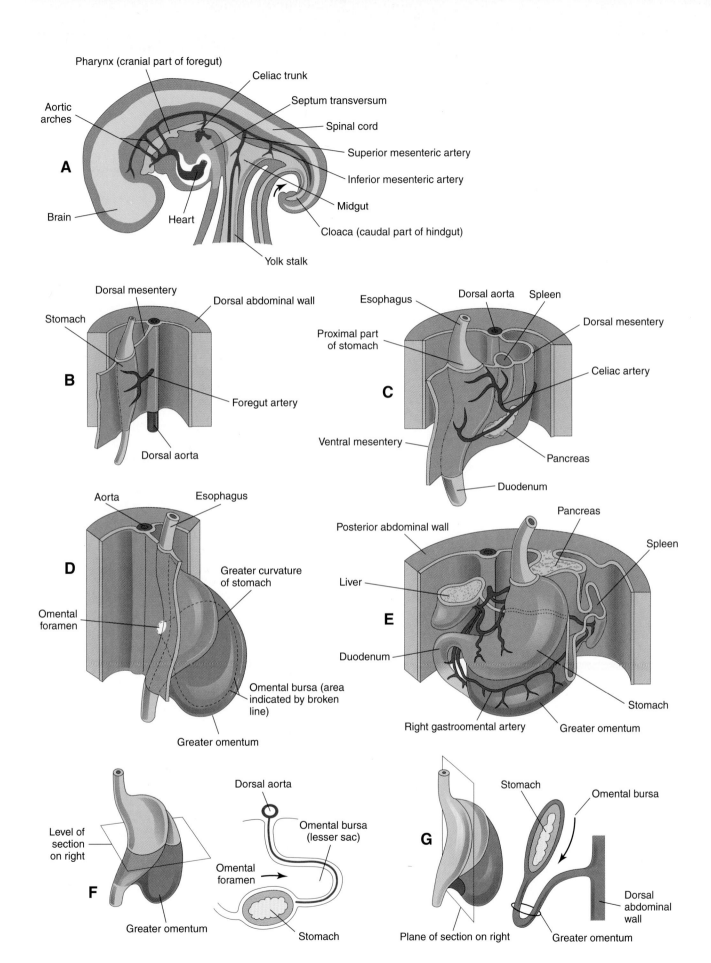

FIG. 9-4

For legend see opposite page.

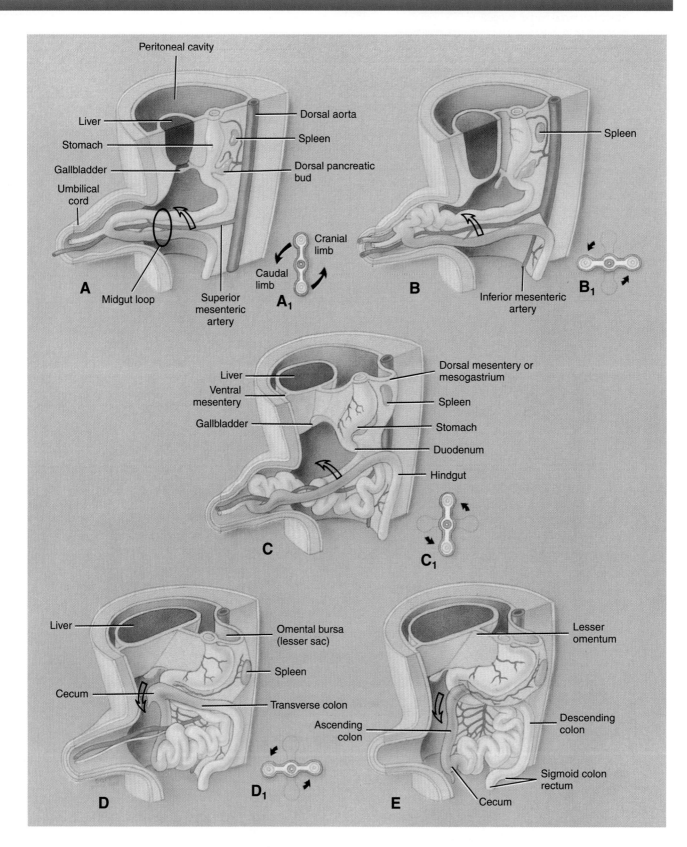

A
- Peritoneal cavity
- Liver
- Stomach
- Gallbladder
- Umbilical cord
- Dorsal aorta
- Spleen
- Dorsal pancreatic bud
- Midgut loop
- Superior mesenteric artery

A₁
- Cranial limb
- Caudal limb

B
- Spleen
- Inferior mesenteric artery

B₁

C
- Liver
- Ventral mesentery
- Gallbladder
- Dorsal mesentery or mesogastrium
- Spleen
- Stomach
- Duodenum
- Hindgut

C₁

D
- Liver
- Cecum
- Omental bursa (lesser sac)
- Spleen
- Transverse colon

D₁

E
- Lesser omentum
- Ascending colon
- Descending colon
- Sigmoid colon rectum
- Cecum

FIG. 9-5
For legend see opposite page.

FIG. 9-5

Schematic drawings illustrating rotation of the midgut as seen from the left. **A**, Around the beginning of the sixth week, showing the midgut loop partially within the umbilical cord. Note the elongated, double-layered dorsal mesentery containing the superior mesenteric artery. **A1**, Transverse section through the midgut loop illustrating the initial relationship of the limbs of the midgut loop to the artery. **B**, Later stage showing the beginning of midgut rotation *(arrows)*. Note that the cranial limb of the midgut has developed into intestines. **B1**, Illustrates the 90-degree counterclockwise rotation that carries the cranial limb of the midgut to the right. **C**, About 10 weeks, showing the intestines returning to the abdomen. **C1**, Illustrates a further rotation of 90 degrees. **D**, About 11 weeks, after return of intestines to the abdomen. **D1**, Shows a further 90-degree rotation of the gut, for a total of 270 degrees. **E**, Late fetal period, showing the cecum rotating to its normal position in the lower right quadrant of the abdomen.

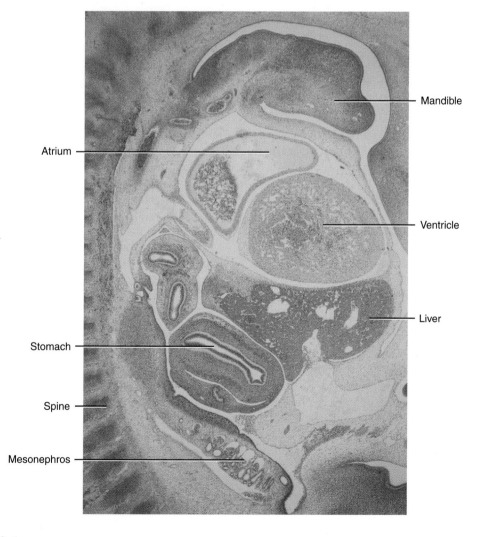

FIG. 9-6

Photomicrograph of a sagittal section of an embryo at Carnegie stage 17. The liver is differentiating in the septum transversum.

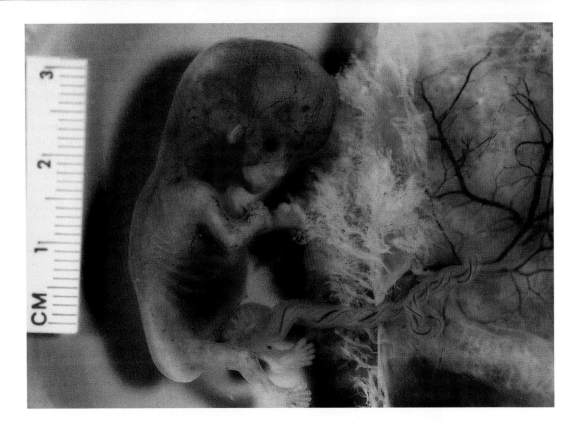

FIG. 9-7

Physiological hernia in embryo (58 days of development) attached to its chorionic sac. Note the herniated intestine derived from the midgut loop in the proximal part of the umbilical cord. Also note the umbilical blood vessels. Because the abdomen and pelvis are poorly developed at this stage (8 weeks) the intestines herniate into the umbilical cord. They return during the tenth week. (Courtesy of Dr. D.K. Kalousek, Department of Pathology, University of British Columbia, Children's Hospital, Vancouver, B.C., Canada.)

tine result from failure of return (Figs. 9-10 to 9-12; see also Fig. 9-7) or incomplete rotation of the intestine in the abdomen. Because the gut is normally occluded during the fifth and sixth weeks because of rapid mitotic activity of its epithelium, *stenosis* (partial obstruction), *atresia* (complete obstruction), and duplications result if recanalization fails to occur or occurs abnormally (Fig. 9-9). Various remnants of the yolk stalk may persist. *Ileal (Meckel's) diverticula* are common, but only a few of them become inflamed and produce pain. Most ileal diverticula develop from remnants of the yolk stalk (Figs. 9-13 and 9-14).

The **hindgut** gives rise to the left one third to one half of the transverse colon, the descending and sigmoid colon, the rectum, and the superior part of the anal canal (Fig. 9-5). The inferior part of the anal canal develops from the proctodeum (anal pit). The expanded caudal part of the hindgut, known as the *cloaca,* is divided by the *urorectal septum* into the urogenital sinus and rectum (Fig. 9-15). The urogenital sinus gives rise to the urinary bladder and urethra (see Chapter 10). At first the rectum and the superior part of the anal canal are separated from the exterior by the *anal membrane,* but this membrane normally breaks down by the end of the eighth week.

Anorectal anomalies usually result from abnormal partitioning of the cloaca by the urorectal septum into the rectum and anal canal posteriorly and the urinary bladder and urethra anteriorly (Fig. 9-15). Arrested growth and/or deviation of the urorectal septum in a dorsal direction causes most of the anorectal abnormalities, such as imperforate anus (Fig. 9-16), rectal atresia and abnormal connections (fistulas) between the rectum and the urethra, urinary bladder, or vagina (Fig. 9-17).

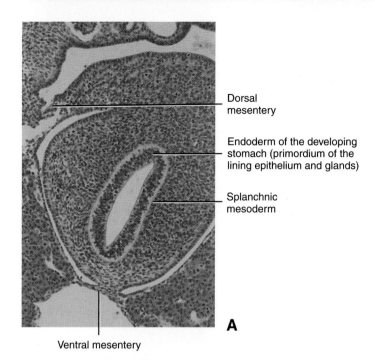

Dorsal mesentery

Endoderm of the developing stomach (primordium of the lining epithelium and glands)

Splanchnic mesoderm

A

Ventral mesentery

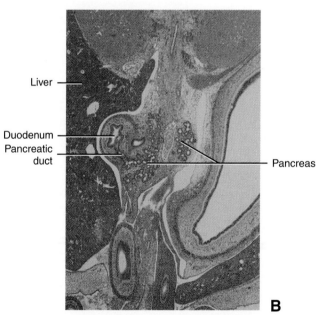

Liver

Duodenum
Pancreatic duct

Pancreas

B

Liver   Duodenum   Pancreas   Splenic vein

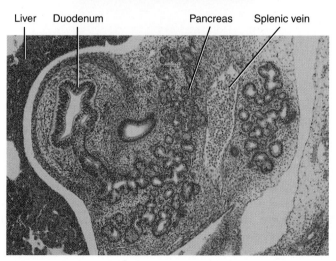

C

FIG. 9-8

Photomicrographs of sections of the developing stomach, duodenum, and pancreas in an embryo at Carnegie stage 21, about 52 days. A, The stomach and its mesenteries (×160). B, The duodenum and pancreas (×20). C, Higher power view of the structures shown in *B* (×50).

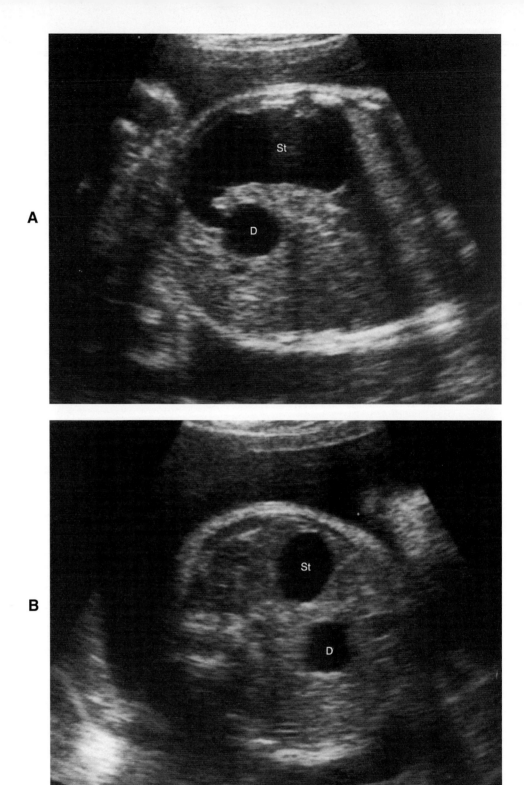

FIG. 9-9

Ultrasound scans of a fetus at 33 weeks of gestation (31 weeks after fertilization) showing duodenal atresia. **A,** An oblique section showing the dilated, fluid-filled stomach *(St)* entering the proximal duodenum *(D),* which is also enlarged as a result of the atresia (blockage) distal to it. **B,** Transverse section illustrating the characteristic double bubble appearance of the stomach and duodenum when there is duodenal atresia. Duodenal atresia occurs in 1 in 10,000 live births. This anomaly is due to failure of recanalization of the duodenum that normally occurs at 10 weeks of gestation (8 weeks after fertilization). Duodenal atresia is associated with other anomalies in 48% of cases: 30% in infants with Down syndrome; 22% in cases of gut malrotation; 20% in infants with congenital heart defects. Duodenal atresia is associated with polyhydramnios in 45% of cases resulting from the failure of absorption of swallowed amniotic fluid. (Courtesy of Dr. Lyndon M. Hill, Magee-Womens Hospital, Pittsburgh, Pa).

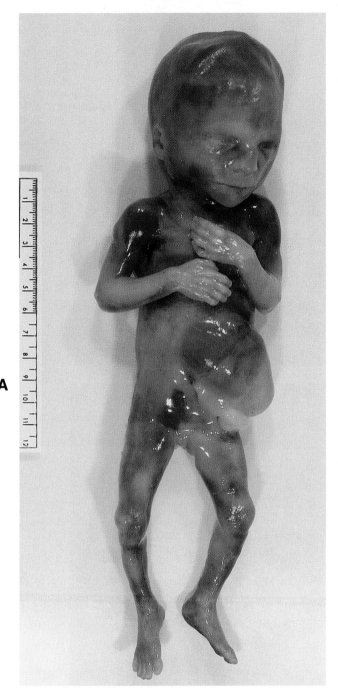

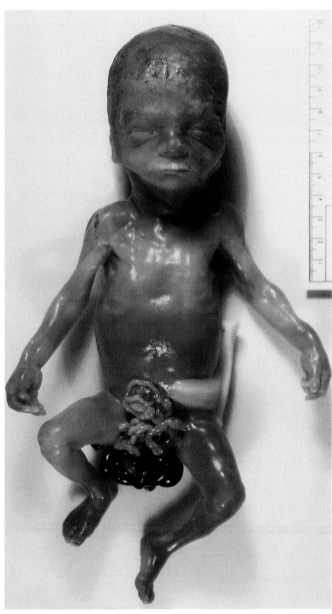

FIG. 9-10

A, Female fetus (19 weeks of development) with a large omphalocele containing intestines and a part of the liver. **B,** Gastroschisis in a female fetus of 20 developmental weeks. Note the normal insertion of the umbilical cord and the abdominal wall defect on the right side. (Courtesy of Dr. D.K. Kalousek, Department of Pathology, University of British Columbia, Children's Hospital, Vancouver, B.C., Canada.)

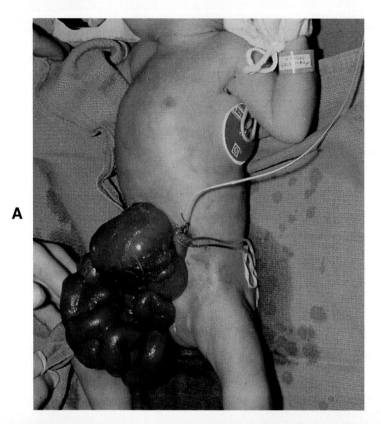

A

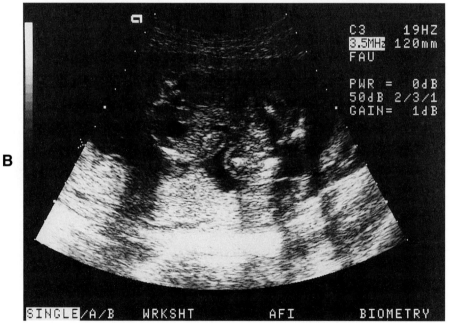

B

FIG. 9-11

A, Neonate with an anterior abdominal wall defect known as gastroschisis. The defect was relatively small (2 to 4 cm) and involved all layers of the abdominal wall. It was located to the right of the umbilicus. The generally accepted etiology of gastroschisis is that the defect is due to abnormal involution of the right umbilical vein that occurs during the fifth week. Most infants with this severe anomaly now survive because of improved perinatal management. Gastroschisis should not be confused with omphalocele (Fig. 9-10). **B,** Sonogram of fetus (21 weeks gestation) with gastroschisis. Note loops of intestine herniating out of the defect; immediately to the right of umbilical cord insertion, and freely floating in the amniotic fluid anterior to the fetal abdomen. The "stomach bubble" is on the left. (**A,** Courtesy of Dr. A.E. Chudley, Department of Pediatrics and Child Health, University of Manitoba, Children's Hospital, Winnipeg, Manitoba, Canada. **B,** Courtesy of Dr. G.J. Reid, Department of Obstetrics, Gynecology and Reproductive Sciences, University of Mantioba, Women's Hospital, Winnipeg, Manitoba, Canada.)

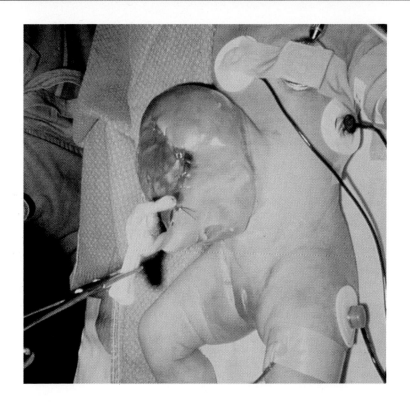

FIG. 9-12

Neonate with a giant-type omphalocele resulting from a median defect of the abdominal muscles, fascia, and skin at the umbilicus that resulted in the herniation of intraabdominal structures (liver and intestine) into the proximal end of the umbilical cord. It is covered by a membrane composed of peritoneum and amnion. In some cases, omphalocele may be a persistence of the normal embryonic stage of umbilical herniation (Fig. 9-7). (Courtesy of Dr. N.E. Wiseman, Pediatric Surgeon, Children's Hospital, Winnipeg, Manitoba, Canada.)

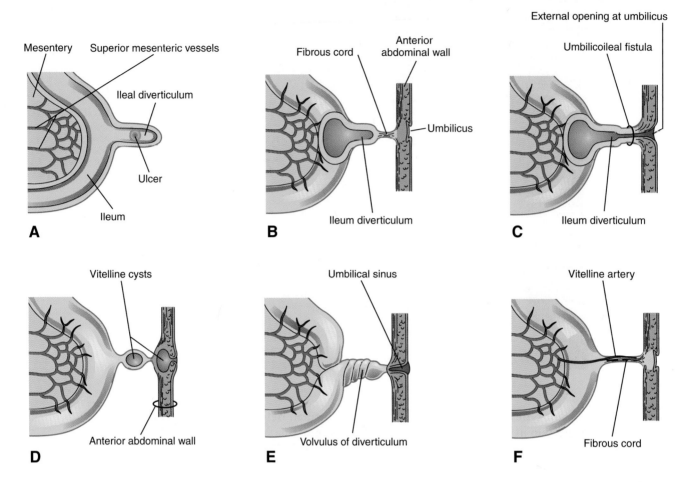

FIG. 9-13

Drawings illustrating ileal (Meckel's) diverticula and other remnants of the yolk stalk. A, Section of ileum and a diverticulum with an ulcer. B, A diverticulum connected to the umbilicus by a fibrous cord. C, Umbilicoileal fistula resulting from persistence of the entire intra-abdominal portion of the yolk stalk. D, Vitelline cysts at the umbilicus and a fibrous remnant of the yolk stalk. E, Umbilical sinus resulting from the persistence of the yolk stalk near the umbilicus. F, The yolk stalk has persisted as a fibrous cord connecting the ileum with the umbilicus. A persistent vitelline artery extends along the fibrous cord to the umbilicus.

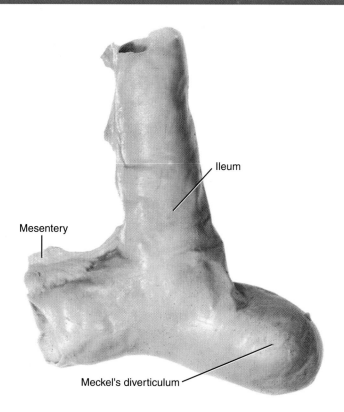

Ileum

Mesentery

Meckel's diverticulum

FIG. 9-14

Photograph of a typical ileal diverticulum, referred to clinically as a Meckel's diverticulum. Only a small percentage of these diverticula produce symptoms. Ileal diverticula are one of the most common anomalies of the digestive tract. They occur in 2% to 4% of people and are three to five times more prevalent in males than females. The embryologic basis of these diverticula is illustrated in Fig. 9-13.

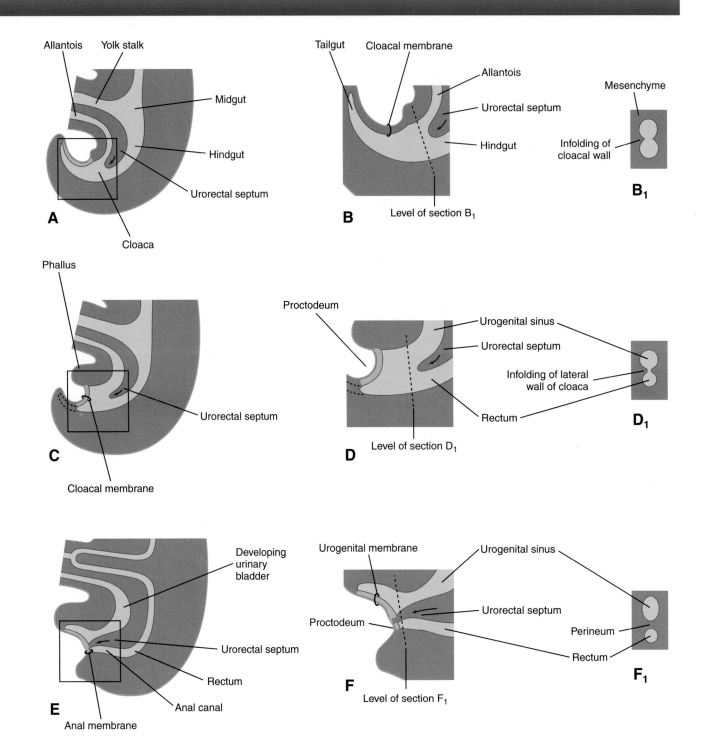

FIG. 9-15

Successive stages in the partitioning of the cloaca into the rectum and urogenital sinus by the urorectal septum. A, C, and **E,** Views from the left side at 4, 6, and 7 weeks, respectively. **B, D,** and **F,** Enlargements of the cloacal region. **B₁, D₁,** and **F₁,** Transverse sections of the cloaca at the levels shown in *B, D,* and *F,* respectively. Note that the tailgut (shown in *B*) degenerates and disappears as the rectum forms from the dorsal part of the cloaca (shown in *C*).

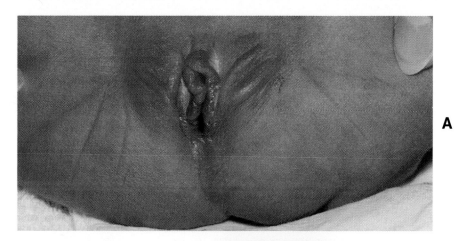

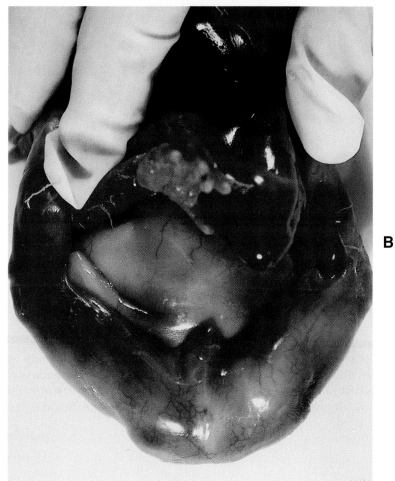

FIG. 9-16

Imperforate anus. **A,** Female neonate with membranous anal atresia (imperforate anus). A tracheoesophageal fistula was also present (see Fig. 8-5). In most cases of anal atresia, a thin layer of tissue separates the anal canal from the exterior (Fig. 9-17, C). This anomaly is due to failure of the anal membrane to perforate at the end of the eighth week. Some form of imperforate anus occurs about once in every 5000 neonates; it is more common in males. **B,** Imperforate anus in a male fetus, 16 developmental weeks with multiple developmental anomalies. (**A,** Courtesy of Dr. A.E. Chudley, Department of Pediatrics and Child Health, University of Manitoba, Children's Hospital, Winnipeg, Manitoba, Canada. **B,** Courtesy of Dr. D.K. Kalousek, Department of Pathology, University of British Columbia, Children's Hospital, Vancouver, B.C., Canada.)

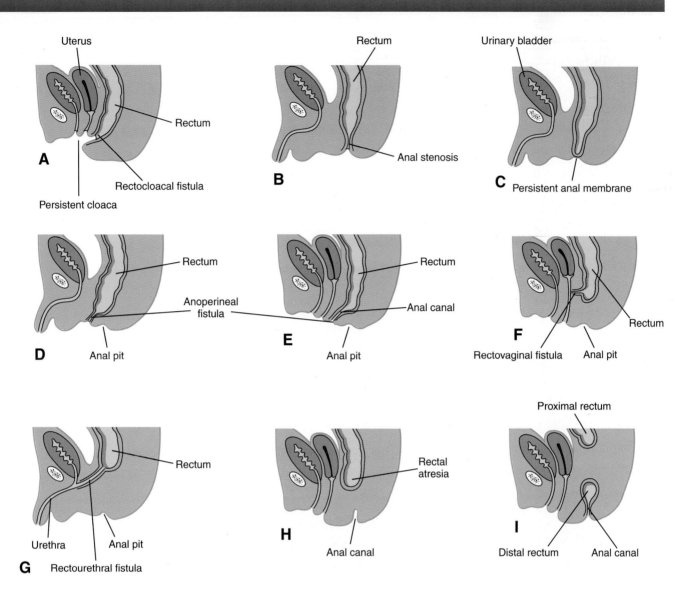

FIG. 9-17

Various types of anorectal anomaly. A, Persistent cloaca. Note the common outlet for the intestinal, urinary, and reproductive tracts. **B,** Anal stenosis. **C,** Membranous anal atresia (covered anus). **D** and **E,** Anal agenesis with a perianal fistula. **F,** Anorectal agenesis with a rectovaginal fistula. **G,** Anorectal agenesis with a rectourethral fistula. **H** and **I,** Rectal atresia.

10

The Urogenital System

The urogenital system develops from three sources: (1) intermediate mesoderm, (2) mesothelium (coelomic epithelium) lining the peritoneal cavity, and (3) endoderm of the urogenital sinus (Fig. 10-1). Three successive sets of **kidneys** develop: (1) the nonfunctional *pronephroi*, (2) the *mesonephroi*, which serve as temporary excretory organs, and (3) the functional *metanephroi* or permanent kidneys (Fig. 10-2).

The metanephroi develop from two sources: (1) the *metanephric diverticulum* or *ureteric bud*, which gives rise to the ureter, renal pelvis, calices, and collecting tubules, and (2) the *metanephric mesoderm*, which gives rise to the nephrons (Figs. 10-2 to 10-4). At first the **kidneys** are located in the pelvis but they gradually ascend to the abdomen. This apparent migration results from disproportionate growth of the lumbar and sacral regions.

The **urinary bladder** develops from the urogenital sinus and the surrounding splanchnic mesenchyme (see Fig. 9-15). The female urethra and almost all of the male urethra have a similar origin. The cortex and medulla of the suprarenal or adrenal glands have different origins (Figs. 10-5 to 10-7). The cortex develops from mesoderm and the medulla develops from neural crest cells.

Exstrophy of the bladder results from a defect in the ventral body wall, through which the posterior wall of the urinary bladder protrudes onto the abdominal wall.

Developmental abnormalities of the kidneys and urinary tract are common (Fig. 10-8 to 10-13). Incomplete division of the metanephric diverticulum results in partial or complete *duplication of the ureter* (Fig. 10-12) and/or a supernumerary kidney. Failure of the kidney to ascend from its embryonic pelvic position results in *ectopic kidney* that is abnormally rotated, for example, **pelvic kidney** (Fig. 10-8). Congenital polycystic disease of the kidneys may result from failure of the first formed rudimentary nephrons to degenerate; later these remnants may accumulate fluid and form cysts. Cysts may also form from detached parts of metanephric tissue. It is now believed that these cysts are dilatations of the nephrons, particularly of the loops of Henle. Ultrasonography remains the most valuable prenatal diagnostic technique for detecting renal and urinary tract anomalies.

Text continued on p. 184

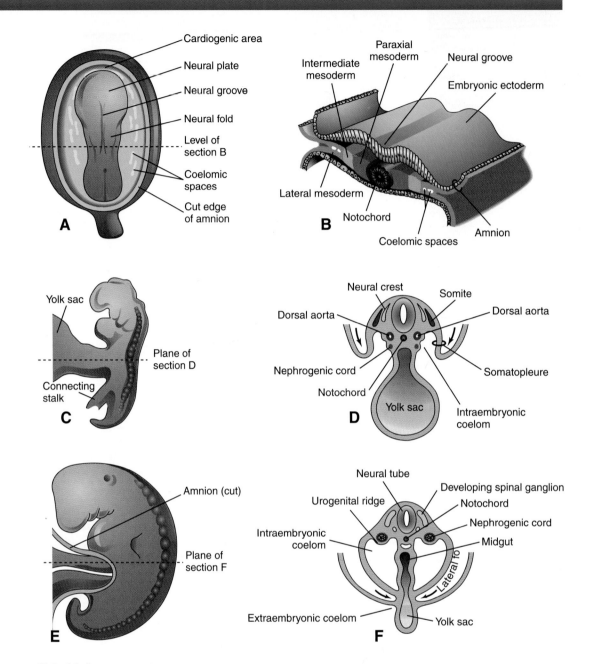

FIG. 10-1

A, Dorsal view of an embryo during the third week (about 18 days). **B,** Transverse section of the embryo showing the position of the intermediate mesoderm before lateral folding of the embryo. **C,** Lateral view of an embryo during the fourth week (about 24 days). **D,** Transverse section of the embryo after the commencement of folding, showing the nephrogenic cords of mesoderm. **E,** Lateral view of an embryo later in the fourth week (about 26 days). **F,** Transverse section of the embryo showing the lateral folds meeting each other ventrally. Observe the position of the urogenital ridges and nephrogenic cords.

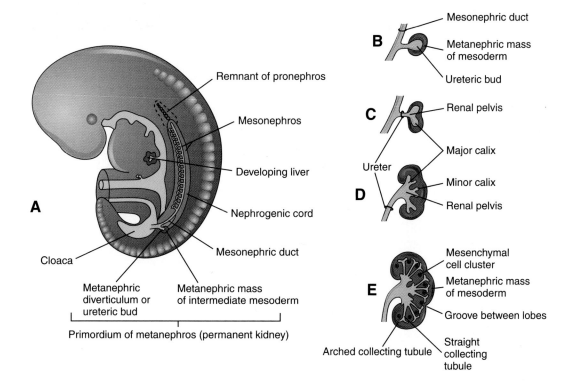

FIG. 10-2

Development of the metanephros or permanent kidney. A, Lateral view of a 5-week embryo, showing the primordium of the metanephros. **B to E,** Sketches showing successive stages in the development of the metanephric diverticulum or ureteric bud (fifth to eighth weeks). Observe the development of the ureter, renal pelvis, calices, and collecting tubules.

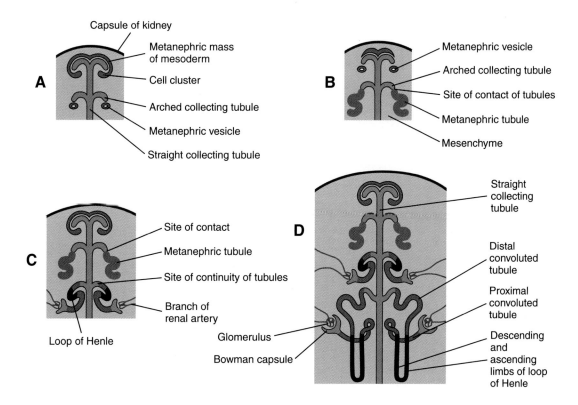

FIG. 10-3

Diagrammatic sketches illustrating stages in nephrogenesis—the development of nephrons. A, Nephrogenesis commences around the beginning of the eighth week. **B and C,** Note that the metanephric tubules, the primordia of the nephrons, become continuous with the collecting tubules to form uriniferous tubules. **D,** The number of nephrons more than doubles from 20 weeks to 38 weeks. Observe that nephrons are derived from the metanephric mass of mesoderm and that the collecting tubules are derived from the metanephric diverticulum.

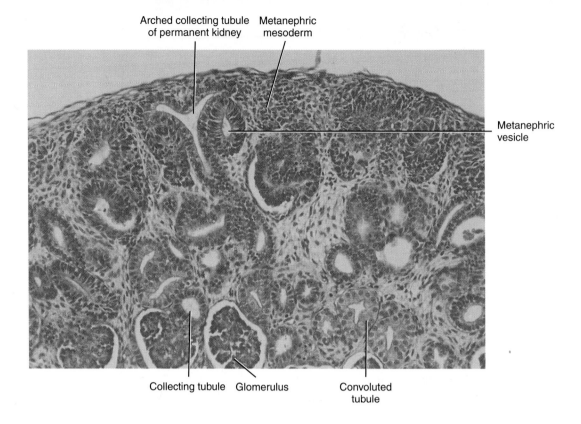

Arched collecting tubule of permanent kidney

Metanephric mesoderm

Metanephric vesicle

Collecting tubule   Glomerulus   Convoluted tubule

FIG. 10-4

Photomicrograph of a section of the metanephric kidney of an 11-week fetus (×200). These kidneys begin to develop late in the fifth week (Fig. 10-2).

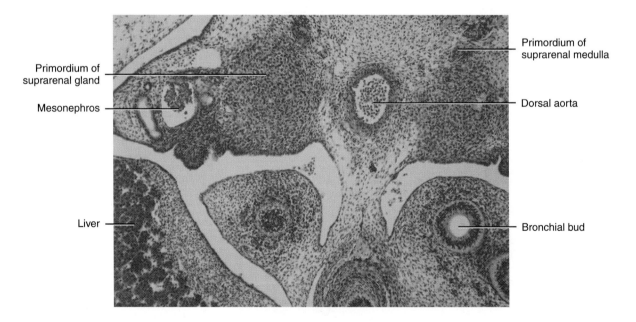

Primordium of suprarenal gland

Mesonephros

Liver

Primordium of suprarenal medulla

Dorsal aorta

Bronchial bud

FIG. 10-5

Photomicrograph of a section of an embryo at Carnegie stage 17, about 42 days, primarily to show the developing suprarenal (adrenal) glands. Observe that the developing cortex of each gland is large, whereas the small medulla lies dorsal to the cortex (see also Fig. 10-14). The medullary cells, derived from neural crest cells, are later engulfed by the cortex and are located inside the cortex.

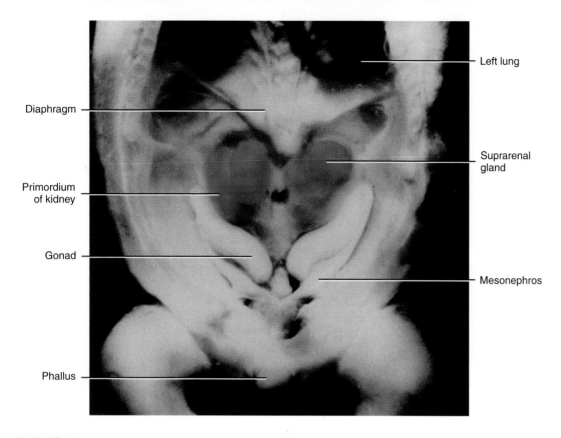

Left lung

Diaphragm

Suprarenal gland

Primordium of kidney

Gonad

Mesonephros

Phallus

FIG. 10-6

Dissection of the thorax, abdomen, and pelvis of an embryo at Carnegie stage 22, about 54 days. (For the external appearance and size of an embryo at this stage, see Fig. 2-25.) Observe the large suprarenal (adrenal) glands and the elongated mesonephros (mesonephric kidney). Also observe the gonads (testes or ovaries). The sex of these glands is not obvious in an external view such as this (see Fig. 10-17). External evidence of sex is not recognizable either. The phallus will develop into a penis or a clitoris depending on the genetic sex of the embryo. (From Nishimura H [editor]: *Atlas of human prenatal histology,* Tokyo, 1983, Igaku-Shoin.)

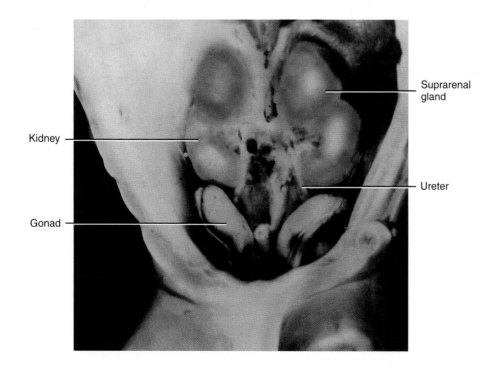

Kidney

Gonad

Suprarenal gland

Ureter

FIG. 10-7

Dissection of the abdomen of a 9-week fetus, (CRL 41 mm). Note the large size of the suprarenal or adrenal glands. These glands normally reduce to their normal size during the first 2 weeks after birth.

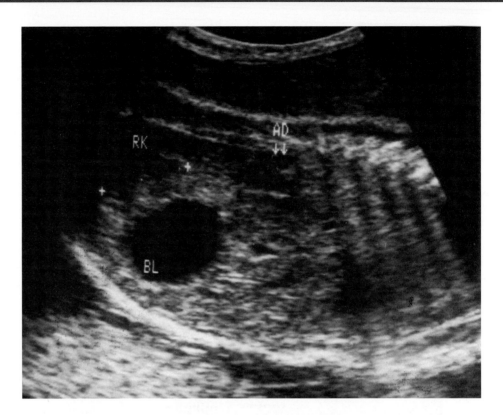

FIG. 10-8

Sonogram of the pelvis of a fetus at 31 weeks of gestation (*29 weeks after fertilization*). Observe the abnormally low position of the right kidney *(RK)* near the urinary bladder *(BL)*. This abnormal pelvic kidney resulted from its failure to ascend during the sixth to ninth weeks. Also observe the suprarenal or adrenal gland *(AD)*, which develops separately from the kidney. When the kidneys ascend into the abdomen, these glands lie at their superior poles (Fig. 10-7). (Courtesy of Dr. Lyndon M. Hill, Director of Ultrasound, Magee-Womens Hospital, Pittsburgh, Pa.)

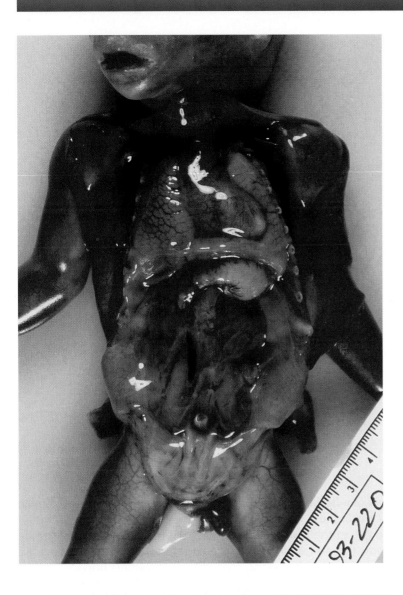

FIG. 10-9

Bilateral renal agenesis. Note prominent adrenal glands. Male fetus of 19.5 developmental weeks. (Courtesy of Dr. D.K. Kalousek, Department of Pathology, University of British Columbia, Children's Hospital, Vancouver, B.C., Canada.)

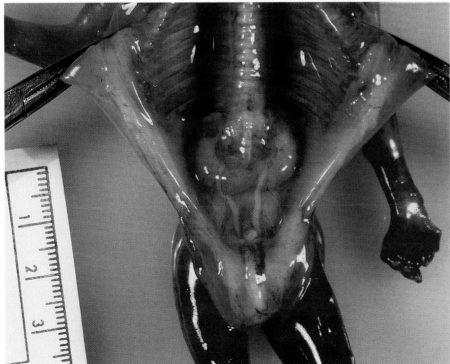

FIG. 10-10

Horseshoe kidney in a female fetus, 13 developmental weeks, with trisomy 18 syndrome. (Courtesy of Dr. D.K. Kalousek, Department of Pathology, University of British Columbia, Children's Hospital, Vancouver, B.C., Canada.)

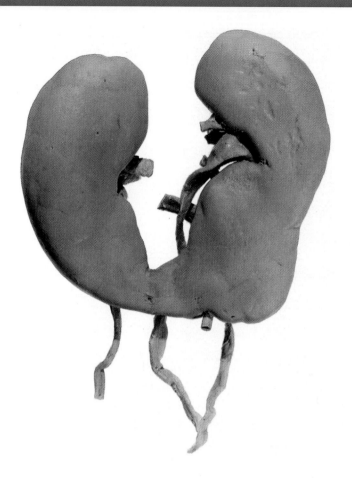

FIG. 10-11

Photograph of a posterior view of a horseshoe kidney. This odd-shaped organ resulted from fusion of the inferior poles of the kidneys while they were in the pelvis. Because the bridge between the kidneys gets caught on the root of the inferior mesenteric artery, a horseshoe kidney is unable to ascend into the abdomen. The larger right kidney has a bifid ureter. Horseshoe kidney, present in 1 of about 500 persons, is asymptomatic unless urinary outflow is impeded. About 7% of people with Down syndrome have a horseshoe kidney. A horseshoe kidney usually produces no symptoms.

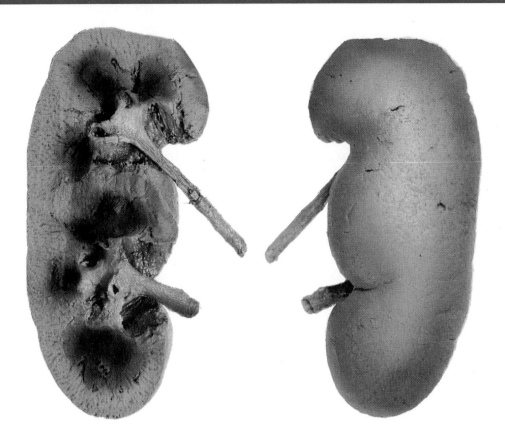

FIG. 10-12

Photographs of a kidney with two ureters and renal pelves. This congenital anomaly results from incomplete division of the metanephric diverticulum or ureteric bud (Fig. 10-2). **A,** Longitudinal section through the kidney showing two renal pelves. **B,** Anterior surface. Both ureters opened into the urinary bladder.

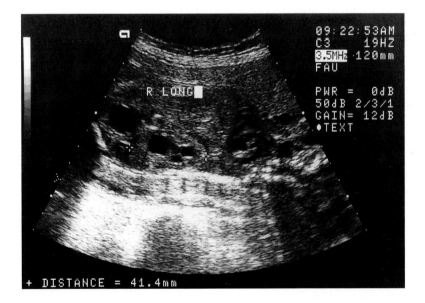

FIG. 10-13

Infantile polycystic kidneys. Sonogram at 34 weeks gestation showing enlarged kidneys with multiple small cysts producing white echoes. (Courtesy of Dr. G.J. Reid, Department of Obstetrics, Gynecology and Reproductive Sciences, University of Manitoba, Women's Hospital, Winnipeg, Canada.)

The genital or reproductive system develops in close association with the urinary or excretory system (Figs. 10-14 and 10-18). *Genetic sex* is established at fertilization, but the gonads do not begin to attain sexual characteristics until the seventh week (Figs. 10-15 to 10-17). The *primordial germ cells* form in the wall of the yolk sac during the fourth week and migrate into the developing gonads and differentiate into the definitive germ cells (oogonia/spermatogonia). The external genitalia do not acquire distinct masculine or feminine characteristics until the twelfth week (Figs. 10-17 and 10-20).

The reproductive organs develop from primordia that are identical in both sexes. During this indifferent or *undifferentiated stage* an embryo has the potential to develop into either a male or a female (Figs. 10-14 and 10-18). Gonadal sex is determined by the *testis-determining factor (TDF) on the Y chromosome.* TDF is located in the sex-determining region of the short arm of the Y chromosome (SRY).

TDF directs testicular differentiation. Embryos with a Y chromosome usually develop testes. By about the eighth week, the interstitial cells (of Leydig) produce testosterone that stimulates development of the mesonephric ducts into male genital ducts (Figs. 10-14 and 10-18). These androgens also stimulate development of the indifferent external genitalia into the penis and scrotum (Fig. 10-17). A glycoprotein, known as *antimüllerian hormone* (AMH) or *müllerian inhibiting substance* (MIS), produced by the Sertoli cells of the testes, inhibits development of the paramesonephric ducts (Fig. 10-18).

In embryos with abnormal sex chromosome complexes, such as XXX or XXY, the number of X chromosomes appears to be unimportant in sex determination. If a *normal* Y chromosome is present, the embryo develops as a male. If no Y chromosome is present, or the testis-determining region of the Y chromosome has been lost, female development occurs. The loss of an X chromosome does not appear to interfere with the migration of primordial germ cells to the gonadal ridges, because some germ cells have been observed in the fetal gonads of 45, X females with Turner syndrome. However, two X-chromosomes are needed to bring about complete ovarian development.

In the absence of a Y chromosome (i.e., TDF and MIS) and the presence of two X chromosomes, **ovaries** develop (Fig. 10-14), the mesonephric ducts regress (Fig. 10-18), the paramesonephric ducts develop into the uterus and uterine tubes (Figs. 10-18 and 10-19), the vagina develops from the vaginal plate derived from the urogenital sinus, and the indifferent external genitalia develop into the clitoris and labia (majora and minora [Figs. 10-20 and 10-22; see also Figs. 10-21 and 10-27]).

Most types of uterine and vaginal anomalies result from arrests of development of the uterovaginal primordium during the eighth week. **Double uterus** (uterus didelphys) results from failure of fusion of the inferior parts of the paramesonephric ducts. It may be associated with a double or a single vagina. In some cases the uterus appears normal externally but is divided internally by a thin septum. If the duplication involves only the superior part of the body of the uterus, the condition called **bicornuate uterus with a rudimentary horn** (cornu) develops. The rudimentary horn may not communicate with the cavity of the uterus. A **unicornuate uterus** develops when one paramesonephric duct fails to develop: this results in a uterus with one uterine tube.

Once in about every 4000 to 5000 female births, absence of the vagina occurs. This results from failure of the sinovaginal bulbs to develop and form the vaginal plate. When the vagina is absent, the uterus is usually absent also because the developing uterus (uterovaginal primordium) induces the formation of sinovaginal bulbs, which fuse to form the vaginal plate. Other anomalies involving the urogenital tract and the skeletal system may also be present.

Failure of canalization of the vaginal plate results in blockage of the vagina. A transverse vaginal septum occurs in approximately 1 in 80,000 women. Usually the septum is located at the junction of the middle and superior thirds of the vagina. Failure of the inferior end of the vaginal plate to perforate results in an **imperforate hymen.** Variations in

Text continued on p. 194

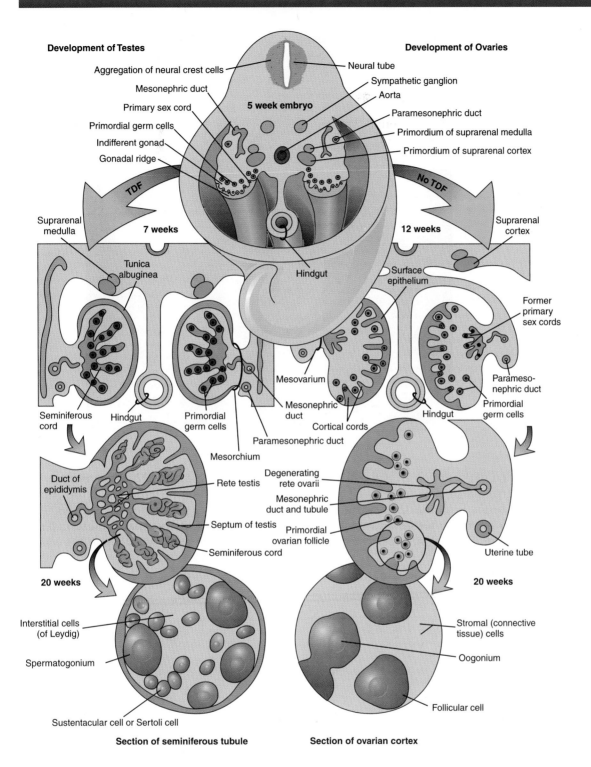

Development of Testes

Aggregation of neural crest cells
Mesonephric duct
Primary sex cord
Primordial germ cells
Indifferent gonad
Gonadal ridge

5 week embryo

Neural tube
Sympathetic ganglion
Aorta
Paramesonephric duct
Primordium of suprarenal medulla
Primordium of suprarenal cortex

Development of Ovaries

TDF

No TDF

Suprarenal medulla

7 weeks

12 weeks

Suprarenal cortex

Tunica albuginea

Hindgut

Surface epithelium

Former primary sex cords

Mesovarium

Mesonephric duct

Paramesonephric duct

Primordial germ cells

Seminiferous cord
Hindgut
Primordial germ cells

Cortical cords

Hindgut

Mesorchium

Paramesonephric duct

Duct of epididymis

Rete testis

Degenerating rete ovarii

Mesonephric duct and tubule

Septum of testis
Primordial ovarian follicle

Seminiferous cord

Uterine tube

20 weeks

20 weeks

Interstitial cells (of Leydig)

Stromal (connective tissue) cells

Spermatogonium

Oogonium

Follicular cell

Sustentacular cell or Sertoli cell

Section of seminiferous tubule

Section of ovarian cortex

FIG. 10-14

Differentiation of the indifferent gonads of a 5-week embryo (top) into ovaries or testes. Left side shows the development of testes resulting from the effects of the testis-determining factor (TDF) located on the Y chromosome. Note that the primary sex cords become seminiferous cords, the primordia of the seminiferous tubules. The parts of the primary sex cords that enter the medulla of the testis for the rete testis. In the section of the testis at the bottom left, observe that there are two kinds of cells, spermatogonia, derived from the primordial germ cells, and sustentacular or Sertoli cells, derived from mesenchyme. The right side shows the development of ovaries in the absence of TDF. Cortical cords have extended from the surface epithelium of the gonad and primordial germ cells have entered them. They are the primordia of the oogonia. Follicular cells are derived from the mesenchyme (primitive connective tissue) separating the oogonia.

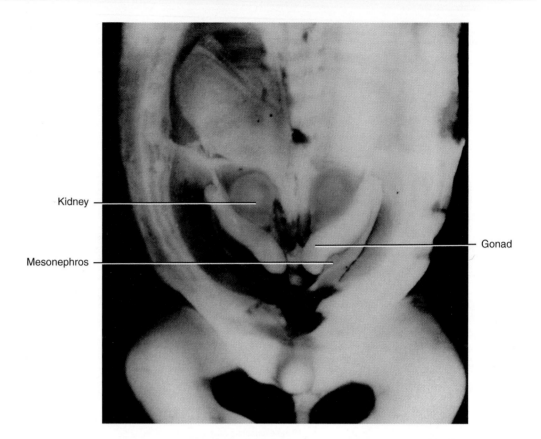

FIG. 10-15

Dissection of the abdomen and pelvis of an embryo at Carnegie stage 22, about 54 days. The suprarenal glands shown in Fig. 10-6 have been removed. Note the large size of the gonads (future testes or ovaries). Note the presence of the temporary mesonephric kidneys. They function for a few weeks and degenerate around the end of the final trimester. (From Nishimura H [editor]: *Atlas of human prenatal histology*, Tokyo, 1983, Igaku-Shoin.)

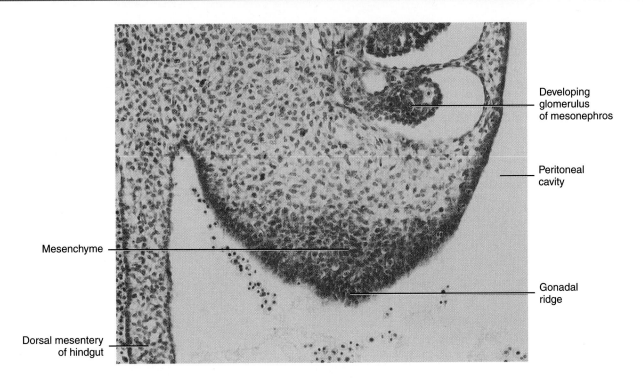

FIG. 10-16

Photomicrograph of a transverse section of the abdomen of an embryo at Carnegie stage 16, about 40 days, showing the gonadal (genital) ridge that will develop into a testis or an ovary depending on the genetic sex of the embryo. The sex of the embryo is not evident morphologically at this stage. (For the external appearance and size of an embryo at this stage, see Fig. 2-19.) Most of the developing gonad is composed of mesenchyme derived from the coelomic epithelium of the gonadal ridge.

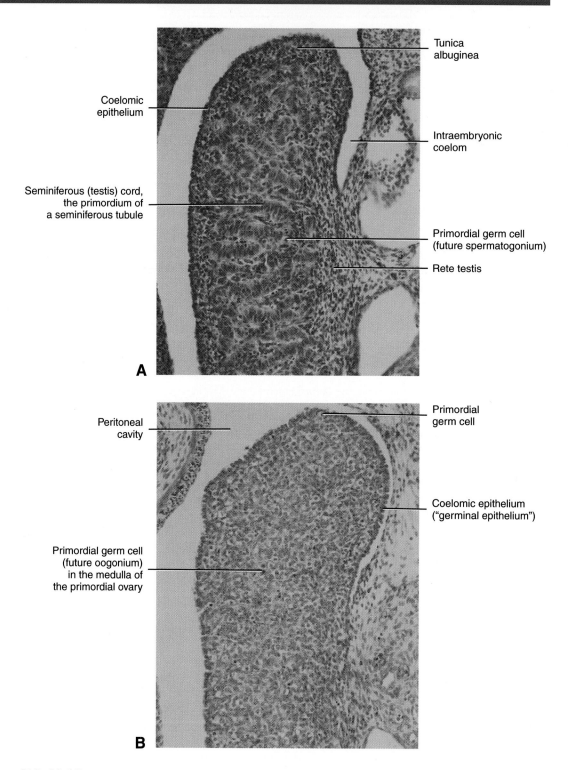

FIG. 10-17

Transverse sections of the gonads of human embryos. **A,** Developing testis from an embryo at Carnegie stage 20, about 51 days. Observe the prominent seminiferous or testis cords, the primordia of the seminiferous tubules. The large cells within them with dark nuclei are primordial germ cells, primordia of spermatogonia (see also Fig. 10-14). **B,** Developing ovary from an embryo at the same stage. The absence of seminiferous cords is a diagnostic characteristic of ovaries. The large cells with dark nuclei are primordial germ cells, the primordia of oogonia.

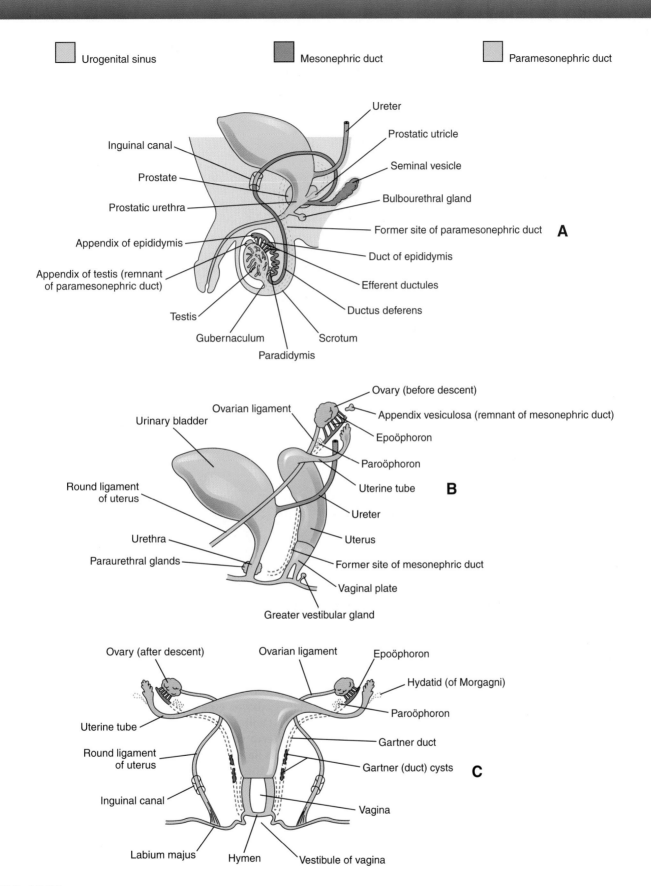

Urogenital sinus **Mesonephric duct** **Paramesonephric duct**

Ureter
Prostatic utricle
Seminal vesicle
Bulbourethral gland
Former site of paramesonephric duct **A**
Duct of epididymis
Efferent ductules
Ductus deferens

Inguinal canal
Prostate
Prostatic urethra
Appendix of epididymis
Appendix of testis (remnant of paramesonephric duct)

Testis
Gubernaculum
Paradidymis
Scrotum

Ovary (before descent)
Appendix vesiculosa (remnant of mesonephric duct)
Epoöphoron
Paroöphoron
Uterine tube **B**
Ureter
Uterus
Former site of mesonephric duct
Vaginal plate

Ovarian ligament
Urinary bladder
Round ligament of uterus
Urethra
Paraurethral glands
Greater vestibular gland

Ovary (after descent)
Ovarian ligament
Epoöphoron
Hydatid (of Morgagni)
Paroöphoron
Gartner duct
Gartner (duct) cysts **C**
Vagina

Uterine tube
Round ligament of uterus
Inguinal canal
Labium majus
Hymen
Vestibule of vagina

FIG. 10-18

Development of the male and female reproductive systems from the genital ducts and urogenital sinus. Vestigial structures are also shown. A, Reproductive system in a newborn male. B, Female reproductive system in a 12-week fetus. C, Reproductive system in a newborn female.

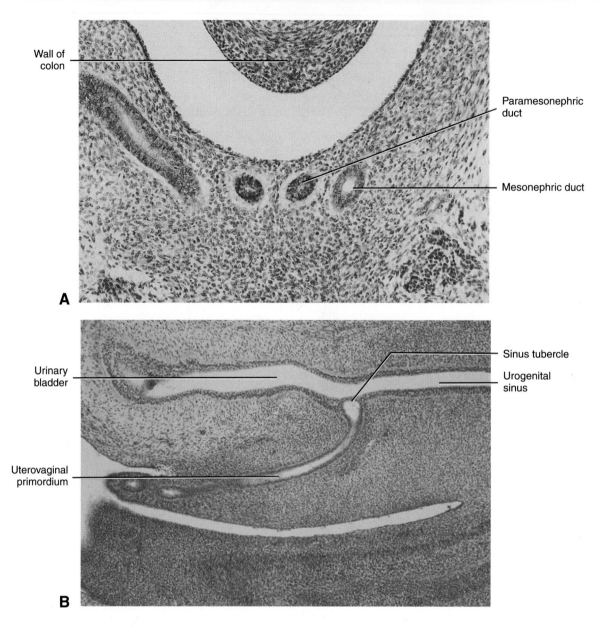

Wall of colon

Paramesonephric duct

Mesonephric duct

A

Sinus tubercle

Urinary bladder

Urogenital sinus

Uterovaginal primordium

B

FIG. 10-19

Photomicrographs of sections of human embryos. A, Transverse section of an embryo at Carnegie stage 22, about 54 days (×200) showing the mesonephric and paramesonephric ducts that are present in male and female embryos (see Fig. 10-15). In female fetuses, the paramesonephric ducts form the uterine (fallopian) tubes and then fuse to form the uterovaginal canal, the primordium of the uterus and vagina. B, Longitudinal section of a female embryo at Carnegie stage 23, about 56 days (×175), showing the uterus developing from the uterovaginal primordium formed by the fused paramesonephric (Müllerian) ducts.

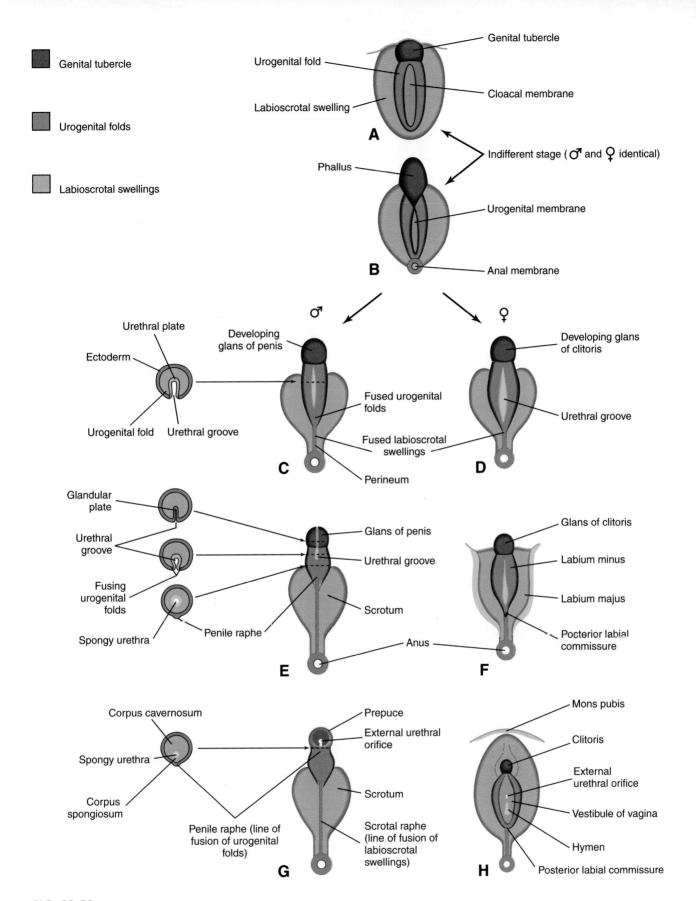

FIG. 10-20

Development of the external genitalia. A and **B,** Diagrams illustrating the appearance of the genitalia during the indifferent stage (fourth to seventh weeks). **C, E,** and **G,** Stages in the development of male external genitalia at 9, 11, and 12 weeks, respectively. To the left are schematic transverse sections of the developing penis, illustrating formation of the spongy urethra. **D, F,** and **H,** Stages in the development of female external genitalia at 9, 11, and 12 weeks, respectively.

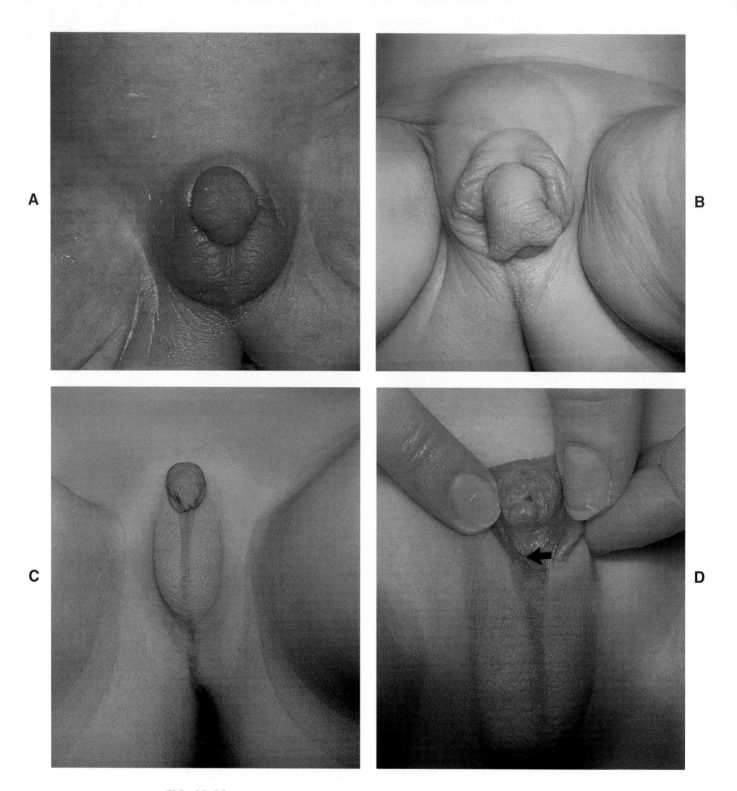

FIG. 10-21

Photographs of the external genitalia of female pseudohermaphrodites resulting from congenital adrenal hyperplasia (CAH). The degree of labioscrotal fusion and clitoral hypertrophy depends on the stage of differentiation at which the fetus is exposed to the masculinizing hormones, as well as on the biologic potency of the androgens produced by the hyperplastic suprarenal or adrenal glands. **A,** External genitalia of a newborn female, exhibiting enlargement of the clitoris and fusion of the labia majora. **B,** External genitalia of a female infant showing considerable enlargement of the clitoris. The unfused labia majora are rugose as in a scrotum. **C** and **D,** External genitalia of a 6-year-old girl, showing an enlarged clitoris and fused labia majora that have formed a scrotumlike structure. In *D* the clitoris has been elevated to show the location of the opening of the urogenital sinus *(arrow),* the primordium of the vestibule of the vagina.

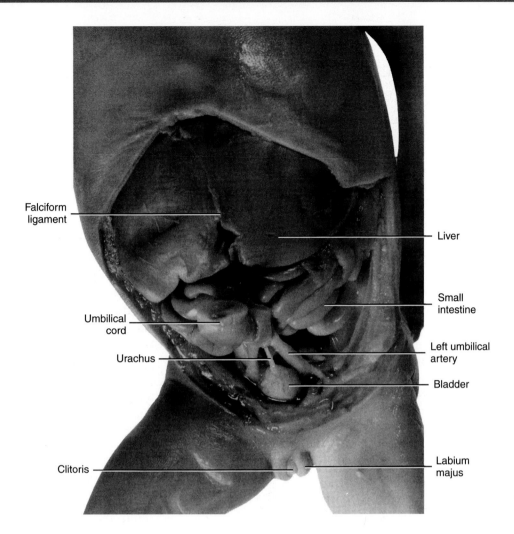

Falciform
ligament

Liver

Small
intestine

Umbilical
cord

Urachus

Left umbilical
artery

Bladder

Clitoris

Labium
majus

FIG. 10-22

Photograph of a dissection of an 18-week female fetus, primarily to show the relationship of the urachus, a derivative of the allantois, to the urinary bladder and umbilical arteries. The urachus becomes the median umbilical ligament in adults. The umbilical arteries carry poorly oxygenated blood to the placenta. They are represented in adults by the medial umbilical ligaments. Observe that the clitoris is still relatively large at this stage. It becomes smaller as full term is approached.

the appearance of the hymen are common. The vaginal orifice varies in diameter from very small to large, and there may be more than one orifice.

Cryptorchidism and ectopic testes result from abnormalities of testicular descent. Cryptorchidism occurs in up to 30% of premature males and in about 3% to 4% of full-term males. Cryptorchidism may be unilateral or bilateral. In most cases the testes descend into the scrotum by the end of the first year. If both testes remain within or just outside the abdominal cavity, they fail to mature and sterility is common. Undescended testes are often histologically normal at birth, but failure of development and atrophy are detectable by the end of the first year.

Cryptorchid testes may be in the abdominal cavity or anywhere along the usual path of descent of the testis, but they are usually in the inguinal canal (Fig. 10-23). The cause of most cases of cryptorchidism is unknown, but a deficiency of androgen production by the fetal testes is an important factor. Men with a history of cryptorchidism have a 20% to 44% increase in risk of developing testicular cancer. After traversing the inguinal canal, the testis may deviate from its usual path of descent and lodge in various abnormal locations: interstitial (external to aponeurosis of external oblique muscle), in the proximal part of the medial thigh, dorsal to the penis, and on the opposite side (crossed ectopia).

All types of ectopic testis are rare, but **interstitial ectopia** occurs most frequently. Ectopic testis occurs when a part of the gubernaculum passes to an abnormal location and the testis follows it.

If the communication between the tunica vaginalis and the peritoneal cavity fails to close, a **persistent processus vaginalis** exists. A loop of intestine may herniate through it into the scrotum or labium majus (Fig. 10-24). Embryonic remnants resembling the ductus deferens or epididymis are often found in inguinal hernial sacs. Congenital inguinal hernia is much more common in males, especially when there are undescended testes. Congenital inguinal hernias are also common with ectopic testes and in females with the androgen insensitivity syndrome.

Occasionally the abdominal end of the processus vaginalis remains open but is too small to permit herniation of intestine. Peritoneal fluid passes into the patent processus vaginalis and forms a **hydrocele of the testis.** If the middle part of the processus vaginalis canal remains open, fluid may accumulate and give rise to a **hydrocele of the spermatic cord** (Figs. 10-24 and 10-25).

In males, failure of the urogenital folds to fuse normally results in various types of *hypospadias*. Hypospadias is the most common anomaly of the penis. In one of every 300

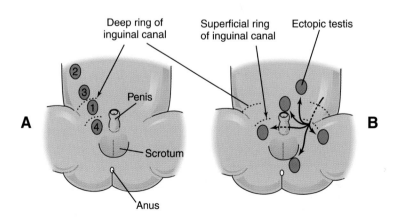

FIG. 10-23

Possible sites of cryptorchid and ectopic testes. A, Positions of cryptorchid testes, numbered in order of frequency. B, Usual locations of ectopic testes.

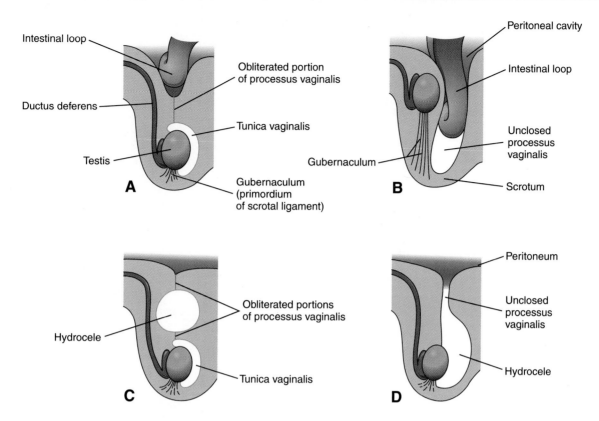

FIG. 10-24

Diagrams of sagittal sections illustrating conditions resulting from failure of closure of the processus vaginalis. **A,** Incomplete congenital inguinal hernia resulting from persistence of the proximal part of the processus vaginalis. **B,** Complete congenital inguinal hernia into the scrotum resulting from persistence of the proximal part of the processus vaginalis. Cryptorchidism, a commonly associated anomaly, is also illustrated. **C,** Large cyst or hydrocele that arose from an unobliterated portion of the processus vaginalis. **D,** Hydrocele of the testis and spermatic cord resulting from peritoneal fluid passing into an unclosed processus vaginalis.

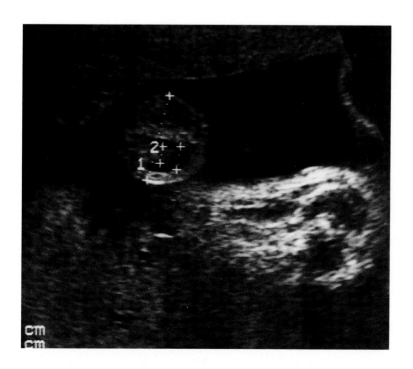

FIG. 10-25

Unilateral hydrocele in a 33-week gestation fetus. Calipers: Widest (1) set indicates the size of the scrotum (27 mm); medium set indicates size of the hydrocele (7 mm); smallest set (2) indicates the size of the testis (5 mm). (From Pretorius DH, Halsted MJ, Abels W, et al: *J Ultrasound Med* 17:49-52, 1998.)

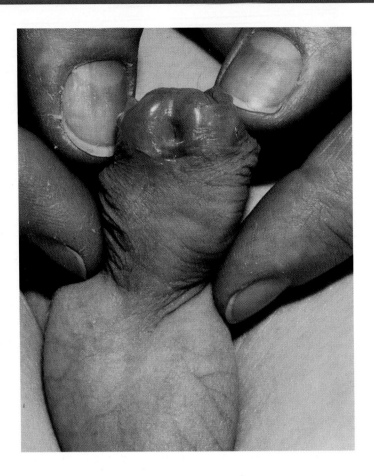

FIG. 10-26

Glandular hypospadia in an infant. The external urethral orifice is on the ventral surface of the glans penis. (Courtesy of Dr. A.E. Chudley, Department of Pediatrics and Child Health, University of Manitoba, Children's Hospital, Winnipeg, Manitoba, Canada.)

male births, the external urethral orifice is on the ventral surface of the glans penis (**glandular hypospadias;** Fig. 10-26), or on the ventral surface of the body of the penis **(penile hypospadias).** Less common sites are penoscrotal, scrotal, or perineal. In **penoscrotal hypospadias** the urethral orifice is at the junction of the penis and scrotum. Because the external genitalia in this severe type of hypospadias are ambiguous, persons with perineal hypospadias and cryptorchidism (undescended testes) are sometimes diagnosed as male pseudohermaphrodites. Hypospadias results from inadequate production of androgens by the fetal testes and/or inadequate receptor sites for the hormones. Genetic factors and environmental teratogens have also been suggested in the etiology of hypospadias.

In one of every 30,000 male infants, the urethra opens on the dorsal surface of the penis. It is *often associated with exstrophy of the bladder.* Epispadias may result from inadequate ectodermal-mesenchymal interactions during development of the genital tubercle. As a consequence, the genital tubercle develops more dorsally than in normal embryos. Consequently, when the urogenital membrane ruptures, the urogenital sinus opens on the dorsal surface of the penis. Urine is expelled at the root of the malformed penis.

Persons with *true hermaphroditism* have both ovarian and testicular tissue and variable internal and external genitalia. Errors in sexual differentiation cause pseudohermaphroditism. *Male pseudohermaphroditism* results from failure of the fetal testes to pro-

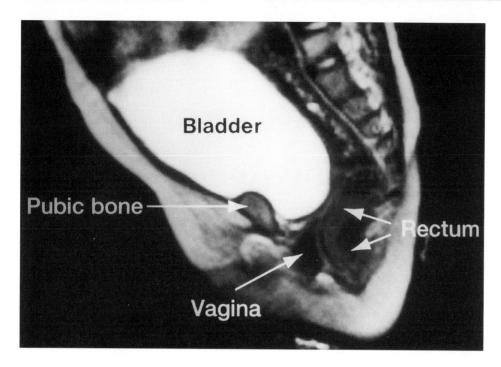

FIG. 10-27

Magnetic resonance imaging (sagittal view) of the pelvic region. Vagina ends blindly, and the uterus is absent. This condition is probably due to developmental failure of both gonads and the Müllerian ducts. (From Ohro Y, Tsutsumi Y, Ogata T: *Clin Genet* 54:52-55, 1998.)

duce adequate amounts of masculinizing hormones or from the tissue insensitivity of the sexual structures. *Female pseudohermaphroditism* usually results from congenital adrenal hyperplasia (CAH), a disorder of the fetal suprarenal (adrenal) glands that causes excessive production of androgens and masculinization of the external genitalia (Fig. 10-21). Commonly there is clitoral hypertrophy, partial fusion of the labia majora, and a persistent urogenital sinus. Female pseudohermaphrodites who do not have CAH are very rare. Administration of *androgenic agents* to women during pregnancy may cause similar anomalies of the fetal external genitalia. *Masculinizing maternal tumors* can also cause virilization of female fetuses (e.g., benign adrenal adenoma and ovarian tumors, especially *arrhenoblastoma*).

Masculinization of some male fetuses fails to occur because of a resistance to the action of testosterone at the cellular level in the labioscrotal and urogenital folds (Fig. 10-20). As a result these fetuses appear as normal female infants. The developmental defect is in the androgen receptor mechanism. Testes are present in these females but they are not functional. This condition, called the *androgen insensitivity syndrome,* was formerly referred to as the testicular feminization syndrome. The infants develop into women whose appearance and psychosexual orientation is female; however they are sterile. Patients with **partial AIS** (androgen insensitivity syndrome) exhibit some masculinization at birth, such as ambiguous external genitalia, and may have an enlarged clitoris. The vagina ends blindly and the uterus is absent (see Fig. 10-7). Testes are in the inguinal canals or the labia majora. Androgen insensitivity syndrome follows X-linked recessive inheritance, and the gene encoding the androgen receptor has been localized.

11

The Cardiovascular System

The cardiovascular system begins to develop toward the end of the third week, and the **primordial heart** starts to beat at 21 to 22 days. Mesenchymal cells derived from splanchnic mesoderm proliferate and form isolated cell clusters, which soon develop into two endothelial tubes that join to form the primitive vascular system (Figs. 11-1 to 11-3). Paired endothelial tubes form and fuse into a single endothelial heart tube. This primitive or primordial heart tube is soon surrounded by myoblasts (muscle-forming cells), which form the *myocardium* (Fig. 11-3).

The primordium of the heart consists of four chambers: sinus venosus, atrium, ventricle, and bulbus cordis. The *truncus arteriosus* is continuous caudally with the *bulbus cordis* and enlarges cranially to form the *aortic sac* (Fig. 11-1). As the heart grows, it bends to the right and soon acquires the general external appearance of the adult heart. The heart becomes partitioned into four chambers between the fourth and seventh weeks (Figs. 11-4 and 11-5). Three systems of paired veins drain into the primordial heart (Fig. 11-1).

FATE OF THE SINUS VENOSUS. This sinus venous is initially a separate chamber of the heart that opens into the right atrium (Figs. 11-1 and 11-3, *C*). As development of the heart proceeds, the left horn of the sinus venosus becomes the *coronary sinus* and the right horn is incorporated into the wall of the right atrium where it forms the smooth portion of the adult right atrial wall. The right half of the primitive atrium persists as the *right auricle,* an appendage of the atrium.

FORMATION OF THE LEFT ATRIUM. Most of the adult left atrium is formed by incorporation of the *primitive pulmonary vein.* As the atrium enlarges, parts of this vein and its branches are absorbed, with the result that four pulmonary veins eventually enter the adult atrium. The smooth-walled part of the left atrium is derived from absorbed pulmonary vein tissue, whereas the left auricle (auricular appendage) is derived from the primitive atrium.

During the fourth and fifth weeks, the primordial heart is divided into a four-chambered organ (Figs. 11-4 and 11-5).

DIVISION OF THE PRIMITIVE ATRIUM. Two localized proliferations of mesenchyme called *endocardial cushions* develop on the ventral and dorsal walls of the atrioven-

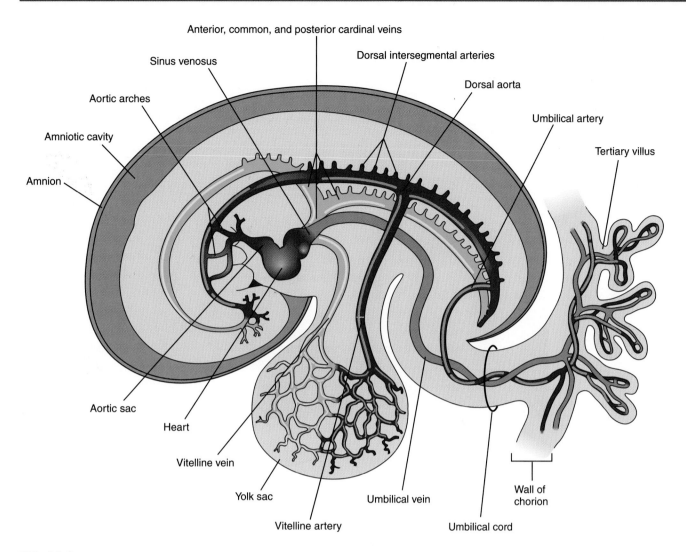

FIG. 11-1

Diagram of the primordial cardiovascular system in an embryo of about 21 days, viewed from the left side. Observe the transitory stage of paired symmetrical vessels. Each heart tube continues dorsally into a dorsal aorta that passes caudally. Branches of the aortae are: (1) umbilical arteries, establishing connections with vessels in the chorion; (2) vitelline arteries to the yolk sac; and (3) dorsal intersegmental arteries to the body of the embryo. The umbilical vein returns well-oxygenated blood from the chorion. Vessels on the yolk sac form a vascular plexus that is connected to the heart tubes by vitelline veins. The cardinal veins return blood from the body of the embryo. The umbilical vein carries oxygenated blood and nutrients from the chorion. The arteries carry poorly oxygenated blood and waste products to the chorionic villi for transfer to the mother's blood.

tricular canal of the heart (Fig. 11-5, *A*). These cushions grow toward each other and fuse, dividing the atrioventricular canal into right and left atrioventricular (AV) canals (Fig. 11-5, *B*). Before the **septum primum** fuses with these cushions, a communication exists between the right and left halves of the primitive atrium through the ostium primum initially and later through the *foramen secundum* and *foramen ovale* (Fig. 11-5, *A* to *C*).

As the septum primum fuses with the endocardial cushions, obliterating the foramen primum, the superior part of the septum primum breaks down, creating another opening called the *foramen secundum* (Fig. 11-5, *B* to *D*). As this round foramen develops, another sickle-shaped membranous fold, called the **septum secundum,** grows into the

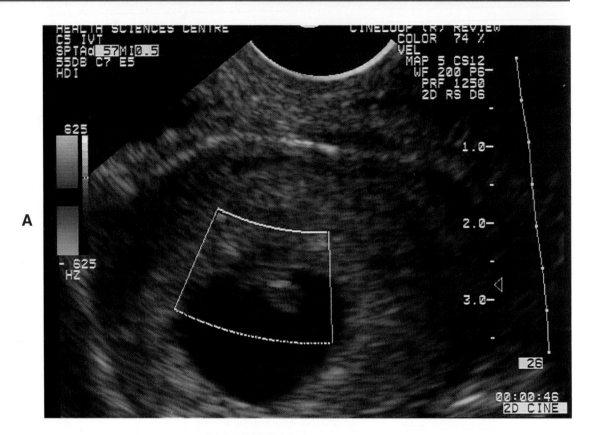

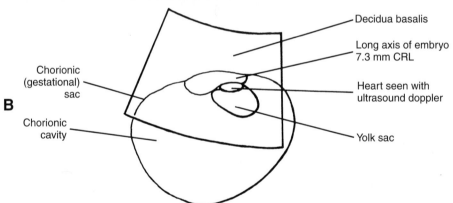

FIG. 11-2

A, Sonogram of a 5-week embryo (7.2 mm) and its attached yolk sac within its chorionic (gestational) sac. The red pulsating heart of the embryo was visualized using Doppler ultrasound. (For a photograph of an embryo at this stage, see Fig. 2-17.) **B,** Sketch of the sonogram for orientation and identification of structures. (Courtesy of Dr. E.A. Lyons, Professor of Radiology and Obstetrics and Gynecology, Department of Radiology, University of Manitoba, Health Sciences Centre, Winnipeg, Manitoba, Canada.)

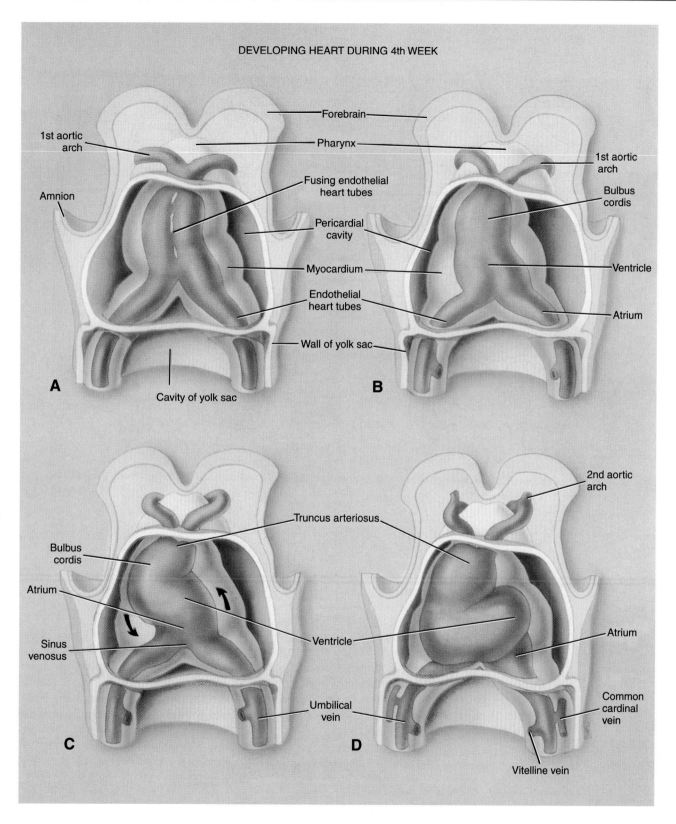

DEVELOPING HEART DURING 4th WEEK

FIG. 11-3

Drawings of ventral views of the developing heart during the fourth week. Note that the endothelial heart tubes gradually fuse to form a single tubular heart. The fusion begins at the cranial ends of the tubes and extends caudally until a single tubular heart is formed (**A** and **B**). The endothelial heart tubes form the endocardium of the heart. They are derived from splanchnic mesenchyme (embryonic connective tissue), as is the myocardium or muscular wall of the heart. As the heart elongates, it bends upon itself (**C**), forming an S-shaped heart (**D**), and establishes its regional divisions.

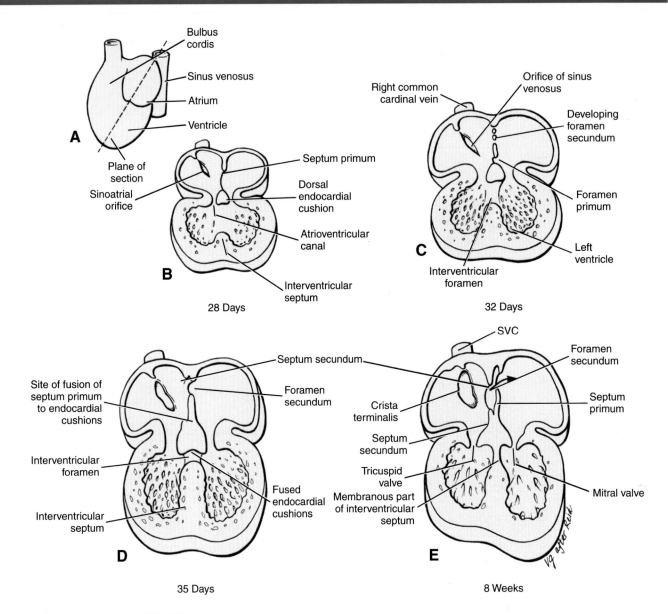

FIG. 11-4

Drawings of the developing heart, showing partitioning of the atrioventricular canal, primitive atrium, and ventricle. **A,** Sketch showing the plane of the coronal sections. **B,** During the fourth week (about 28 days), showing the early appearance of the septum primum, interventricular septum, and dorsal endocardial cushion. **C,** Section of the heart (about 32 days), showing perforations in the dorsal part of the septum. **D,** Section of the heart (about 35 days) showing the foramen secundum. **E,** About 8 weeks, showing the heart after it is partitioned into four chambers.

atrium to the right of the septum primum (Fig. 11-5, *D* to *H*). The septum secundum overlaps the foramen secundum, the opening in the septum primum. There is also an opening between the free edge of the septum secundum and the dorsal wall of the atrium, called the **foramen ovale** (Fig. 11-5, *E* to *H*). By this stage, the remains of the septum primum have formed the flaplike valve of the foramen ovale.

The *conduction system of the heart* begins to develop in the fifth week and is well developed by the end of the eighth week. Recent experimental studies suggest that neural crest cells may contribute to the formation of the conducting system.

Atrial septal defects (ASDs) result from abnormal development of the interatrial septum (Fig. 11-6). The common defect is characterized by a large opening in the septum between the right and left atria **(persistent foramen ovale).** This defect results from (1) excessive resorption of the septum primum, (2) underdevelopment of the septum secundum, or (3) a combination of these abnormalities.

FORMATION OF THE VENTRICLES (FIGS. 11-7 AND 11-8). The primordial ventricle gives rise to most of the left ventricle, whereas the bulbus cordis forms most of the right ventricle. The *interventricular septum* begins as a ridge in the floor of the primitive ventricle (Fig. 11-7, *A*) and slowly grows toward the endocardial cushions. Until the end of the seventh week, the future right and left ventricles communicate through a large **interventricular foramen** (Figs. 11-7, *B*, and 11-8). Closure of the interventricular foramen results in the formation of the membranous part of the interventricular septum. This part is derived from the fusion of tissue from the endocardial cushions and bulbar ridges (Fig. 11-7, *C* to *E*).

PARTITIONING OF THE BULBUS CORDIS AND TRUNCUS ARTERIOSUS. Division of these parts of the primordial heart results from the development and fusion of the truncal ridges and bulbar ridges (Fig. 11-7, *C*). Neural crest cells, which migrate into the truncus arteriosus and bulbus cordis, play an important role in the partitioning of the outflow tract. The fused mesenchymal ridges form an aorticopulmonary septum that divides the truncus arteriosus and bulbus cordis into the *ascending aorta* and *pulmonary trunk.* Abnormalities in the formation of the aorticopulmonary septum result in the following major congenital anomalies: transposition of the great arteries (vessels), persistent truncus arteriosus, and ventricular septal defects. Ventricular septal defects (VSDs) are the most common congenital heart anomalies.

Cardiac anomalies are the most common birth defects, with an incidence of about 8 in 1000 live births and close to 30 per 1000 in fetuses at autopsy. The critical period of heart development is from day 20 to day 50 after fertilization. It has been suggested that retinoic acid is essential for normal cardiac development, and that abnormal levels may result in cardiac defects. Genetic predisposition plays an important role in the etiology of many congenital cardiac defects. Numerous critical events occur during cardiac development, and deviation from the normal pattern at any time may produce one or more congenital heart defects (e.g., ASDs and VSDs). Because partitioning of the primordial heart results from complex processes, defects of the cardiac septa are relatively common (Figs. 11-9 to 11-11). Many structural heart defects can be diagnosed in utero by ultrasound techniques (Figs. 11-12 to 11-14).

Because the lungs are nonfunctional during prenatal life, the fetal cardiovascular system is structurally designed so that the blood is oxygenated in the placenta and largely bypasses the lungs (Fig. 11-15). The modifications that establish the postnatal circulatory pattern at birth are not abrupt but extend into infancy (Figs. 11-16 to 11-18). Failure of these changes in the circulatory system to occur at birth results in two of the most common congenital abnormalities of the heart and great vessels: *patent foramen ovale* (Figs. 11-6 and 11-10) and *patent ductus arteriosus* (Fig. 11-19; see also Figs. 14-15 and 14-16).

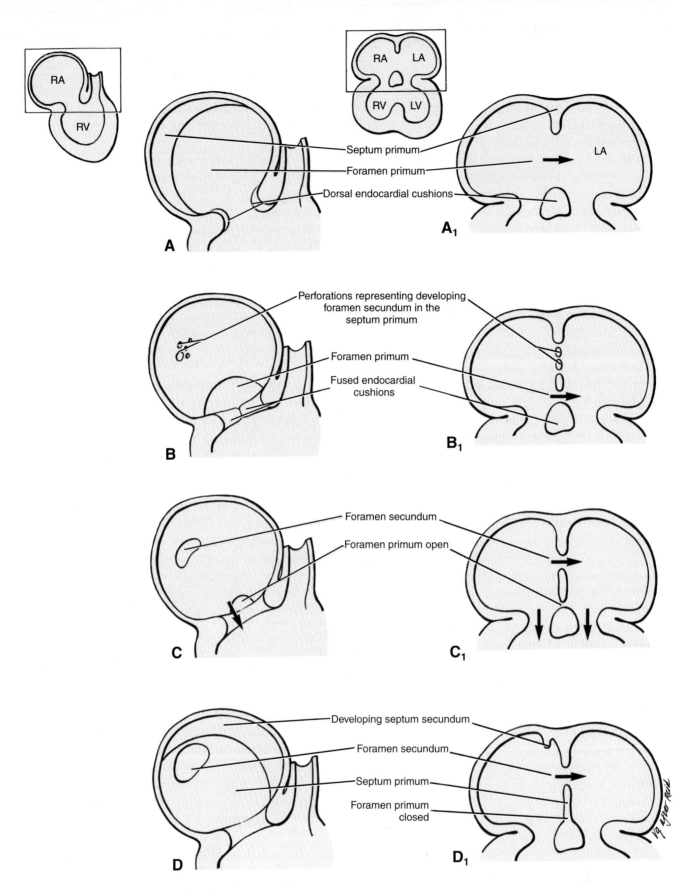

FIG. 11-5

Diagrammatic sketches illustrating partitioning of the primordial atrium. **A₁** to **H₁** are coronal sections of the developing interatrial septum. Note that as the septum secundum grows, it overlaps the opening in the septum primum (foramen secundum). The valvelike nature of the foramen ovale is illustrated in **G₁** and **H₁**. When pressure in the right atrium exceeds that in the left atrium, blood passes from the right to the left side of the heart (**H₁**). When the pressures are equal or higher in the left atrium, the septum primum closes the foramen ovale (**G₁**).

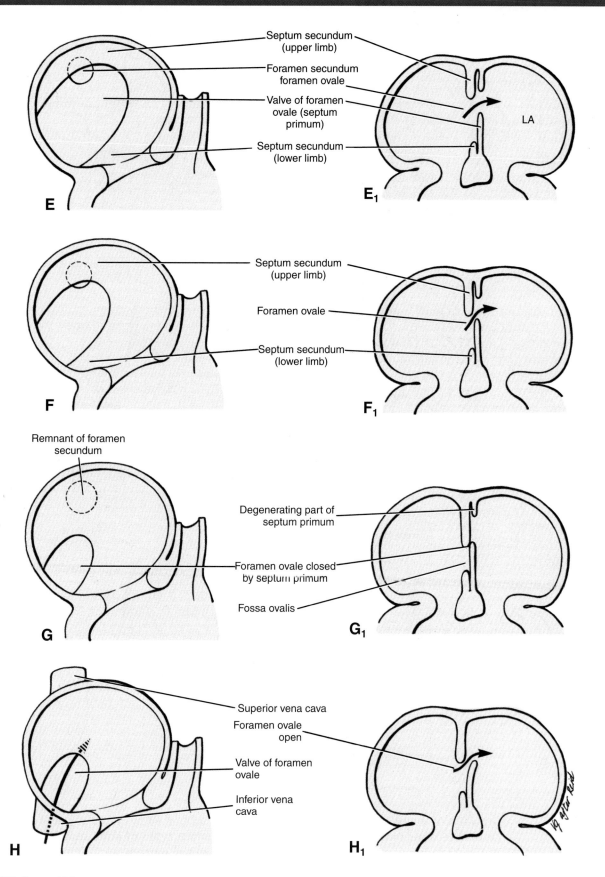

Septum secundum (upper limb)

Foramen secundum foramen ovale

Valve of foramen ovale (septum primum)

Septum secundum (lower limb)

LA

E   **E₁**

Septum secundum (upper limb)

Foramen ovale

Septum secundum (lower limb)

F   **F₁**

Remnant of foramen secundum

Degenerating part of septum primum

Foramen ovale closed by septum primum

Fossa ovalis

G   **G₁**

Superior vena cava

Foramen ovale open

Valve of foramen ovale

Inferior vena cava

H   **H₁**

FIG. 11-5, cont'd

For legend see opposite page.

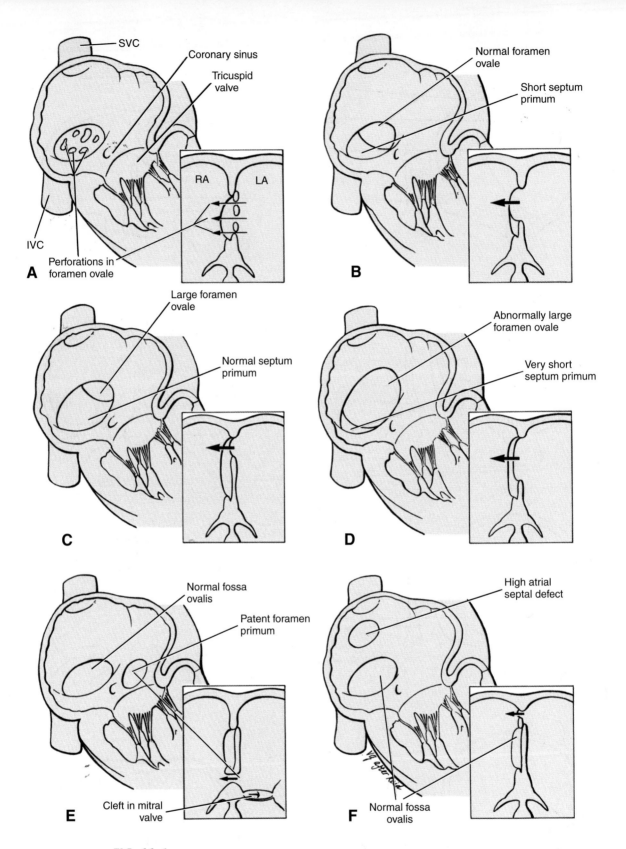

FIG. 11-6

Drawings of the right atrial aspect of the interatrial septum (**A** to **F**) and adjacent sketches of coronal sections through the septum illustrating various types of atrial septal defect (ASD). **A**, Patent foramen ovale resulting from resorption of the septum primum in abnormal locations. **B**, Patent foramen ovale caused by excessive resorption of the septum primum, sometimes called the short flap defect. **C**, Patent foramen ovale resulting from an abnormally large foramen ovale. **D**, Patent foramen ovale resulting from an abnormally large foramen ovale and excessive resorption of the septum primum. **E**, Endocardial cushion defect with primum-type atrial septal defect. **F**, Sinus venosus ASD resulting from abnormal absorption of the sinus venosus into the right atrium. In the sections *E* and *F*, note that the fossa ovalis has formed normally.

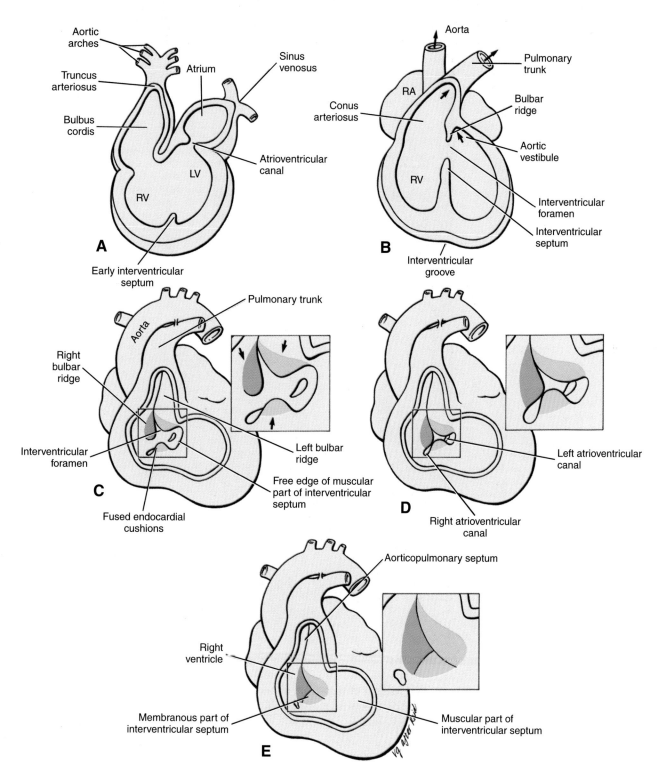

FIG. 11-7

A and **B**, Sketches of the developing heart showing incorporation of the bulbus cordis into the ventricles and partitioning of the bulbus cordis and truncus arteriosus into the aorta and pulmonary trunk. **A**, Sagittal section at 5 weeks, showing the bulbus cordis as one of the five primordial chambers of the heart. **B**, Schematic coronal section at 6 weeks, after the bulbus cordis has been incorporated into the ventricles to form the conus arteriosus (infundibulum) of the right ventricle and the aortic vestibule of the left ventricle. **C** to **E**, Schematic drawings illustrating closure of the interventricular foramen and formation of the membranous part of the interventricular septum. The walls of the truncus arteriosus, bulbus cordis and right ventricle have been removed. **C**, 5 weeks, showing the bulbar ridges and the fused endocardial cushions. **D**, 6 weeks, showing how proliferation of subendocardial tissue diminishes the interventricular foramen. **E**, 7 weeks, showing the fused bulbar ridges and the membranous part of the interventricular septum formed by extensions of tissue from the right side of the endocardial cushions.

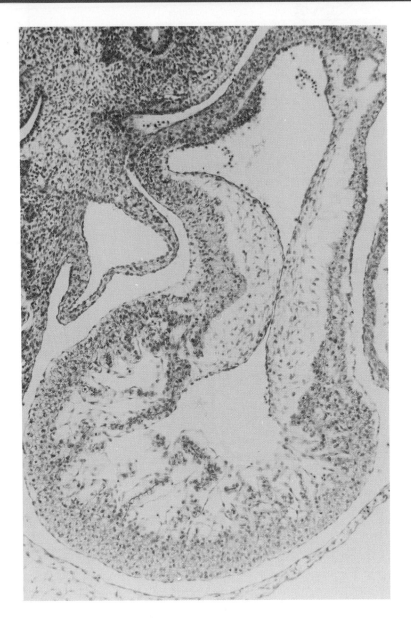

FIG. 11-8

Photomicrograph of a section of the heart of an embryo at Carnegie stage 13. Developing endocardial cushions divide the primitive atrium and ventricle. Myocardial tissue is differentiating in the wall of the ventricle.

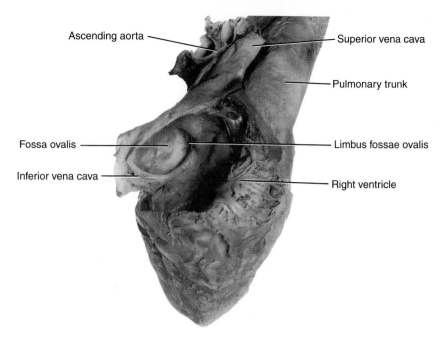

Ascending aorta — Superior vena cava

Pulmonary trunk

Fossa ovalis — Limbus fossae ovalis

Inferior vena cava — Right ventricle

FIG. 11-9

Photograph of a dissection of the adult heart, particularly to show the right atrial aspect of the interatrial septum. Observe the fossa ovalis and the limbus fossa ovalis. The floor of the fossa is formed by the septum primum, whereas the limbus fossa ovalis is formed by the free edge of the septum secundum (see Fig. 11-5, *G* and *G₁*). Aeration of lungs at birth is associated with a dramatic fall in pulmonary vascular resistance and a marked increase in pulmonary flow. As a result of the increased pulmonary blood flow, the pressure in the left atrium is raised above that in the right atrium. This increased left atrial pressure closes the foramen ovale by pressing the valve of the foramen ovale against the septum secundum (see Fig. 11-5, *G₁*). This forms the fossa ovalis, a landmark of the interatrial septum.

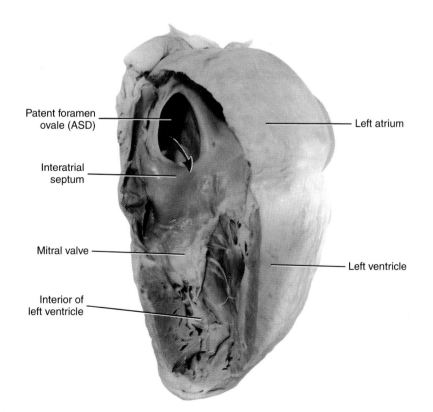

Patent foramen ovale (ASD)

Left atrium

Interatrial septum

Mitral valve

Left ventricle

Interior of left ventricle

FIG. 11-10

Photograph of a dissection of an adult male heart with a large patent foramen ovale. The arrow passes through a large atrial septal defect (ASD), which resulted from an abnormally large foramen ovale and excessive resorption of the septum primum (see Fig. 11-6, *D*). This is referred to as a secundum-type ASD and is one of the most common types of congenital cardiac defect. The right ventricle and atrium are enlarged.

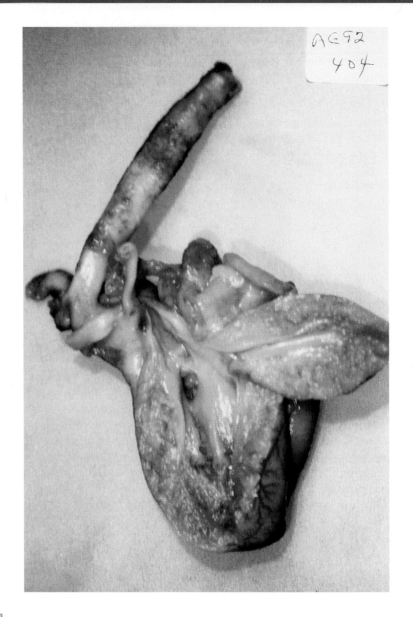

FIG. 11-11

Ventricular septal defect in 15-week female fetus. (Courtesy of Dr. D.K. Kalousek, Department of Pathology, University of British Columbia, Children's Hospital, Vancouver, B.C., Canada.)

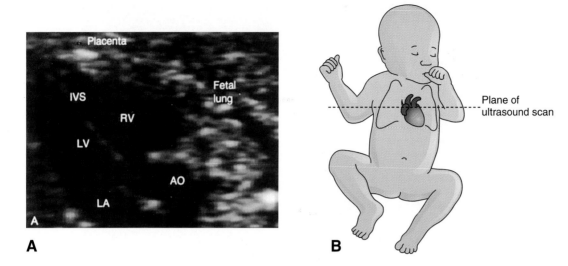

FIG. 11-12

A, Ultrasound image of the heart of a 20-week fetus with tetralogy of Fallot. Note that the large overriding aorta *(AO)* straddles the interventricular septum. As a result it receives blood from the left *(LV)* and right *(RV)* ventricles. *(IVS,* Interventricular septum; *LA,* left atrium.) **B,** Orientation drawing. (Courtesy of Dr. B. Benacerraf, Diagnostic Ultrasound Associates, P.C., Boston, Ma.)

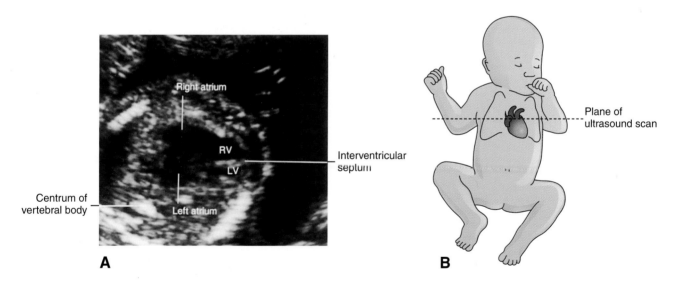

FIG. 11-13

A, Ultrasound image of the heart of a second-trimester fetus with a hypoplastic left heart. Note that the left ventricle *(LV)* is much smaller than the right ventricle *(RV)*. This is an oblique scan of the fetal thorax through the long axis of the ventricles. **B,** Orientation drawing. (Courtesy of Dr. B. Benacerraf, Diagnostic Ultrasound Associates, P.C., Boston, Ma.)

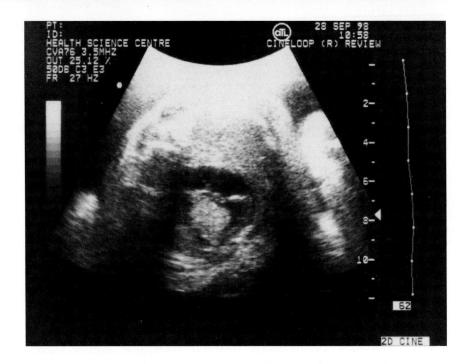

FIG. 11-14

Sonogram at 38 weeks of gestation showing cardiac rhabdomyomas (neoplasm of striated muscle fibers) in the interventricular septum and in the left ventricular free wall, associated with tuberous sclerosis. (Courtesy of Dr. G.J. Reid, Department of Obstetrics, Gynecology and Reproductive Sciences, University of Manitoba, Women's Centre, Winnipeg, Canada.)

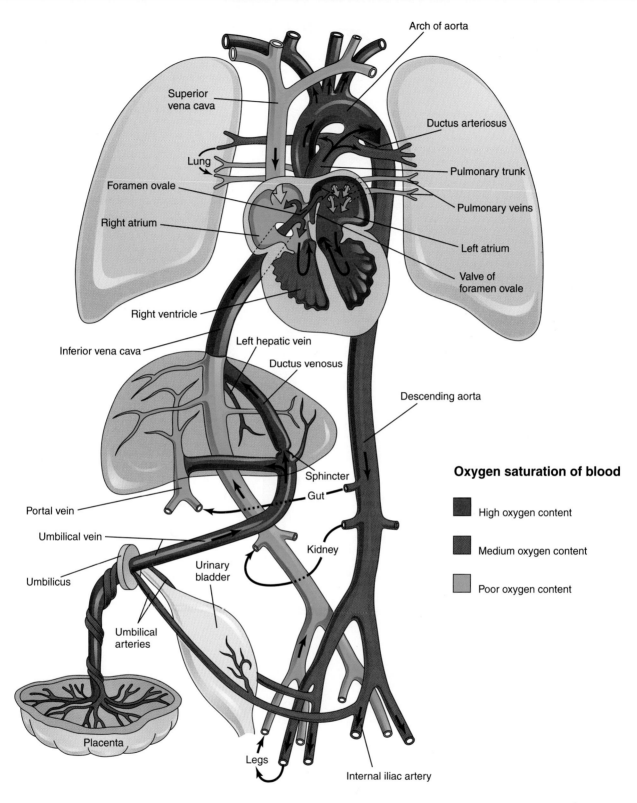

FIG. 11-15

Schematic illustration of the fetal circulation. The colors indicate the oxygen saturation of the blood, and the arrows show the course of the blood from the placenta to the heart. The organs are not drawn to scale. Observe that three shunts permit most of the blood to bypass the liver and lungs: (1) ductus venosus; (2) foramen ovale; and (3) ductus arteriosus. The poorly oxygenated blood returns to the placenta for oxygen and nutrients through the umbilical arteries.

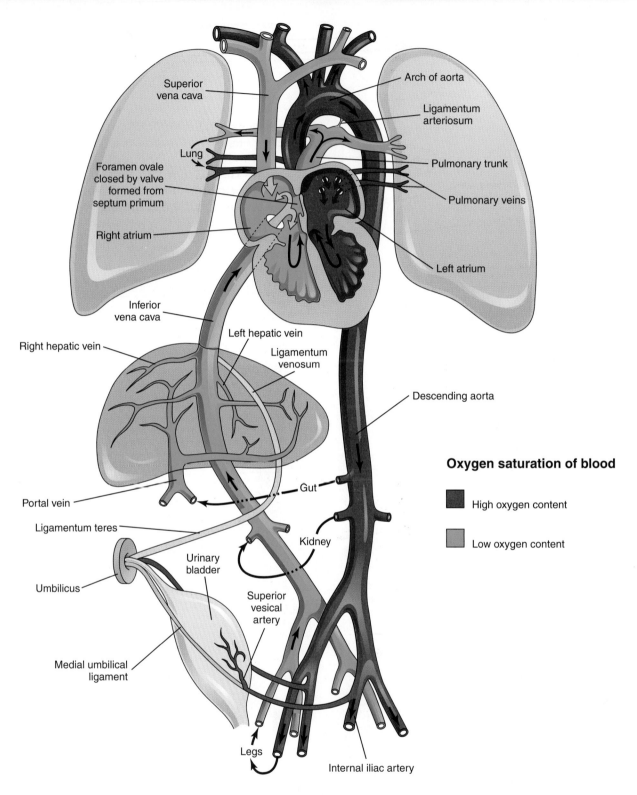

FIG. 11-16

Schematic illustration of the neonatal circulation. The adult derivatives of the fetal vessels and structures that become nonfunctional at birth are also shown. The arrows indicate the course of the blood in the infant. The organs are not drawn to scale. After birth the three shunts that short-circuited the blood during fetal life cease to function, and the pulmonary and systemic circulations become separated.

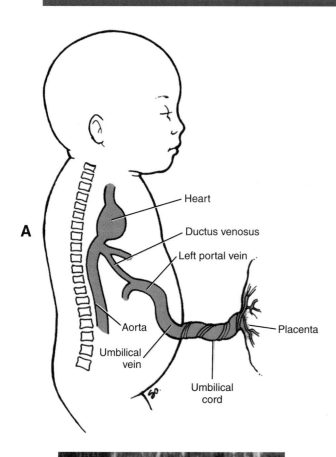

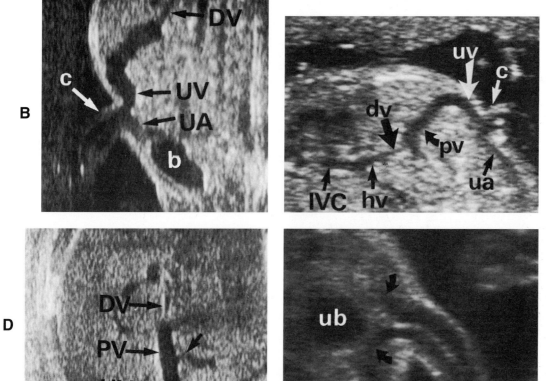

FIG. 11-17

A, Schematic illustration of the course of the umbilical vein from the umbilical cord to the liver (see also Fig. 11-12, *B*). **B,** Fetus with placental chorioangioma. The umbilical vein appears prominent. *c,* umbilical cord; *b,* bladder; *UV,* umbilical vein; *UA,* umbilical artery; *DV,* ductus venosus. **C,** Sagittal view of the fetal abdomen. *c,* Umbilical cord insertion; *ua,* umbilical artery. The umbilical vein *(uv)* courses cranially (cephalad) to the left portal vein *(pv)*. The ductus venosus *(dv)* is a narrow channel that connects the left portal vein to the left hepatic vein *(hv)* or inferior vena cava *(IVC)*. It shunts blood from the umbilical vein to the IVC, thereby bypassing the liver. **D,** This ultrasound scan shows the umbilical vein *(UV)* as it becomes the left portal vein *(PV)*. The branch vessel *(arrow)* distinguishes this vessel *(PV)* from the umbilical vein. *DV,* ductus venosus (see also Fig. 11-12, *B*). **E,** The umbilical cord insertion demonstrates the proximity of the distal umbilical arteries *(arrows)* to the wall of the urinary bladder *(ub)*. The ductus venosus *(DV)* joins the inferior vena cava as shown in *C*. (From Goldstein RB: Ultrasound evaluation of the fetal abdomen. In Callen PW [editor]: *Ultrasonography in obstetrics and gynecology*, ed 3, Philadelphia, 1994, Saunders.)

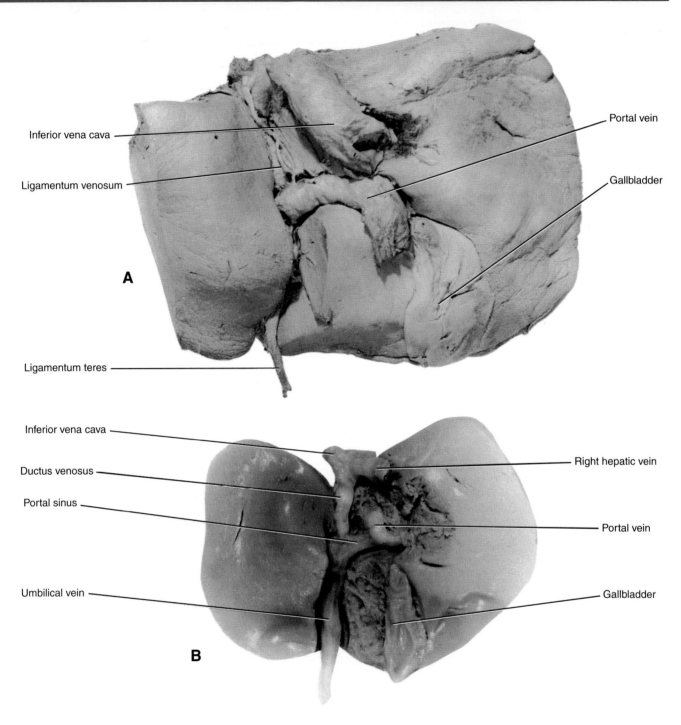

Inferior vena cava

Ligamentum venosum

Portal vein

Gallbladder

A

Ligamentum teres

Inferior vena cava

Ductus venosus

Portal sinus

Right hepatic vein

Portal vein

Umbilical vein

Gallbladder

B

FIG. 11-18

Photographs of dissections of the visceral surface of the liver. A, Adult. B, Fetus. Note that the umbilical vein is represented in the adult by the ligamentum teres and the ductus venosus by the ligamentum venosum (also see Fig. 11-10).

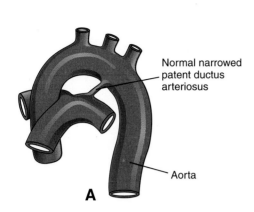
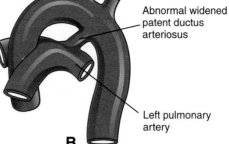

FIG. 11-19

Closure of the ductus arteriosus. **A,** The ductus arteriosus (DA) of a newborn infant. **B,** Abnormal patent DA in a 6-month-old infant. The large ductus is nearly the same size as the left pulmonary artery. **C,** The ligamentum arteriosum in a 6-month-old infant.

12

The Musculoskeletal System

Most parts of the muscular and skeletal systems, including the limbs, are derived from mesoderm (Figs. 12-1 to 12-3). The skeleton mainly develops from condensed mesenchyme (embryonic connective tissue), which undergoes chondrification to form hyaline cartilage models of the bones. Ossification centers appear in these models by the end of the embryonic period (eight weeks) and the bones ossify by *endochondral ossification* (Figs. 12-4 to 12-7). Some bones (e.g., the flat bones of the skull) develop by *intramembranous ossification.*

The **vertebral column and ribs** develop from sclerotomal cells that arise from the somites (Figs. 12-1 and 12-2; see also Fig. 2-7). Initially, the mesenchymal column retains traces of its segmental origin from the somites as the sclerotomal blocks are separated by less dense areas (Fig. 12-2). The **notochord** regresses in the area of the developing vertebral bodies, but it persists and enlarges in the region of the developing intervertebral discs. Here it gives rise to the *nucleus pulposus* of the disc, which is later surrounded by the circular fibers of the *anulus fibrosis.* The combination of these structures forms the *intervertebral disc.* The vertebral (neural) arch is formed from mesenchymal cells surrounding the neural tube. Mesenchymal cells in the body wall form the costal processes, from which the ribs develop in the thoracic region. Ossification of typical vertebrae begins during the embryonic period and usually ends by the twenty-fifth year. The ribs become cartilaginous during the embryonic period and ossify during the fetal period.

The **skull** develops from cells that are derived from paraxial mesoderm and the *neural crest.* The skull consists of a neurocranium and a viscerocranium, each of which has membranous and cartilaginous components. The *neurocranium* is divided into two parts: (1) a membranous part consisting of flat bones which surround the brain and form the calvaria (cranial vault), and (2) a cartilaginous part (chondrocranium), which forms the bones of the base of the skull (Fig. 12-8). The *viscerocranium* consists of the bones of the face and is formed mainly by the cartilages of the first two pairs of pharyngeal (branchial) arches (Fig. 12-3; see also Figs. 7-2 and 7-4).

The **limb buds** appear toward the end of the fourth week as slight elevations of the ventrolateral body wall (Fig. 12-9). The *apical ectodermal ridge* (AER), a thickening of ectoderm at the distal end of the limb bud, exerts an inductive influence on the mesenchyme in the limb buds that promotes growth and development of the limbs. The upper limb buds develop two days before the lower limb buds. The tis-

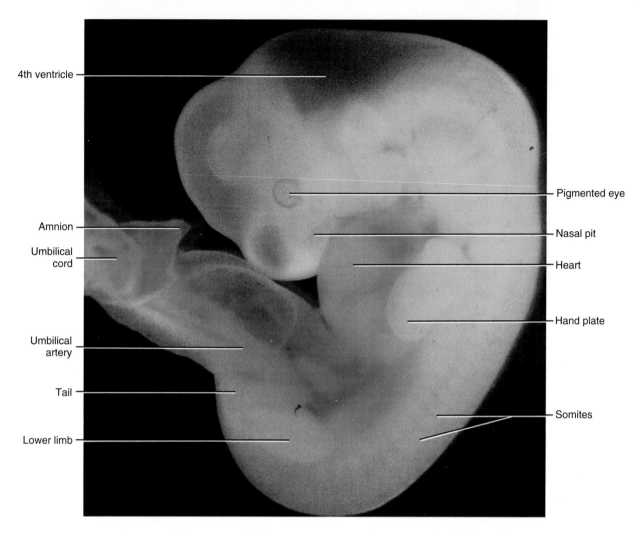

4th ventricle

Pigmented eye

Amnion

Nasal pit

Umbilical cord

Heart

Umbilical artery

Hand plate

Tail

Lower limb

Somites

FIG. 12-1

Photograph of a lateral view of an embryo at Carnegie stage 15, about 36 days (see also Fig. 2-17). Mesenchymal models of the limb bones (not visible) have begun to form in a proximodistal sequence (i.e., the humerus appears before the forearm bones).

sues of the limb buds are derived from three sources, the somatic layer of lateral mesoderm, the somitic mesoderm (Figs. 12-3, A_1, and 12-4), and the ectoderm. The nerves grow into the limb buds during the fifth week (Fig. 12-3, *B*). The upper and lower limbs rotate in opposite directions and to different degrees.

Most **skeletal muscle** is derived from the myotome regions of the somites (Fig. 12-3), but some head and neck muscles are derived from pharyngeal arch (branchial) mesenchyme, which is of neural crest origin (Chapter 7). The limb muscles develop from myogenic precursor cells, which are derived from somites. The earliest indication of myogenesis is the elongation of the nuclei and the cell bodies of mesenchymal cells as they differentiate into myoblasts. These primordial muscle cells fuse to form elongated, multinucleated, cylindrical myotubules. Muscle growth during development results from the fusing of myoblasts and myotubules. Cardiac muscle and most smooth muscle are mainly derived from splanchnic mesoderm. Cardiac myoblasts are derived from the primordial myocardium, and by the fourth week heart muscle is recognizable. Whereas cardiac muscle fibers arise by differentiation and growth of single cells, striated skeletal muscle fibers develop by fusion of cells. The splanchnic mesenchyme

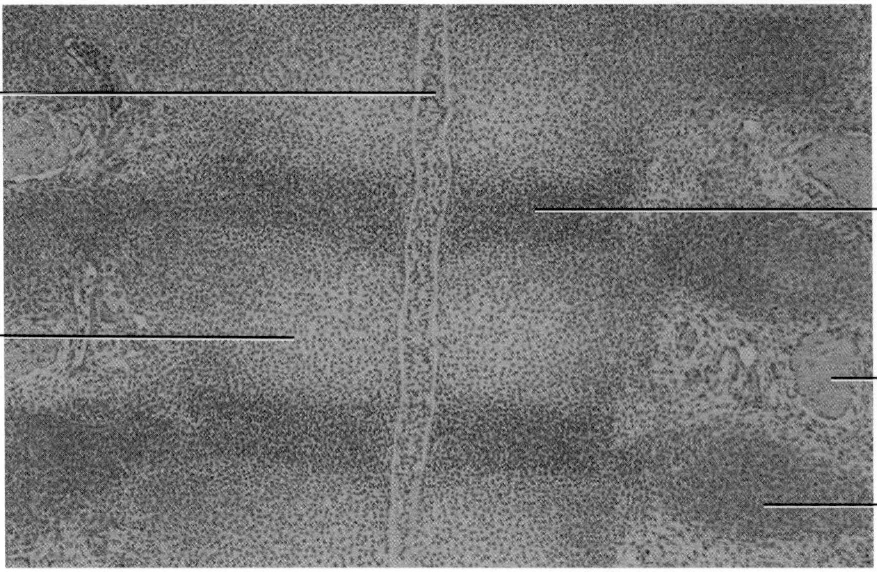

FIG. 12-2

Coronal section of the axial region of an embryo at Carnegie stage 18, about 44 days. Observe the cartilaginous primordia of the vertebral bodies and ribs. Also observe the notochord in the center of the developing vertebrae. It will disappear except for the portion that forms the nucleus pulposus of the intervertebral disc. (From Nishimura H [editor]: *Atlas of human prenatal histology,* Tokyo, 1983, Igaku-Shoin.)

surrounding the primitive gut and its derivatives gives rise to its smooth muscle fibers (Fig. 12-3, *A*). Absence or variation of some muscles is common and is usually of little consequence.

Anomalies of the musculoskeletal system, including those of the limbs, are usually caused by genetic factors; however, many congenital anomalies result from an interaction of genetic and environmental factors (multifactorial inheritance). *Limb defects vary greatly* (Figs. 12-10 to 12-14). The most critical period of limb development is from 24 to 36 days after fertilization. In the most extreme form, one or more of the limbs are absent *(amelia).* More commonly, part of a limb is absent (e.g., a hand) producing a defect that is known as *meromelia* (Fig. 12-10, *A*). If there are extra digits (fingers or toes), the condition is called *polydactyly* (Fig. 12-11). The extra digit is often nonfunctional because of inadequate muscular connections. Polydactyly may be inherited as a dominant trait. Abnormal fusion of the digits is called *syndactyly.* Normally, the mesenchyme between the developing digit breaks down as they develop by means of programmed cell death (apoptosis) (see Figs. 2-22 to 2-25). Failure of the process to occur results in fusion of one or more fingers or toes. Failure of bones to develop also occurs (Fig. 12-10, *B* and *C*). Syndactyly occurs in about 1 of 2200 births (Fig. 12-12). Lack of fetal movement (e.g., caused by neuromuscular abnormalities) may result in abnormal development of joints (arthrogryposis or joint contractures) (Fig. 12-10, *D*). An abnormal cleft in the hands (Fig. 12-13) or feet results from aplasia of the central digits.

Clubfoot is a common anomaly, occurring about once in 1000 births. It is characterized by an abnormal position of the foot that prevents normal weight bearing (Fig. 12-14). In the most common type, *talipes equinovarus,* the sole of the foot is turned medially and inverted. This defect is often a solitary anomaly, but not infrequently it is associated with congenital dislocation of the hip, myelomeningocele (see Fig. 13-15), arthrogryposis (Fig. 12-10, *D*), or other defects. There is much uncertainty about the cause of clubfoot. Hered-

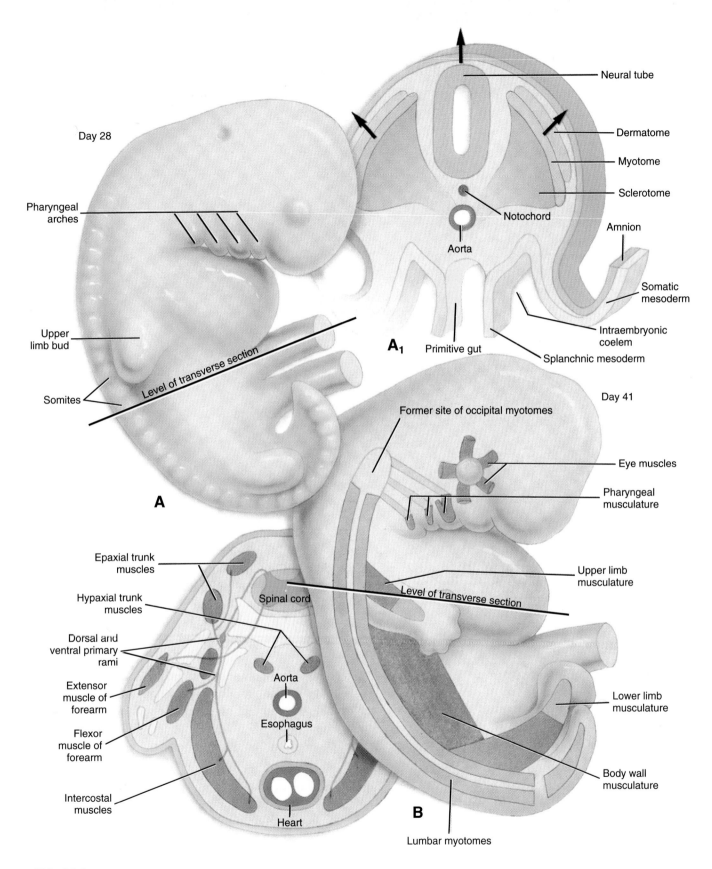

FIG. 12-3

Drawings of embryos illustrating differentiation of the somites and formation of muscles. **A,** Embryo at 28 days. The arrows in **A₁** indicate the directions of the somite remnants and the neural tube in relation to the notochord. **B,** Embryo at 41 days showing the muscle layers formed from the myotome regions of the somites. The limb muscles develop from myogenic precursor cells, derived from somites.

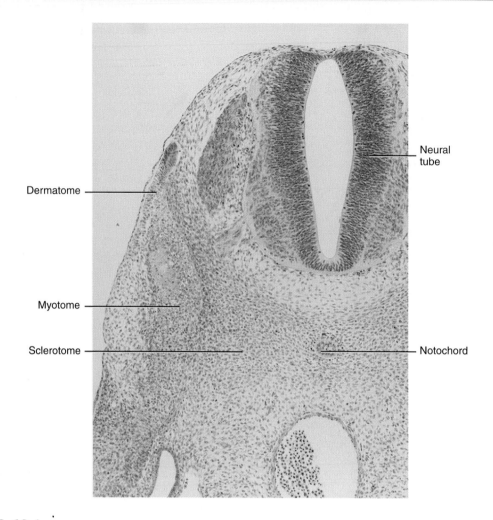

FIG. 12-4

Photomicrograph of a section of an embryo at Carnegie stage 15. The somite differentiates into dermatome, myotome, and sclerotome. Sclerotomal cells are migrating toward the notochord to form the primordial spine.

itary factors are involved in some cases, and it appears that environmental factors are involved in most cases. Clubfoot appears to follow a multifactorial pattern of inheritance. Clubfoot may be due to in utero postural-induced compression (positional deformation), especially if the fetus is genetically predispositioned to this deformity. Clubfoot is bilateral in 50% of cases; the male to female ratio is about 21.

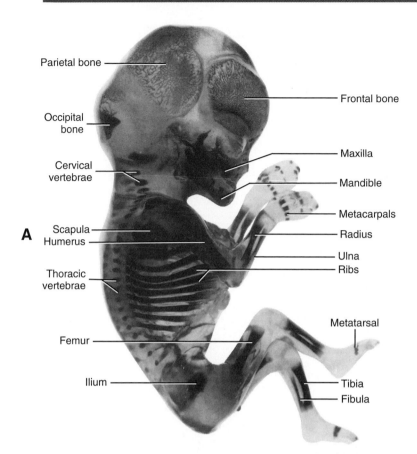

A

Parietal bone

Occipital bone

Cervical vertebrae

Scapula

Humerus

Thoracic vertebrae

Femur

Ilium

Frontal bone

Maxilla

Mandible

Metacarpals

Radius

Ulna

Ribs

Metatarsal

Tibia

Fibula

FIG. 12-5

Alizarin-stained and cleared human fetuses. **A**, 12-week fetus. Observe the degree of progression of ossification from the primary centers of ossification, which is endochondral in the appendicular and axial parts of the skeleton except for most of the cranial bones (i.e., those that form the calvaria or cranial vault). Observe that the carpus and tarsus are wholly cartilaginous at this stage, as are the epiphyses of all long bones. **B** and **C**, 16-week fetus. The degree of ossification of the cranial and limb bones has progressed further. Note the severe unilateral facial cleft. During processing, the fetus was eviscerated and the brain removed, using a thin-gauge needle placed in the posterior fontanelle. The calvarium appears collapsed. (**A**, Courtesy of Dr. Gary Geddes, Lake Oswego, Ore. **B** and **C**, Courtesy of Dr. R.L. Jordan, Department of Anatomical Sciences, St. George's University School of Medicine, Grenada, West Indies.)

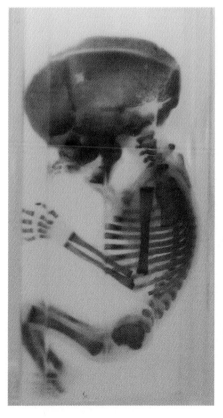

B

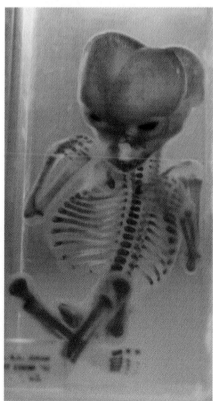

C

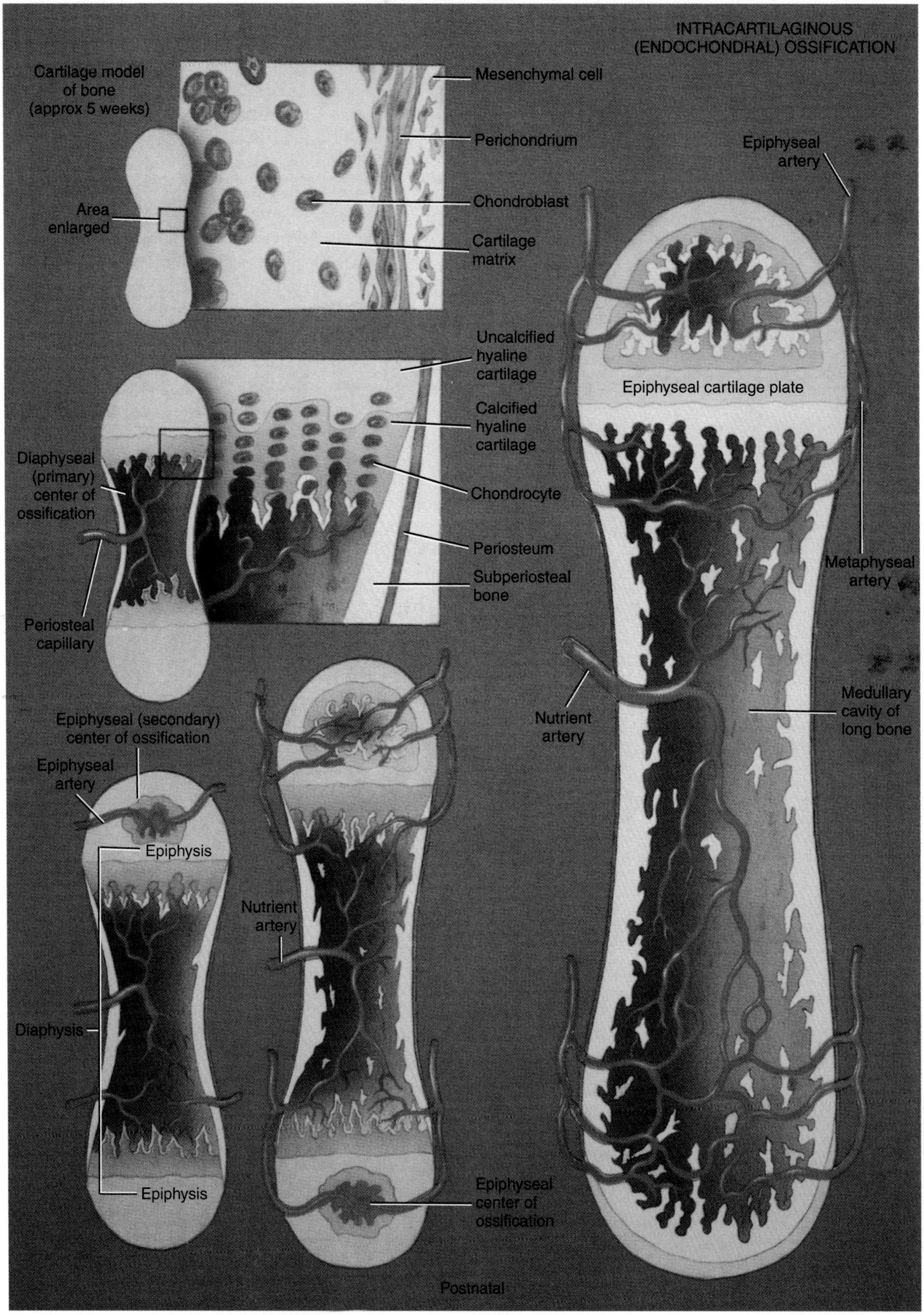

FIG. 12-6

Schematic diagrams illustrating intracartilaginous or endochondral ossification and the development of a typical long bone.

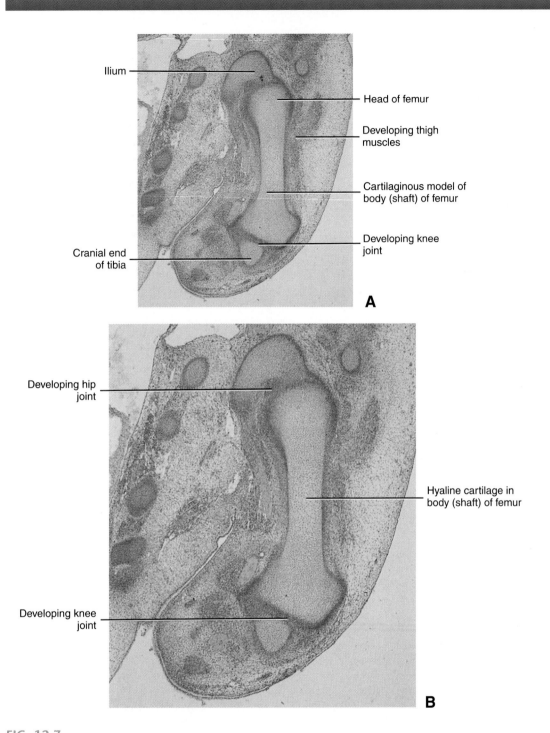

FIG. 12-7

A, Longitudinal section of the lower limb of an embryo at Carnegie stage 19, about 48 days (×75). (See Fig. 2-22 for the appearance and size of an embryo at this stage.) Chondrification has begun in the bone and occurs in a proximodistal sequence. **B,** Higher magnification of this femur (×110).

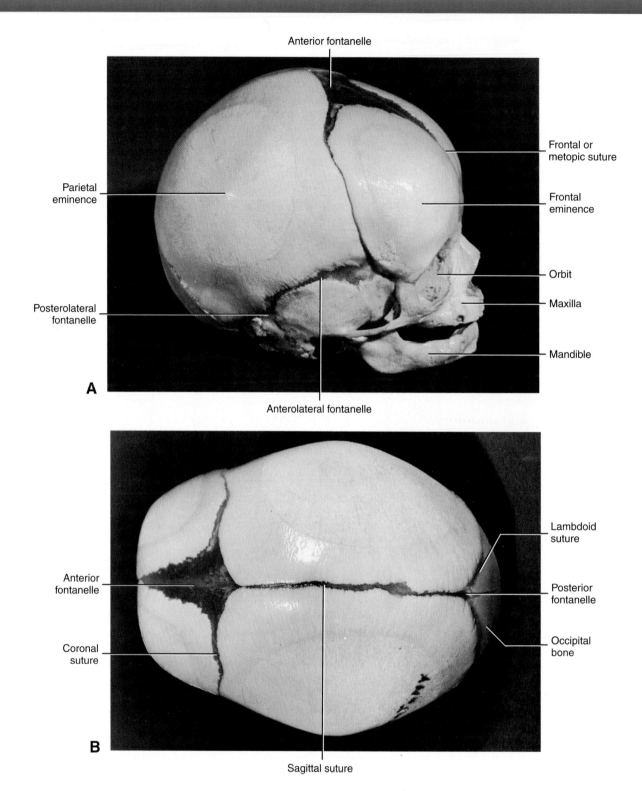

Anterior fontanelle

Frontal or metopic suture

Frontal eminence

Orbit

Maxilla

Mandible

Parietal eminence

Posterolateral fontanelle

A

Anterolateral fontanelle

Anterior fontanelle

Coronal suture

Lambdoid suture

Posterior fontanelle

Occipital bone

B

Sagittal suture

FIG. 12-8

Photographs of a fetal skull showing the bones, fontanelles, and connecting sutures. A, Lateral view. B, Superior view. The posterior and anterolateral fontanelles disappear by growth of surrounding bones within 2 or 3 months after birth, but they remain as sutures for several years. The posterolateral fontanelles disappear in a similar manner by the end of the first year, and the anterior fontanelle by the end of the second year. The two halves of the frontal bone normally begin to fuse during the second year, and the frontal or metopic suture is often obliterated by the eighth year. The other sutures begin to disappear during adult life, but the times when the sutures close are subject to wide variation.

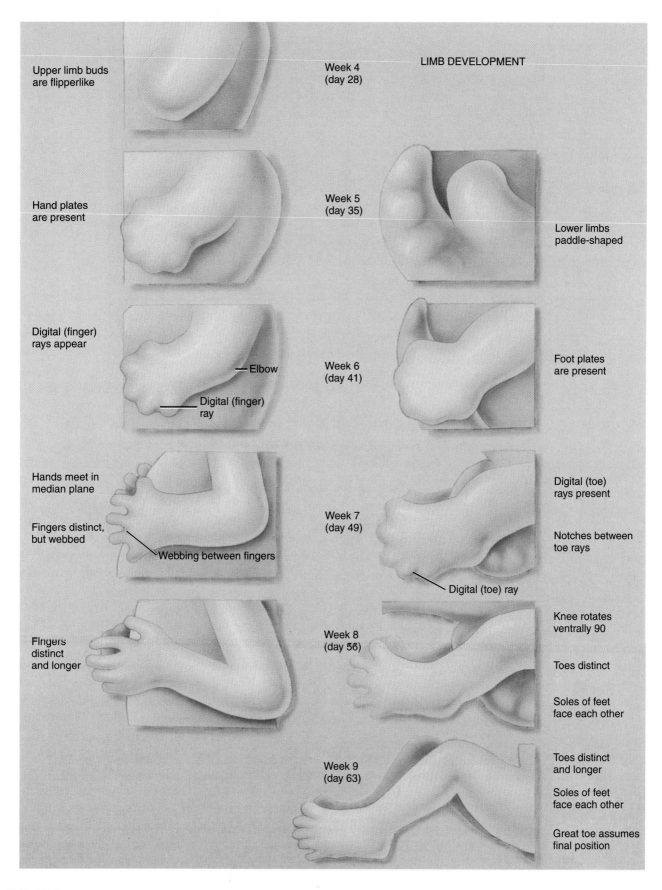

Upper limb buds are flipperlike

Week 4 (day 28)

Hand plates are present

Week 5 (day 35)

Lower limbs paddle-shaped

Digital (finger) rays appear

Elbow

Digital (finger) ray

Week 6 (day 41)

Foot plates are present

Hands meet in median plane

Fingers distinct, but webbed

Webbing between fingers

Week 7 (day 49)

Digital (toe) rays present

Notches between toe rays

Digital (toe) ray

Fingers distinct and longer

Week 8 (day 56)

Knee rotates ventrally 90

Toes distinct

Soles of feet face each other

Week 9 (day 63)

Toes distinct and longer

Soles of feet face each other

Great toe assumes final position

FIG. 12-9

Drawings illustrating development of the limbs. The upper limb buds are visible by day 26 or 27; the lower limb buds appear two days later (see also Figs. 2-13 to 2-27). The stages of limb development are alike for the upper and lower limbs, except that development of the upper limbs precedes that of the lower limbs. Programmed cell death (apoptosis) occurs in the interdigital tissue when digits are separated.

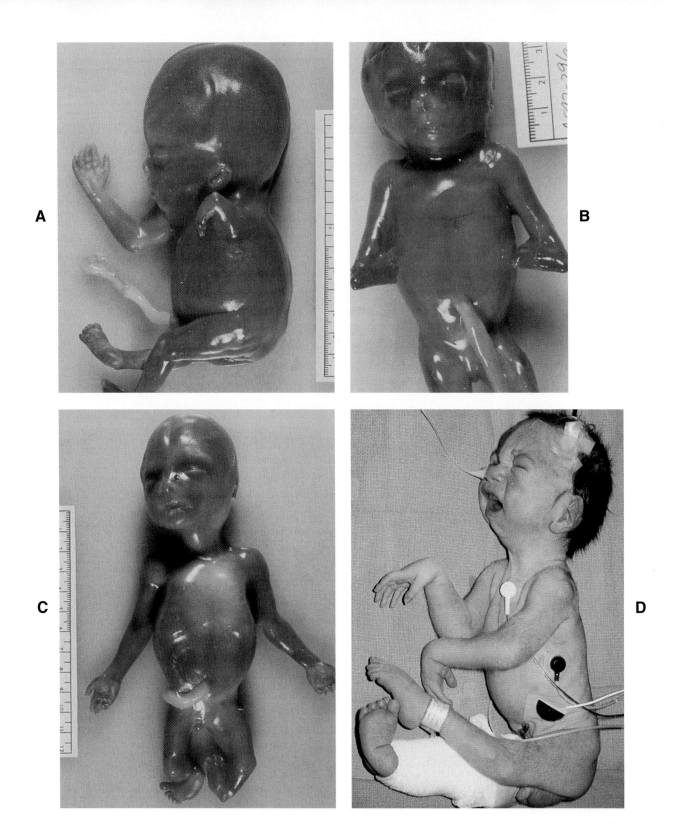

FIG. 12-10

A, Female fetus (16 weeks) with a large head and meromelia (phocomelia) of the left upper limb. In the complete form, the hand arises directly from the trunk (i.e., the arm and forearm are absent). **B,** Absent radii in a 13.5-week female fetus. This anomaly may be associated with thrombocytopenia. **C,** Male fetus (16 weeks) with tibial aplasia on the right and hypoplasia on the left. **D,** Neonate with multiple joint contractures. Observe the elbows, knees, hips, and ankles (arthrogryposis). The common cause of this severe condition is decreased fetal activity resulting from neuromuscular deficiency. Also observe the micrognathia, that is, small jaw. (**A, B,** and **C,** Courtesy of Dr. D.K. Kalousek, Department of Pathology, University of British Columbia, Children's Hospital, Vancouver, B.C., Canada. **D,** Courtesy of Dr. A.E. Chudley, Department of Pediatrics and Child Health, University of Manitoba, Children's Hospital, Winnipeg, Manitoba, Canada.)

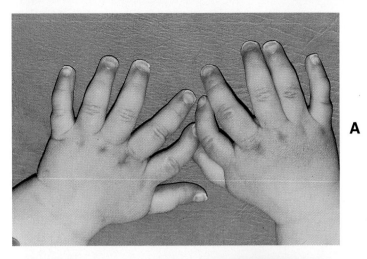

A

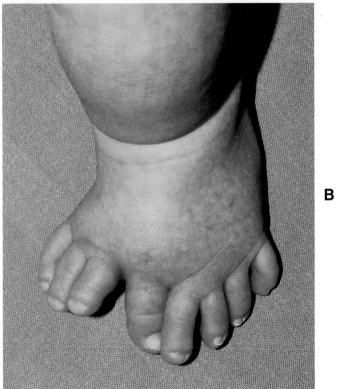

B

FIG. 12-11

Polydactyly of the hands (A), and of the foot (B). This condition results from the formation of one or more extra digital rays during the embryonic period. (Courtesy of Dr. A.E. Chudley, Department of Pediatrics and Child Health, University of Manitoba, Children's Hospital, Winnipeg, Manitoba, Canada.)

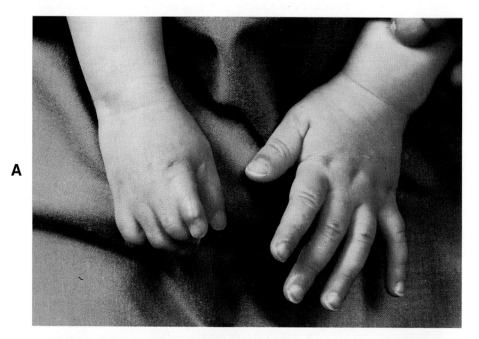

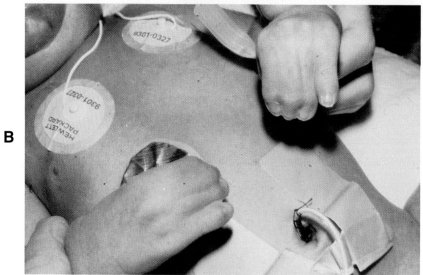

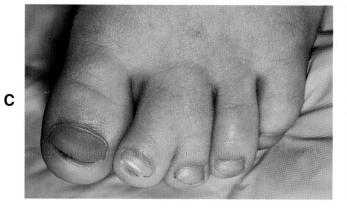

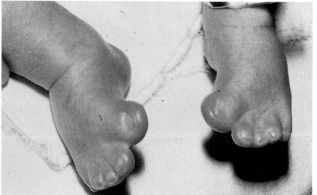

FIG. 12-12

Various forms of syndactyly involving the fingers (**A** and **B**), and toes (**C** and **D**). Cutaneous syndactyly (**A**) is the most common form of this condition and is probably due to incomplete programmed cell death (apoptosis) in the tissues between the digital rays during embryonic life. In osseous syndactyly (**D**), the digital rays merge on account of excessive cell death resulting in fusion of the bones. (Courtesy of Dr. A.E. Chudley, Department of Pediatrics and Child Health, University of Manitoba, Children's Hospital, Winnipeg, Manitoba, Canada.)

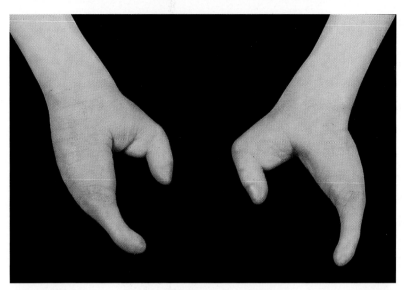

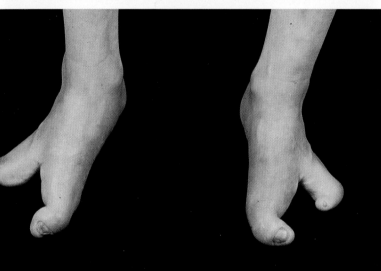

FIG. 12-13

Malformations of the hands and feet. **A,** Ectrodactyly in a child. Note the absence of the central digits of the hands resulting in split hands (lobster claw anomaly). **B,** A similar type of defect involving the feet. These limb defects can be inherited in an autosomal dominant pattern. (Courtesy of Dr. A.E. Chudley, Department of Pediatrics and Child Health, University of Manitoba, Children's Hospital, Winnipeg, Manitoba, Canada.)

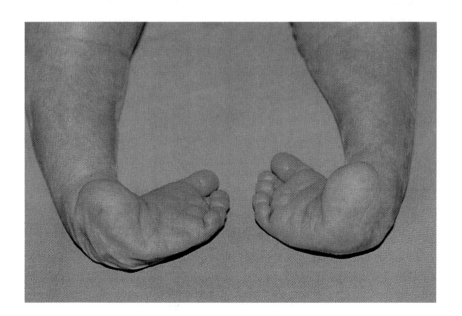

FIG. 12-14

Neonate with bilateral talipes equinovarus deformities (clubfeet). This is the classic type with sharp and tight hyperextension and incurving of the feet. (Courtesy of Dr. A.E. Chudley, Department of Pediatrics and Child Health, University of Manitoba, Children's Hospital, Winnipeg, Manitoba, Canada.)

13

The Nervous System

The central nervous system (CNS) develops from the *neural plate,* a dorsal thickening of ectoderm (Fig. 13-1, *A* and *B*). This slipper-shaped plate appears around the middle of the third week and soon infolds to form a *neural groove* that has neural folds on each side (Figs. 13-1, *C* and *D,* and 13-2). When the *neural folds* fuse to form the *neural tube* during the middle of the fourth week (Figs. 13-1, *C* to *F,* and 13-3), some neuroectodermal cells are not included in it but remain between the **neural tube** and the surface ectoderm as the *neural crest* (Figs. 13-1, *E,* and 13-3).

*Most of the **neural tube** becomes the spinal cord* (Figs. 13-4 and 13-5). The cranial end of the neural tube forms the brain, consisting of the forebrain, midbrain, and hindbrain (Figs. 13-6 to 13-8). The forebrain gives rise to the cerebral hemispheres (telencephalon) and diencephalon. The midbrain becomes the adult midbrain, and the hindbrain gives rise to the pons, cerebellum, and medulla oblongata. The remainder of the neural tube becomes the spinal cord. The lumen of the neural tube becomes the ventricles of the brain and the central canal of the spinal cord. The walls of the neural tube thicken as a result of proliferation of its neuroepithelial cells. These cells give rise to all nerve and macroglial cells in the central nervous system. The microglial cells differentiate from mononuclear leukocytes that penetrate the blood brain barrier and enter the central nervous system. Nerve cells in the cranial, spinal, and autonomic ganglia are derived from the **neural crest** (Figs. 13-1, *E,* and 13-3). Schwann cells, which myelinate the axons external to the spinal cord, also arise from the neural crest. Similarly, most of the autonomic nervous system and all chromaffin tissue, including the suprarenal medulla, develop from neural crest cells.

Hydrocephalus (Fig. 13-9), a progressive increase in ventricular volume, is due to either a relative or complete obstruction of flow of cerebrospinal fluid (CSF) or, much less commonly, to overproduction of CSF. There are three types of congenital anomaly of the nervous system: (1) structural abnormalities resulting from abnormal organogenesis (e.g., **neural tube defects** [NTDs] resulting from failure of the neural tube to close [Figs. 13-10 to 13-19]); (2) disturbances in the organization of the cells of the nervous system that may result in mental retardation; and (3) *errors of metabolism,* which are often inherited and can lead to severe mental retardation resulting from an accumulation of toxic substances (e.g., phenylketonuria) or from a deficiency of essential substances (e.g., congenital hypothyroidism).

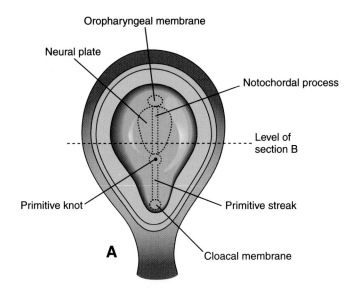

A

Oropharyngeal membrane

Neural plate

Notochordal process

Level of section B

Primitive knot

Primitive streak

Cloacal membrane

FIG. 13-1

Diagrams illustrating the neural plate and folding of it into the neural tube. **A,** Dorsal view of an embryo of about 18 days, exposed by removing the amnion. **B,** Transverse section of the embryo showing the neural plate and early development of the neural groove. The developing notochord is also shown. **C,** Dorsal view of an embryo of about 22 days. The neural folds have fused opposite the fourth to sixth somites but are widely spread apart at both ends. **D to F,** Transverse sections of this embryo at the levels shown in C illustrating formation of the neural tube and its detachment from the surface ectoderm. Note that some neuroectodermal cells are not included in the neural tube but remain between it and the surface ectoderm as the neural crest.

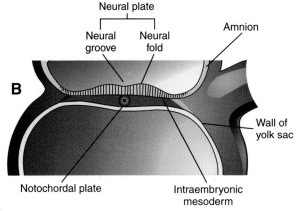

B

Neural plate

Neural groove

Neural fold

Amnion

Wall of yolk sac

Notochordal plate

Intraembryonic mesoderm

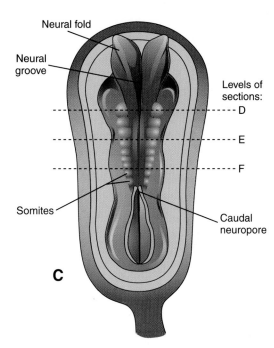

C

Neural fold

Neural groove

Levels of sections:
D
E
F

Somites

Caudal neuropore

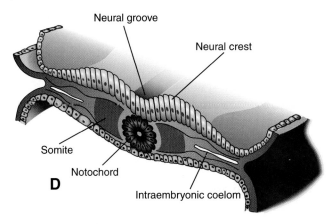

D

Neural groove

Neural crest

Somite

Notochord

Intraembryonic coelom

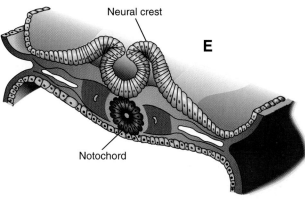

E

Neural crest

Notochord

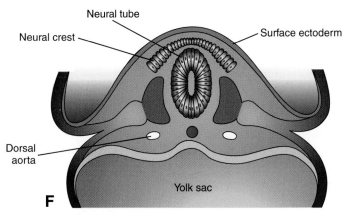

F

Neural tube

Neural crest

Surface ectoderm

Dorsal aorta

Yolk sac

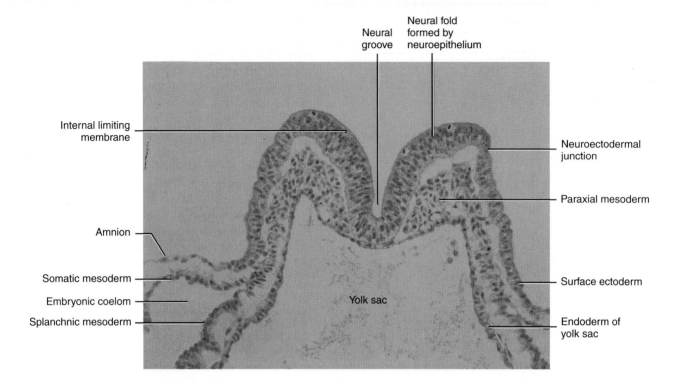

FIG. 13-2

Transverse section of an embryo (×150) at Carnegie stage 10, about 21 days (see Fig. 2-8 for the appearance and size of an embryo at this stage). Observe the dividing cells in the neuroepithelium adjacent to the internal limiting membrane.

Congenital anomalies of the central nervous system are common (about 3 per 1000 births). Defects in the closure of the neural tube (NTDs) account for most anomalies (e.g., **meningomyelocele** [Figs. 13-15 to 13-18]). The anomalies may be limited to the nervous system or they may include the overlying tissues (bone, muscle, and connective tissue). Gross congenital anomalies (e.g., meroanencephaly [Figs. 13-13 and 13-14]) are incompatible with life. Other severe defects (e.g., spina bifida with meningomyelocele) often cause functional disability, (e.g., muscle paralysis of the lower limbs). Central nervous system anomalies can be diagnosed by ultrasound examination of the fetal head and vertebral column.

Mental retardation may result from chromosomal abnormalities arising during gametogenesis, from metabolic disorders, from in utero exposure to drugs and alcohol, or from infections occurring during prenatal life (see Chapter 5). Various postnatal conditions (e.g., cerebral infection or trauma) may also cause abnormal mental development.

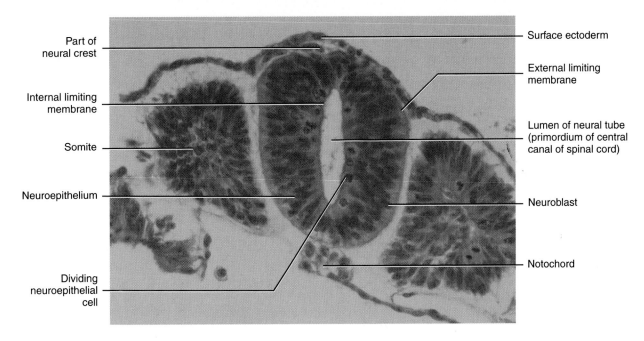

FIG. 13-3

Transverse section of an embryo (×300) at Carnegie stage 11, about 24 days (see Fig. 2-10 for the appearance and size of an embryo at this stage). Observe the neural tube, the primordium of the spinal cord in this region. At this stage, the neural tube is open at its cranial and caudal ends (Fig. 13-1, C). Observe the dividing cells in the neuroepithelium adjacent to the internal limiting membrane. Mitotic cells are also visible in the somite on the left side. Neuroblasts (developing nerve cells) are visible near the external limiting membrane because of their large nuclei.

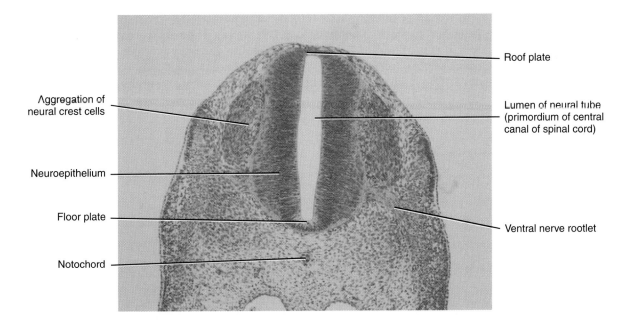

FIG. 13-4

Transverse section of an embryo (×200) at Carnegie stage 13, about 28 days (see Fig. 2-12 for the appearance of an embryo at this stage). The central nervous system is a closed tube at this stage. Observe that the neuroepithelium is pseudostratified (caused by the developing nerve cells at this stage). Aggregations of neural crest cells are located at the sides of the neural tube where they will differentiate into the ganglion cells of the spinal (dorsal root) ganglia.

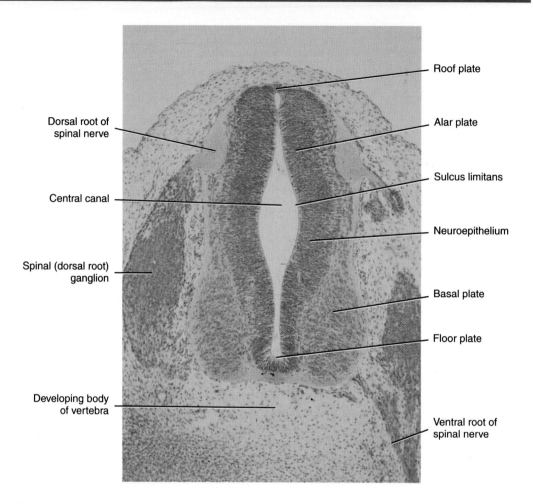

Roof plate

Dorsal root of
spinal nerve

Alar plate

Sulcus limitans

Central canal

Neuroepithelium

Spinal (dorsal root)
ganglion

Basal plate

Floor plate

Developing body
of vertebra

Ventral root of
spinal nerve

FIG. 13-5

Transverse section of an embryo (×100) at Carnegie stage 16, about 40 days (see Fig. 2-18 for the appearance and size of an embryo at this stage). The ventral root of the spinal nerve is composed of nerve fibers arising from neuroblasts (developing nerve cells) in the basal plate (developing ventral horn of the spinal cord), whereas the dorsal root is formed by nerve processes arising from neuroblasts in the spinal (dorsal root) ganglion.

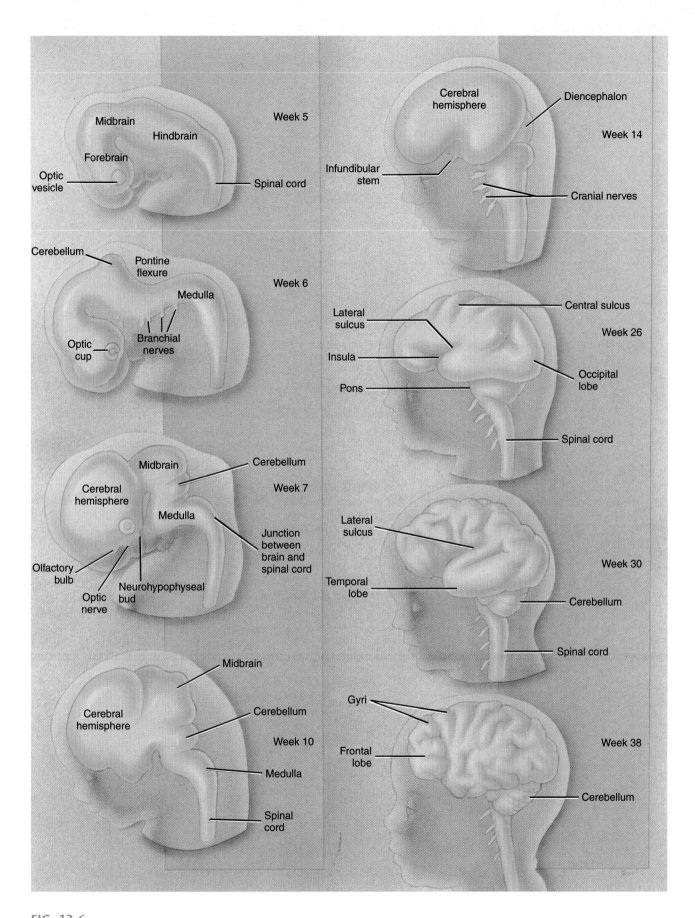

FIG. 13-6

Series of drawings showing the developing brain and spinal cord at the ages indicated. They also demonstrate the changes in size and development of the sulci and gyri of the cerebral hemispheres.

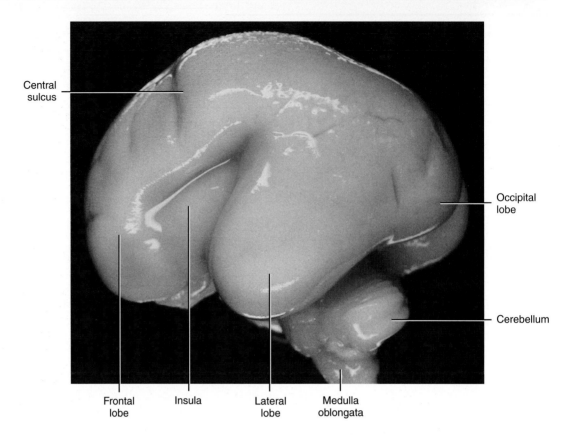

Central
sulcus

Occipital
lobe

Cerebellum

Frontal
lobe

Insula

Lateral
lobe

Medulla
oblongata

FIG. 13-7

Photomicrograph of a lateral view of the brain of a stillborn fetus (20 weeks, CRL 170 mm). (From Nishimura H, Semba R, Tanimura T, Tanaka O: *Prenatal development of the human with special reference to craniofacial structures: an atlas,* **US Department of Health, Education, and Welfare, Bethesda, 1977, National Institutes of Health.)**

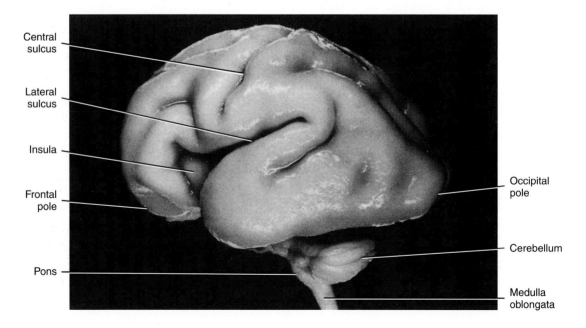

Central
sulcus

Lateral
sulcus

Insula

Frontal
pole

Pons

Occipital
pole

Cerebellum

Medulla
oblongata

FIG. 13-8

Photograph of a lateral view of the brain of a stillborn fetus (25 weeks). See Fig. 3-8 for the appearance of a fetus at this stage. (From Nishimura H, Semba R, Tanimura T, Tanaka O: *Prenatal development of the human with special reference to craniofacial structures: an atlas,* **US Department of Health, Education, and Welfare, Bethesda, 1977, National Institutes of Health.)**

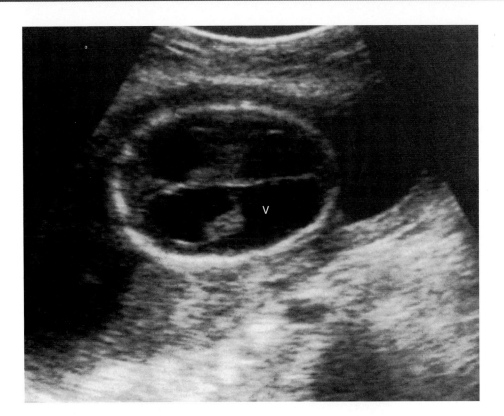

FIG. 13-9

Transverse axial sonogram of a 17-week gestation (15-week fetus) demonstrating hydro-cephalus. Observe the enlarged ventricles *(V)* of the brain. This condition is usually due to a relative or complete obstruction of flow of cerebrospinal fluid (CSF), for example, in the cerebral aqueduct. (Courtesy of Dr. Lyndon M. Hill, Director of Ultrasound, Magee-Womens Hospital, Pittsburgh, Pa.)

FIG. 13-10

A, Photograph of an embryo at Carnegie stage 16, about 38 days, with a defect in the lumbosacral area (see Fig. 2-18 for the appearance of a normal embryo at this stage). The abnormal embryo shown above had the following chromosome constitution: 70,XXY,+18. **B,** Photograph of an abnormal female embryo at Carnegie stage 19, about 45 days (see Fig. 2-22 for the appearance and size of a normal embryo at this stage). This embryo has an occipital encephalocele. (Courtesy of Dr. D.K. Kalousek, Department of Pathology, University of British Columbia, Children's Hospital, Vancouver, B.C., Canada.)

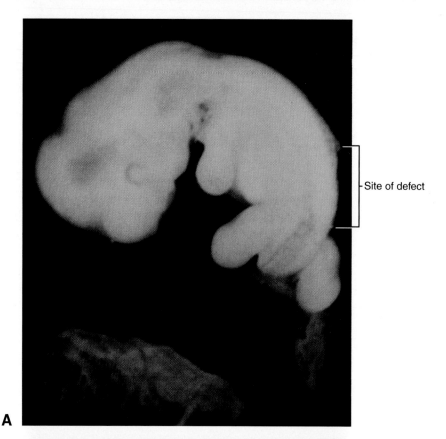

Site of defect

A

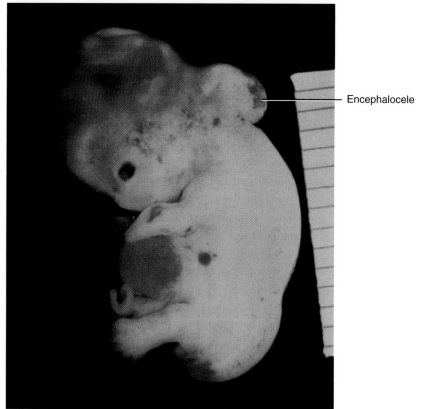

Encephalocele

B

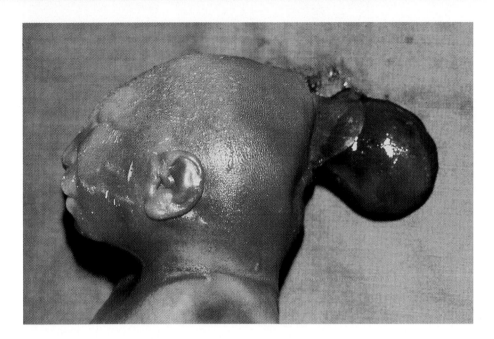

FIG. 13-11

Photograph of an aborted fetus (about 16 weeks) with an occipital encephalocele consisting of a protrusion of the occipital lobe of the brain that is covered with cranial meninges. The ear is abnormally large and low set. (Courtesy of Dr. A.E. Chudley, Department of Pediatrics and Child Health, University of Manitoba, Children's Hospital, Winnipeg, Manitoba, Canada.)

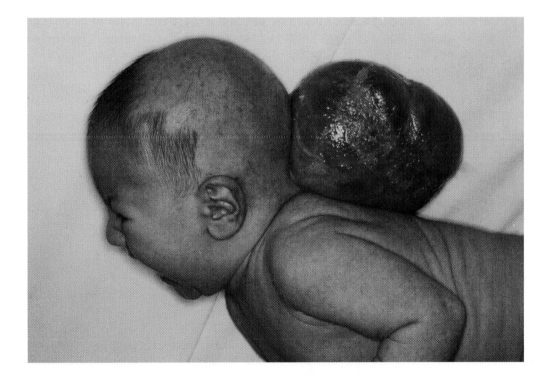

FIG. 13-12

Photograph of a female neonate with a large meningoencephalocele in the occipital area resulting from a large defect in the occipital bone. It consists of a protrusion of the occipital lobe of the brain that is covered with cranial meninges and skin. (Courtesy of Dr. Dwight Parkinson, Department of Surgery, University of Manitoba, Winnipeg, Manitoba, Canada.)

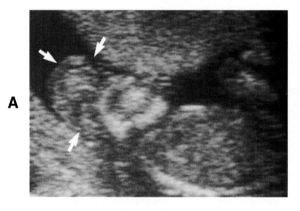
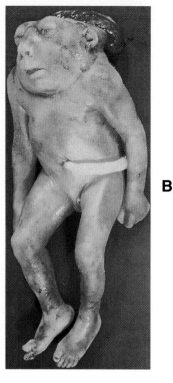

FIG. 13-13

A, Photograph of a female fetus (16 weeks) with meroanencephaly or anencephaly. The remnant of the brain (hindbrain) appears as a spongy, vascular mass. **B,** Stillborn infant with meroanencephaly. As a result of the absence of most of the brain, these infants do not survive. This is the most common of the open neural tube defects and the most common defect affecting the central nervous system. It shows a clear female predominance with a female to male ratio of 4 to 1. This severe defect results from failure of the rostral neuropore to close at the end of the fourth week. (**A,** Courtesy of Dr. D.K. Kalousek, Department of Pathology, University of British Columbia, Children's Hospital, Vancouver, B.C., Canada. **B,** Courtesy of Dr. A.E. Chudley, Department of Pediatrics and Child Health, University of Manitoba, Children's Hospital, Manitoba, Winnipeg, Canada.)

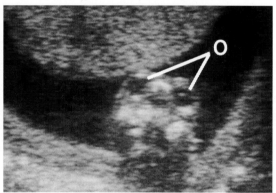

FIG. 13-14

Meroanencephaly, or anencephaly, early in the second trimester. **A,** Sagittal sonogram demonstrating a large mass of angiomatous stroma *(arrows)* cephalad to the skull base. **B,** The coronal image of the face demonstrates the symmetric absence of the calvaria superior to the orbits *(O)*, thus confirming the diagnosis of meroanencephaly. Even though this anomaly is often called anencephaly (without a brain), there is always functioning neural tissue present. For this reason, the term *meroanencephaly* (part brain) describes the anomaly better. The calvaria (cranial vault) is always absent. (From Filly RA: Ultrasound evaluation of the fetal neural axis. In Callen PW [editor]: *Ultrasonography in obstetrics and gynecology,* ed 3, Philadelphia, 1994, Saunders.)

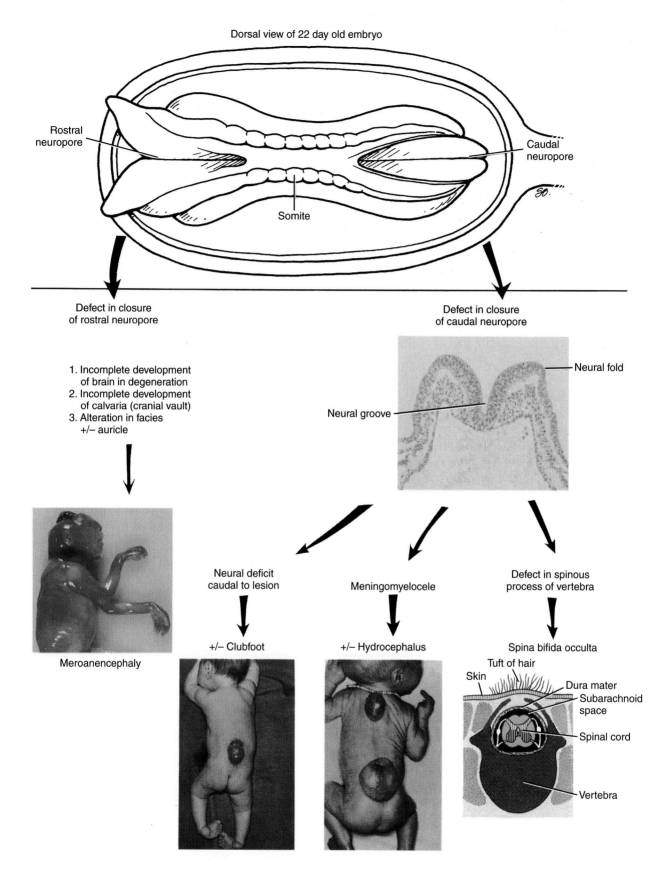

Dorsal view of 22 day old embryo

Rostral neuropore

Caudal neuropore

Somite

Defect in closure of rostral neuropore

Defect in closure of caudal neuropore

1. Incomplete development of brain in degeneration
2. Incomplete development of calvaria (cranial vault)
3. Alteration in facies
   +/− auricle

Neural fold

Neural groove

Meroanencephaly

Neural deficit caudal to lesion

Meningomyelocele

Defect in spinous process of vertebra

+/− Clubfoot

+/− Hydrocephalus

Spina bifida occulta

Tuft of hair

Skin

Dura mater

Subarachnoid space

Spinal cord

Vertebra

FIG. 13-15

Schematic drawings and photographs illustrating and explaining the embryologic basis of neural tube defects (NTDs), such as meroanencephaly (anencephaly) and spina bifida with meningomyelocele. Meroanencephaly is due to defective closure of the rostral neuropore and meningomyelocele is due to defective closure of the caudal neuropore. (Modified from Jones KL: *Smiths recognizable patterns of human malformations*, ed 4, Philadelphia, 1988, Saunders. Photograph of clubfoot is courtesy of Dr. Dwight Parkinson, Department of Surgery, University of Manitoba, Winnipeg, Manitoba, Canada.)

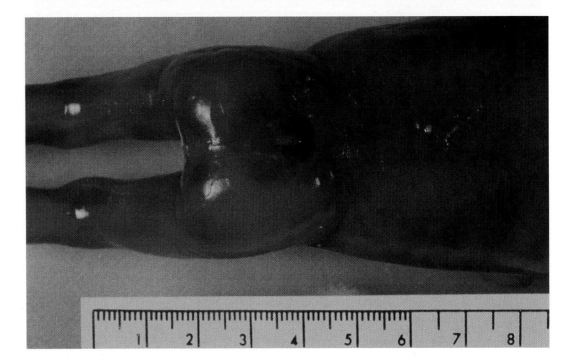

FIG. 13-16

Photograph of the back of a 16.5-week female fetus with a lumbosacral meningomyelocele. A defect in the vertebral (neural) arches of the lower lumbar and upper sacral vertebrae resulted in protrusion of the meninges and defective development of the spinal cord. Meningomyeloceles are often accompanied by a marked neurological deficit inferior to the protruding sac (e.g., paralysis of the lower limbs and sphincter paralysis of the urinary bladder). These defects may be covered by skin or a thin, easily ruptured membrane as in this case. (Courtesy of Dr. D.K. Kalousek, Department of Pathology, University of British Columbia, Children's Hospital, Vancouver, B.C., Canada.)

FIG. 13-17

Ultrasound scan of a 14-week-old fetus, showing a cystlike protrusion representing a meningomyelocele (m) in the sacral region of the vertebral column. The well-formed vertebral (neural) arches of the vertebrae superior to the neural tube defect are clearly visible. (Courtesy Dr. Lyndon, M. Hill, Director of Ultrasound, Magee-Womens Hospital, Pittsburgh, Pa.)

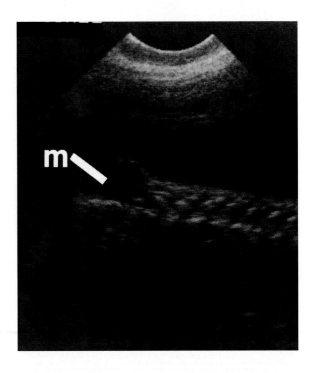

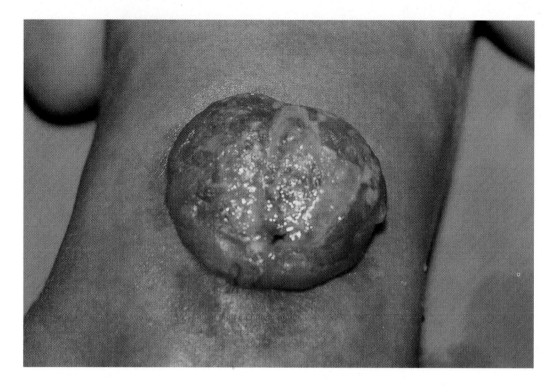

FIG. 13-18

Photograph of the back of a neonate with a large lumbar meningomyelocele. The neural tube defect (NTD) was covered with a thin membrane. These defects may occur anywhere along the vertebral column, but they are most common in the lumbar region. For the embryologic basis of the NTD, see Fig. 13-14. (Courtesy of Dr. A.E. Chudley, Department of Pediatrics and Child Health, University of Manitoba, Children's Hospital, Winnipeg, Manitoba, Canada.)

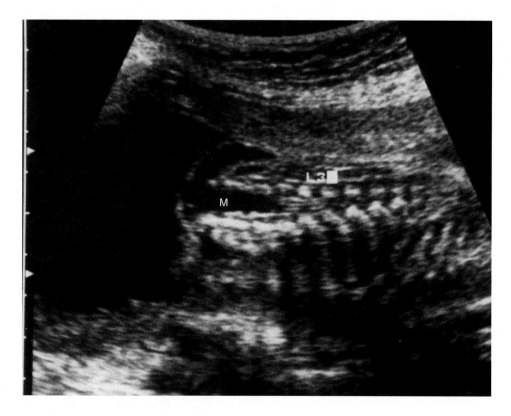

FIG. 13-19

Sonogram of the caudal end of a 20-week fetus (22 weeks gestation) showing myelorachis-chisis of the lower lumbar region of the vertebral column, distal to L3 vertebra. This defect resulted in a meningomyelocele *(M)* of the spinal cord. (Courtesy of Dr. Lyndon Hill, Director of Ultrasound, Magee-Womens Hospital, Pittsburgh, Pa.)

CHAPTER 14

The Eye and Ear

These special sense organs begin to develop during the fourth week. The eyes and ears are very sensitive to the teratogenic effects of drugs, chemicals, and infectious agents (see Table 5-5). The most serious defects result from disturbances during the fourth to sixth weeks of development, but defects of sight and hearing may result from infection of tissues and organs by certain microorganisms during the fetal period (e.g., rubella virus and *Treponema pallidum*, the microorganism that causes syphilis).

THE EYE

The first indication of the eye is the *optic sulcus,* which forms at the beginning of the fourth week. This groove soon deepens to form a hollow *optic vesicle* that projects laterally from the forebrain (Figs. 13-6 and 14-1). The optic vesicle contacts the surface ectoderm and induces development of the *lens placode* (see Fig. 2-12), the primordium of the lens. As the lens placode invaginates to form a *lens pit* and a *lens vesicle* (Figs. 14-2 and 14-4), the optic vesicle invaginates to form an **optic cup.** The retina forms from the two layers of the optic cup.

The **retina,** the optic nerve fibers, the muscles of the iris, and the epithelium of the iris and ciliary body are derived from the *neuroectoderm* of the forebrain (Figs. 14-2 to 14-6). The *surface ectoderm* gives rise to the lens and the epithelium of the lacrimal glands, eyelids, conjunctiva, and cornea. The head mesenchyme and the neural crest give rise to the eye muscles, except those of the iris, and to all connective and vascular tissues of the cornea, iris, ciliary body, choroid, and sclera. The sphincter and dilator muscles of the iris develop from the ectoderm at the rim of the optic cup.

There are many *ocular anomalies* but most of them are uncommon (Fig. 14-7). Most anomalies are caused by defective closure of the optic fissure (Fig. 14-3, *B*) during the sixth week (e.g., coloboma of the iris). *Congenital cataract* and **glaucoma** may result from intrauterine infections (e.g., rubella virus [see Fig. 5-12]), but most congenital cataracts are inherited.

246

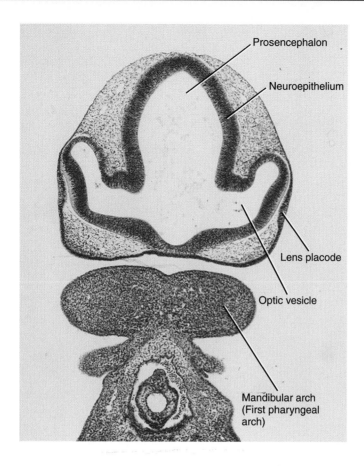

FIG. 14-1

Photomicrograph of a coronal section of the head of an embryo at Carnegie stage 13. Observe the optic vesicles protruding laterally from the prosencephalon. Lens placodes are being induced at the surface ectoderm over the optic vesicle.

THE EAR

The surface ectoderm gives rise to the *otic vesicle* during the fourth week (Figs. 14-8 to 14-10). It develops into the membranous labyrinth of the internal ear. The otic vesicle divides into: (1) a dorsal utricular portion, which gives rise to the utricle, semicircular ducts, and endolymphatic duct; and (2) a ventral saccular portion, which gives rise to the saccule and cochlear duct. The cochlear duct gives rise to the *spiral organ* (of Corti). The *bony labyrinth* develops from the mesenchyme adjacent to the membranous labyrinth (Fig. 14-10).

The epithelium lining the tympanic cavity, mastoid antrum, and auditory tube is derived from the endoderm of the *tubotympanic recess* that develops from the first pharyngeal pouch (Fig. 14-10, *A*). The auditory ossicles (malleus, incus, and stapes) develop from the dorsal ends of the cartilages of the first two pharyngeal arches (Fig. 14-10, *B*).

The epithelium of the *external acoustic meatus* develops from the ectoderm of the first pharyngeal (branchial) groove (Fig. 14-10, *A*). The *tympanic membrane* is derived from three sources: (1) the endoderm of the first pharyngeal pouch, (2) the ectoderm of the first branchial or pharyngeal groove, and (3) the mesenchyme that grows between these layers (Fig. 14-10, *C*).

The auricle develops from six *auricular hillocks*, which result from mesenchymal swellings that develop around the margins of the first branchial or pharyngeal groove (Fig. 14-11). These hillocks fuse to form the definitive auricle (Fig. 4-12).

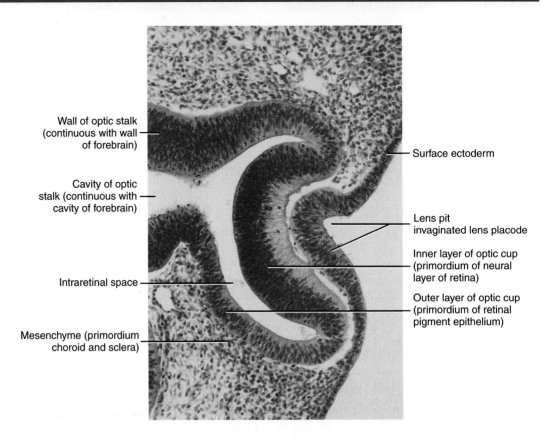

FIG. 14-2

Photomicrograph of a sagittal section of the eye of an embryo (×200) at Carnegie stage 14, about 32 days. (See Fig. 2-15 for the external appearance and size of an embryo at this stage.) Observe the primordium of the lens (invaginated lens placode), the walls of the optic cup (primordium of the retina), and the optic stalk (primordium of the optic nerve).

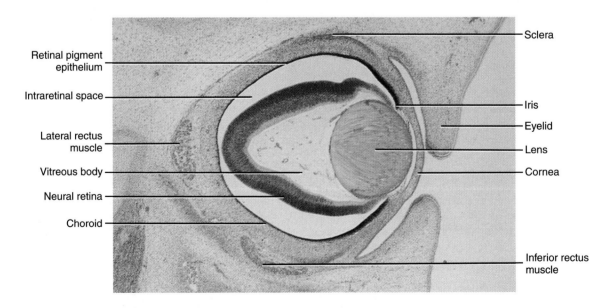

FIG. 14-3

Photomicrograph of a sagittal section of the eye of an embryo (×50) at Carnegie stage 23, about 56 days. (See Fig. 2-26 for the external appearance and size of an embryo at this stage.) Observe the neural retina and the retinal pigment epithelium.

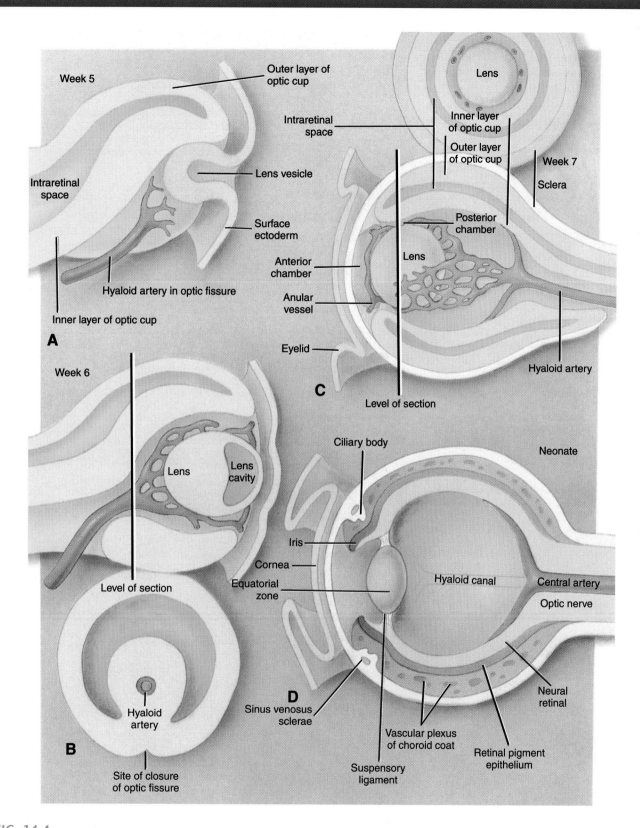

FIG. 14-4

Drawings showing development of the eye from the fifth week to birth. The intraretinal space between the inner (primordium of neural retina) and outer (primordium of the retinal pigment epithelium) layers of the optic cup disappears as the eye develops. Trauma may separate the layers of the retina in this area. The hyaloid artery supplies the developing lens but most of it disappears. Its proximal part forms the central artery of the retina. The hyaloid canal in the vitreous body (shown in *D*) indicates the former site of the distal part of the hyaloid artery.

FIG. 14-5

Photomicrograph of a sagittal section of the eye of an embryo (×100) at Carnegie stage 18, about 44 days. (See Fig. 2-21 for the external appearance and size of an embryo at this stage.) Observe that it is the posterior wall of the lens vesicle that forms the lens fibers. The anterior wall does not change appreciably as it becomes the anterior lens epithelium. (From Nishimura H [editor]: *Atlas of human prenatal histology*, Tokyo, 1983, Igaku-Shoin.)

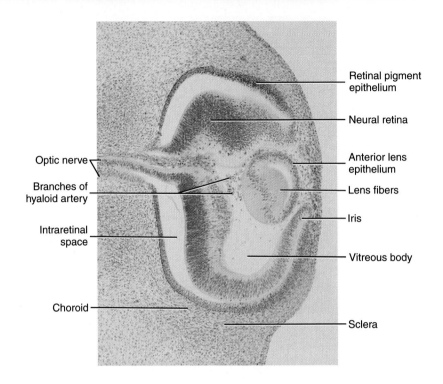

- Retinal pigment epithelium
- Neural retina
- Anterior lens epithelium
- Lens fibers
- Iris
- Vitreous body
- Sclera
- Optic nerve
- Branches of hyaloid artery
- Intraretinal space
- Choroid

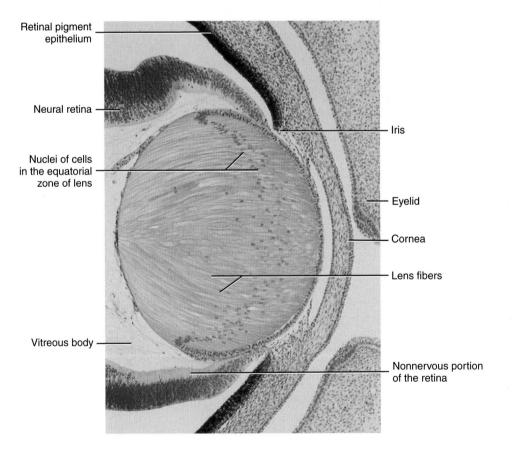

- Retinal pigment epithelium
- Neural retina
- Nuclei of cells in the equatorial zone of lens
- Vitreous body
- Iris
- Eyelid
- Cornea
- Lens fibers
- Nonnervous portion of the retina

FIG. 14-6

Photomicrograph of a sagittal section of a portion of the developing eye of an embryo (×280) at Carnegie stage 23, about 56 days. Observe that the lens fibers have elongated and obliterated the cavity of the lens vesicle. Note that the inner layer of the optic cup has thickened greatly to form the neural retina and that the outer layer is heavily pigmented (retinal pigment epithelium).

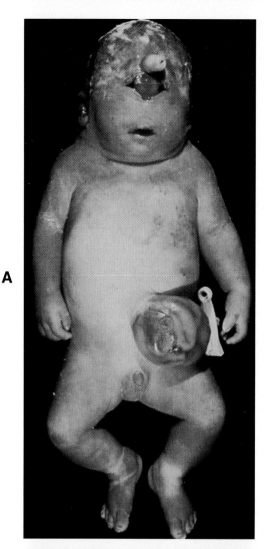

A

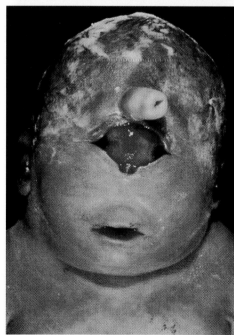

B

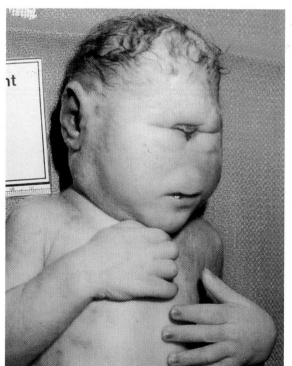

C

FIG. 14-7

A and **B,** Male neonate with cyclopia (synophthalmia) and omphalocele (herniation of the intestines into the proximal part of the umbilical cord). Cyclopia (fusion of the eyes) is a severe, uncommon anomaly of the face and eye associated with a proboscislike appendage located superior to the eye. Several facial bones are absent, for example, nasal bones and ethmoids. **C,** Cyclopia in a neonate with absence of a proboscis. This condition and the one shown in *A* and *B* are due to holoprosencephaly (failure of the forebrain to divide into cerebral hemispheres). This severe anomaly results from faulty interaction between the notochord and the neuroectoderm during the fourth week of development. These infants usually die during the neonatal period because of the presence of other major anomalies (e.g., of the forebrain). Less severe forms of holoprosencephaly include ethmocephaly, cebocephaly, and milder midfacial anomalies with hypotelorism and median cleft lip and palate. (**A** and **B,** Courtesy of Dr. Susan Phillips, Department of Pathology, Health Sciences Centre, Winnipeg, Manitoba, Canada. **C,** Courtesy of Dr. A.E. Chudley, Department of Pediatrics and Child Health, University of Manitoba, Children's Hospital, Winnipeg, Manitoba, Canada.)

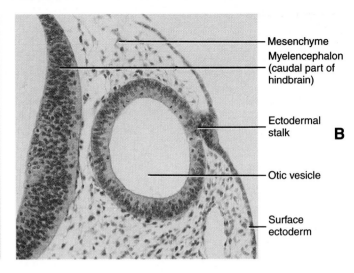

FIG. 14-8

A, Photomicrograph of a transverse section of an embryo (×55) at Carnegie stage 12, about 26 days. (See Fig. 2-11 for the external appearance and size of an embryo at this stage.) Observe the otic vesicles (auditory vesicles), the primordia of the membranous labyrinths, which give rise to the internal ears (Fig. 14-10). **B,** Higher magnification of the right otic vesicle (×120). Note the ectodermal stalk, which is still attached to the remnant of the otic placode (see Fig. 14-10, *C*). (From Nishimura H [editor]: *Atlas of human prenatal histology,* Tokyo, 1983, Igaku-Shoin.)

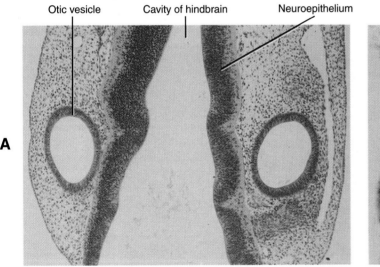
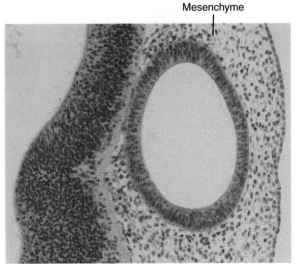

FIG. 14-9

A, Photomicrograph of a transverse section of the embryo (×55), shown in Fig. 14-8, at slightly more caudal level showing the otic vesicles lying free in the mesenchyme adjacent to the hindbrain. **B,** Higher magnification of the right otic vesicle (×120), the primordium of the membranous labyrinth (see Fig. 14-10).

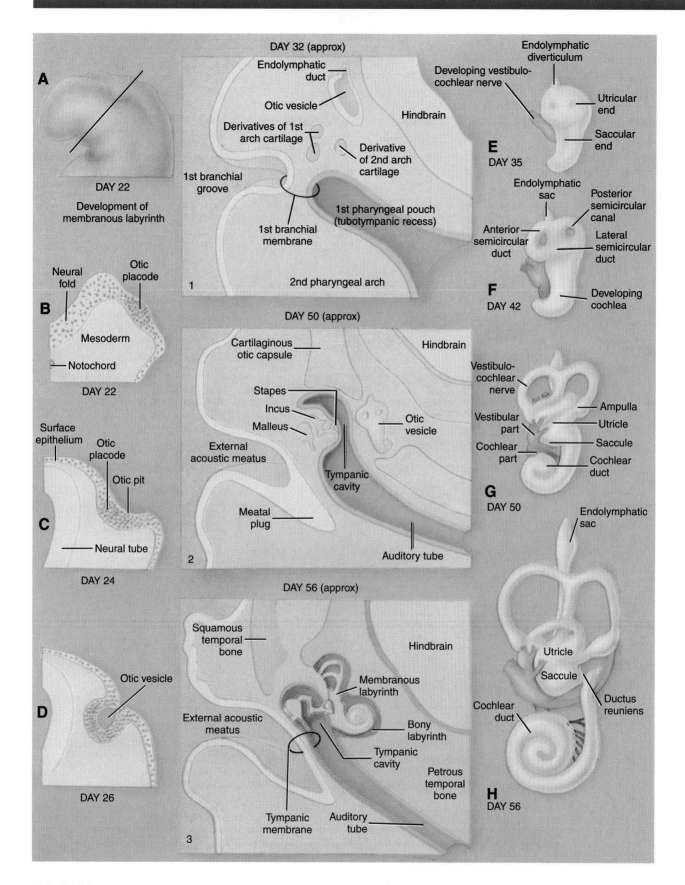

A DAY 22

Development of membranous labyrinth

B

Neural fold

Otic placode

Mesoderm

Notochord

DAY 22

C

Surface epithelium

Otic placode

Otic pit

Neural tube

DAY 24

D

Otic vesicle

DAY 26

DAY 32 (approx)

Endolymphatic duct

Otic vesicle

Hindbrain

Derivatives of 1st arch cartilage

Derivative of 2nd arch cartilage

1st branchial groove

1st branchial membrane

1st pharyngeal pouch (tubotympanic recess)

2nd pharyngeal arch

1

DAY 50 (approx)

Cartilaginous otic capsule

Hindbrain

Stapes

Incus

Malleus

Otic vesicle

External acoustic meatus

Tympanic cavity

Meatal plug

Auditory tube

2

DAY 56 (approx)

Squamous temporal bone

Hindbrain

Membranous labyrinth

External acoustic meatus

Bony labyrinth

Tympanic cavity

Petrous temporal bone

Tympanic membrane

Auditory tube

3

E DAY 35

Endolymphatic diverticulum

Developing vestibulo-cochlear nerve

Utricular end

Saccular end

F DAY 42

Endolymphatic sac

Posterior semicircular canal

Anterior semicircular duct

Lateral semicircular duct

Developing cochlea

G DAY 50

Vestibulo-cochlear nerve

Vestibular part

Cochlear part

Ampulla

Utricle

Saccule

Cochlear duct

H DAY 56

Endolymphatic sac

Utricle

Saccule

Cochlear duct

Ductus reuniens

FIG. 14-10

Drawings showing the development of the three parts of the ear; external, middle, and internal. Note that the otic placode (**B**), the first indication of the internal ear, appears first. The primordia of the middle and external parts of the ear appear about two days later.

FIG. 14-11

Drawings showing development of the auricle of the external ear. A, 6 weeks. Note that three auricular hillocks are located on the first pharyngeal arch and three on the second arch. **B, 8 weeks.** The fused auricular hillocks are located on each side of the first branchial or pharyngeal groove, the primordium of the external acoustic (auditory) meatus. **C, 10 weeks. D, 32 weeks.** As the jaws develop, the auricles move from the neck to the side of the head. (From Moore KL, Persaud TVN: *The developing human,* ed 6, Philadelphia, 1998, Saunders.)

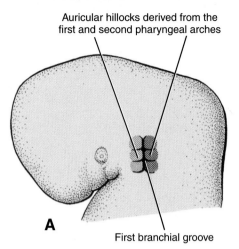

Auricular hillocks derived from the first and second pharyngeal arches

A

First branchial groove

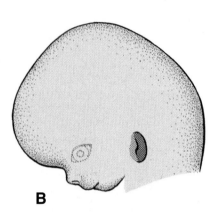

B

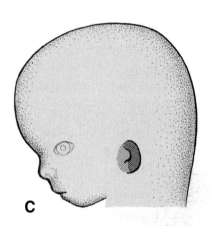

C

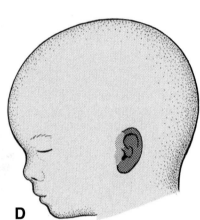

D

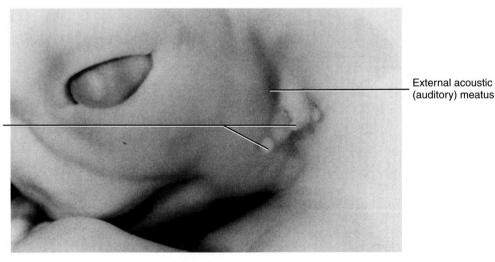

External acoustic (auditory) meatus

Malformed pinna of external ear

FIG. 14-12

Lateral view of the head and neck of an embryo at Carnegie stage 22, about 54 days, showing a severely malformed auricle (pinna). For the normal appearance of the auricle at this stage, see Fig. 2-25. As fusion of the auricular hillocks to form the auricle is rather complicated, anomalies of the auricles (usually minor) are common. Minor deformities of the auricles may be clues to serious anomalies, for example, of the kidneys. (From Nishimura H, Semba R, Tanimura T, Tanaka O: *Prenatal development of the human with special reference to craniofacial structures: an atlas,* US Department of Health, Education, and Welfare, Bethesda, 1977, National Institutes of Health.)

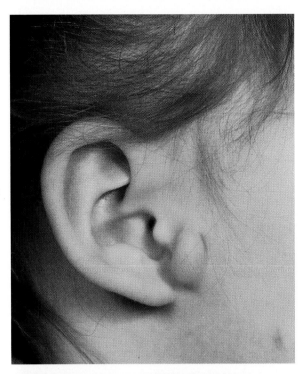

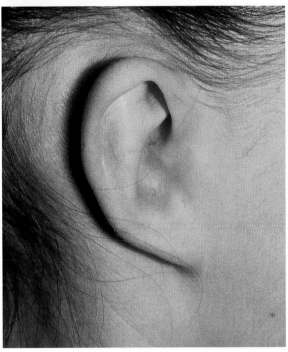

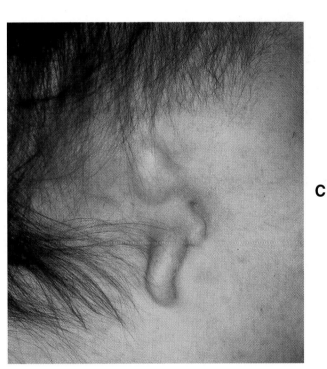

FIG. 14-13

Ear anomalies. **A,** Preauricular tag in a child with oculo-auriculo-vertebral spectrum (first and second branchial arch syndrome). **B,** Child with absence of external auditory canal with slightly malformed auricle. **C,** Severe degree with microtia in an infant with absence of the external auditory canal. (Courtesy of Dr. A.E. Chudley, Department of Pediatrics and Child Health, University of Manitoba, Children's Hospital, Winnipeg, Manitoba, Canada.)

Congenital deafness may result from abnormal development of the membranous labyrinth and/or bony labyrinth, as well as from abnormalities of the auditory ossicles. Recessive inheritance is the most common cause of congenital deafness, but a rubella virus infection near the end of the embryonic period is a major environmental factor known to cause abnormal development of the spiral organ and defective hearing. Congenital aural atresia (abnormal development of the external auditory canal, tympanic membrane, and ear ossicles occurs infrequently (1:10,000 to 1:20,000 live births; Fig. 14-13).

There are many minor, clinically unimportant abnormalities of the auricle (Figs. 14-12 and 14-13), but they alert the clinician to the possible presence of associated major anomalies (e.g., of the heart and kidneys). Low-set, severely malformed ears are often associated with chromosomal abnormalities, particularly trisomy 13 and trisomy 18 (see Chapter 5).

15

The Skin and Related Structures

The skin and its appendages develop from ectoderm and mesoderm (Figs. 15-1 to 15-7). The **epidermis** is derived from ectoderm. The *melanocytes* are derived from *neural crest cells* that migrate into the epidermis. The **dermis** develops from mesenchyme that arises from mesoderm. Cast-off cells from the fetal epidermis mix with secretions of the sebaceous glands to form a whitish, greasy coating for the skin known as *vernix caseosa.* It protects the epidermis, probably making it more waterproof, and facilitates birth because of its slipperiness.

Congenital anomalies of the skin are mainly *disorders of keratinization* (Fig. 15-8) and pigmentation (Figs. 15-9 and 15-10). Abnormal blood vessel development results in various types of angioma (Figs. 15-11 and 15-12).

HAIR

Hairs develop from downgrowths of the epidermis into the dermis (Figs. 15-2 and 15-5). By about 20 weeks the fetus is completely covered with fine, downy hairs called *lanugo.* These hairs are shed by birth or shortly thereafter and are replaced by coarser hairs (see Fig. 15-13). Abnormally excessive hair growth (hypertrichosis) may occur either in patches or extensively (Fig 15-14).

GLANDS

Most *sebaceous glands* develop as outgrowths from the side of hair follicles (Figs. 15-2 and 15-6). Some sebaceous glands develop as downgrowths of the epidermis into the dermis. Hyperplasia of the sebaceous glands is not uncommon (Fig. 15-15). *Sweat glands* also develop from epidermal downgrowths into the dermis (Figs. 15-2 and 15-7). *Mammary glands* develop in a similar manner (Fig. 15-13). Absence of mammary glands is rare, but supernumerary breasts (polymastia) or nipples (polythelia) are relatively common.

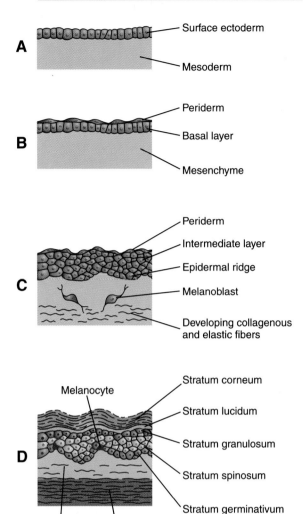

FIG. 15-1

Drawings illustrating successive stages in skin development. A, 4 weeks. B, 7 weeks. C, 11 weeks. The cells of the periderm continually undergo keratinization and desquamation. The exfoliated peridermal cells form part of the vernix caseosa. D, Newborn. Note the position of the melanocytes in the basal layer of the epidermis and the way their branching processes extend between the epidermal cells to supply them with melanin.

TEETH

Teeth develop from ectoderm and mesoderm. The enamel is produced by *ameloblasts,* which are derived from the oral ectoderm; all other dental tissues develop from neural crest–derived mesenchyme of the jaw (Figs. 15-16 to 15-20).

TOOTH ERUPTION (FIG. 15-16, *G* AND *H*). As the teeth develop they begin a continuous movement externally. The mandibular teeth usually erupt before the maxillary teeth, and girls' teeth usually erupt sooner than boys' teeth. The child's dentition contains 20 deciduous teeth (Fig. 15-21). The complete adult dentition consists of 32 teeth.

As the root of the tooth grows, the crown gradually erupts through the oral epithelium (Fig. 15-16, *G* and *H*). The part of the oral mucosa around the erupted crown becomes the *gingiva* (gum). Eruption of the deciduous teeth usually occurs between the sixth and twenty-fourth months after birth. The mandibular medial or central incisors usually erupt 6 to 8 months after birth, but this process may not begin until 12 or 13 months in some normal children. Despite this, all 20 deciduous teeth are usually present by the end of the second year in healthy children.

The permanent teeth develop in a manner similar to that just described for deciduous teeth. As a permanent tooth grows, the root of the corresponding deciduous tooth is gradually resorbed by osteoclasts. Consequently, when the deciduous tooth is shed, it

Text continued on p. 263

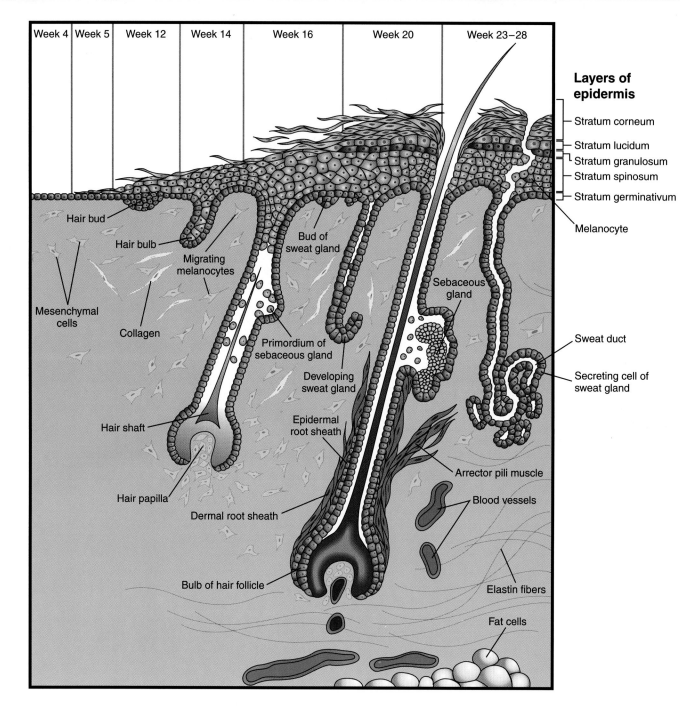

FIG. 15-2

Light micrograph of thick skin (×132). Observe the epidermis and dermis, as well as the dermal ridges interdigitating with the epidermal ridges. (From Gartner LP, Hiatt JL: *Color textbook of histology,* **Philadelphia, 1997, Saunders.)**

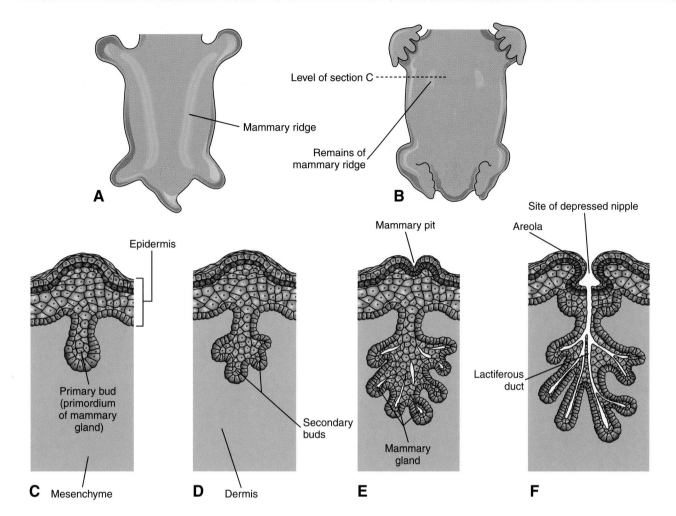

A, Mammary ridge

Level of section C

Remains of mammary ridge

B

Epidermis

Primary bud (primordium of mammary gland)

C Mesenchyme

Secondary buds

D Dermis

Mammary pit

Mammary gland

E

Site of depressed nipple

Areola

Lactiferous duct

F

FIG. 15-3

Drawings illustrating the development of mammary glands. **A,** Ventral view of an embryo of about 28 days, showing mammary ridges. **B,** Similar view at 6 weeks, showing the remains of these ridges. **C,** Transverse section of a mammary ridge at the site of a developing mammary gland. **D, E,** and **F,** Similar sections showing successive stages of breast development between the twelfth week and birth.

FIG. 15-4

Photomicrograph of the skin of an embryo at Carnegie stage 22. The thin periderm covers the single-layered basal layer of the epidermis.

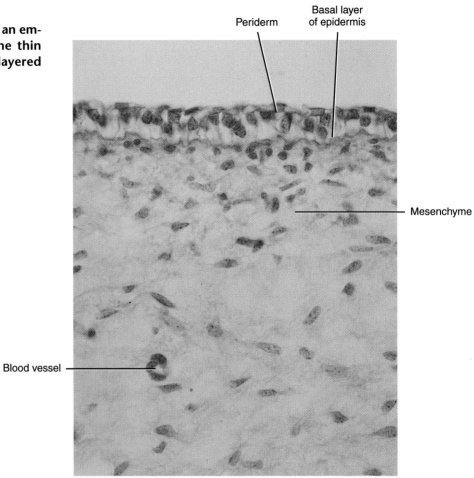

Periderm

Basal layer of epidermis

Mesenchyme

Blood vessel

FIG. 15-5

Photomicrograph of the skin of a 14-week fetus. Hair buds are developing from the epidermis into the dermis. Note the mesenchymal condensation at the deep layer of the hair bud.

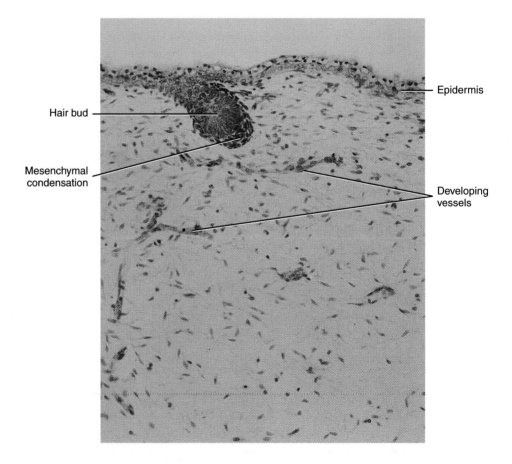

Hair bud

Mesenchymal condensation

Epidermis

Developing vessels

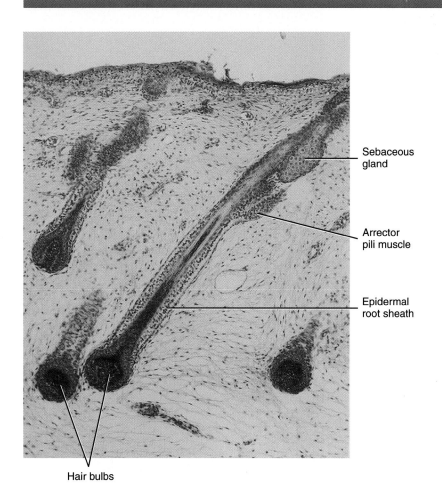

Hair bulbs

Sebaceous
gland

Arrector
pili muscle

Epidermal
root sheath

FIG. 15-6

Photomicrograph of the scalp of a 18-week fetus. Hair bulbs are formed at the tip of hair buds, and the hair and its root sheath are developing. Primordial sebaceous glands and arrector pili muscles are recognized.

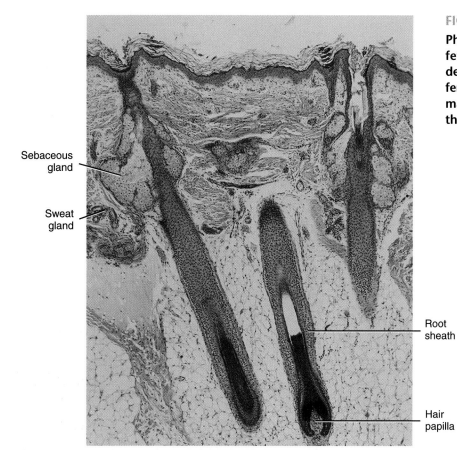

Sebaceous
gland

Sweat
gland

Root
sheath

Hair
papilla

FIG. 15-7

Photomicrograph of the scalp of a term fetus. Sebaceous glands, sweat gland, dermis, and subcutaneous tissue are differentiating. Keratinization and desquamation occur at the superficial layer of the epidermis (Stratum corneum).

FIG. 15-8

A case of epidermolytic hyperkeratosis. This clinical condition may occur sporadically or is autosomal dominantly inherited. It is characterized by severe hyperkeratosis from the time of birth, which persists throughout life. (Courtesy of Dr. Joao Carlos Fernandes Rodrigues, Servico de Dermatologia, Hospital do Desterro, Lisbon, Portugal.)

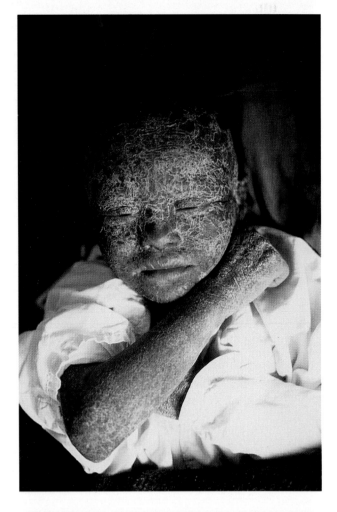

FIG. 15-9

A patient with focal dermal hypoplasia (Goltz syndrome) showing on the right arm multiple linear cutaneous defects, including hyperpigmentation, telangiectasias, and angiofibromas. It has been suggested that this rare congenital disorder may be due to collagen deficiency or heterotopic proliferation of fatty nevi in the dermis. (Courtesy of Dr. Joao Carlos Fernandes Rodrigues, Servico de Dermatologia, Hospital do Desterro, Lisbon, Portugal.)

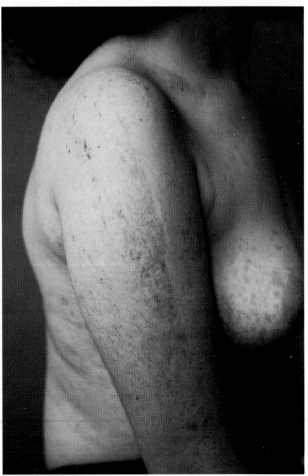

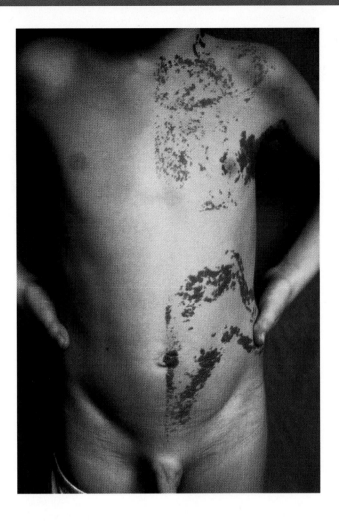

FIG. 15-10

Verrucous epidermal nervus. Observe the extensive hyperpigmentation on the front of the chest, lower abdomen, and groin, resulting from this congenital inherited disorder. This condition is due to an increase of melatonin pigment in the basal keratinocytes. (Courtesy of Dr. Maria Joao Brano Ferreira, Servico de Dermatologia, Hospital do Desterro, Lisbon, Portugal.)

consists of the crown only and the uppermost portion of the root. The permanent teeth usually begin to erupt during the sixth year and continue to appear until early adulthood.

The common congenital anomalies of teeth are defective formation of enamel and dentin, abnormalities in shape, and variations in number and position (Fig. 15-22). All tetracyclines are extensively incorporated into the enamel of developing teeth and produce brownish-yellow discoloration and hypoplasia of the enamel. Consequently, they are not administered during pregnancy and to children.

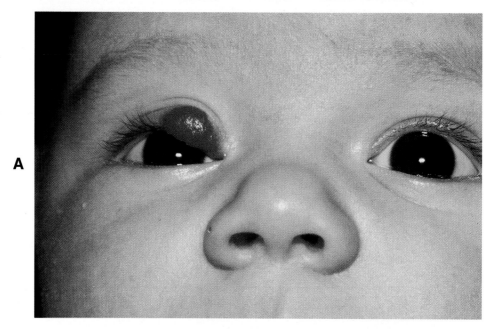

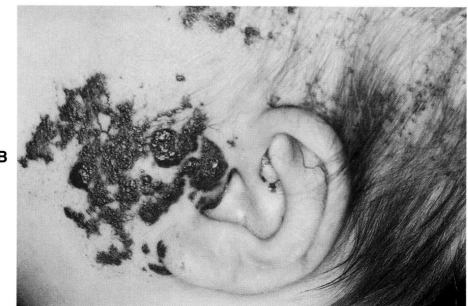

FIG. 15-11

A, An infant with congenital capillary hemangioma of the right upper eyelid. **B,** Capillary hemangioma located in the region of the auricle. This bright red lesion is usually sharply demarcated and may occur on any part of the body. The face and scalp are often affected. (**A,** Courtesy of Dr. G.B. Bartley, Department of Ophthalmology, Mayo Clinic, Mayo Medical School, Rochester, Minn. **B,** Courtesy of Dr. A.E. Chudley, Department of Pediatrics and Child Health, University of Manitoba, Children's Hospital, Winnipeg, Manitoba, Canada.)

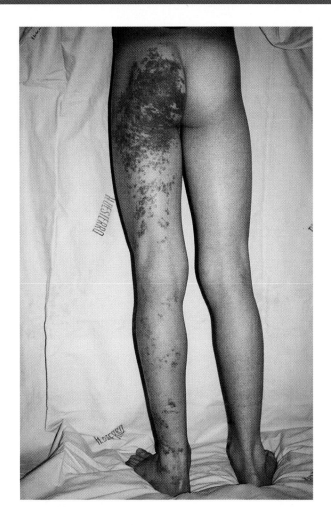

FIG. 15-12

A case of angiokeratoma circumscriptum. These vascular lesions (hemangiomas) on the left gluteal region and lower limb usually appear during infancy. (Courtesy of Dr. Maria Joao Brano Ferreira, Servico de Dermatologia, Hospital do Desterro, Lisbon, Portugal.)

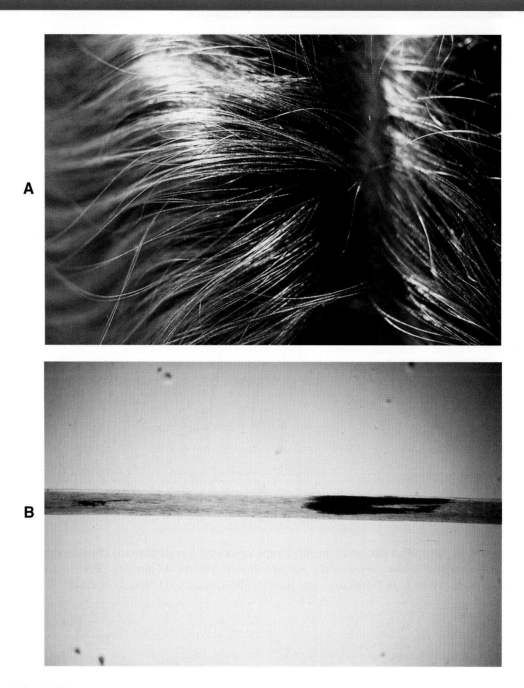

FIG. 15-13

A case of pili annulati. **A,** Observe the varying color of the hair (dark and light) on the scalp. **B,** Microscopic examination of the hair shaft reveals alternating dark and light bands. This disorder may be autosomal dominant. (Courtesy of Dr. Joao Carlos Fernandes Rodrigues, Servico de Dermatologia, Hospital do Desterro, Lisbon, Portugal.)

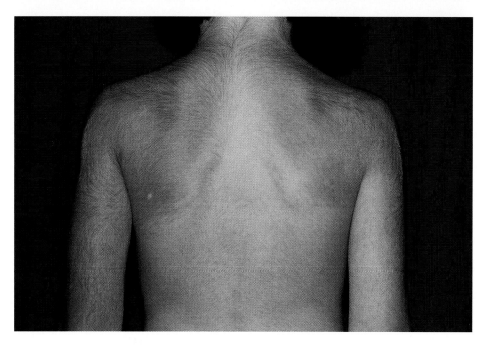

FIG. 15-14

Excessive and diffuse hair growth in unusual locations. (Courtesy of Dr. Maria Joao Brano Ferreira, Servico de Dermatologia, Hospital do Desterro, Lisbon, Portugal.)

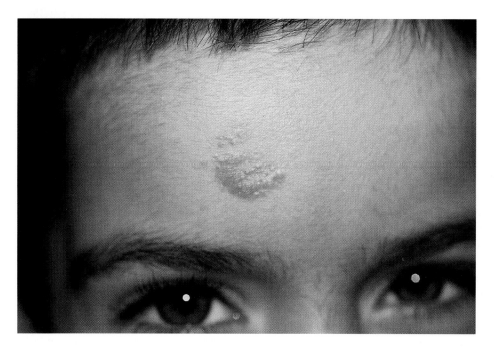

FIG. 15-15

A child with sebaceous nevus. Note the patch of hyperplastic sebaceous glands on the forehead. (Courtesy of Dr. Maria Joao Brano Ferreira, Servico de Dermatologia, Hospital do Desterro, Lisbon, Portugal.)

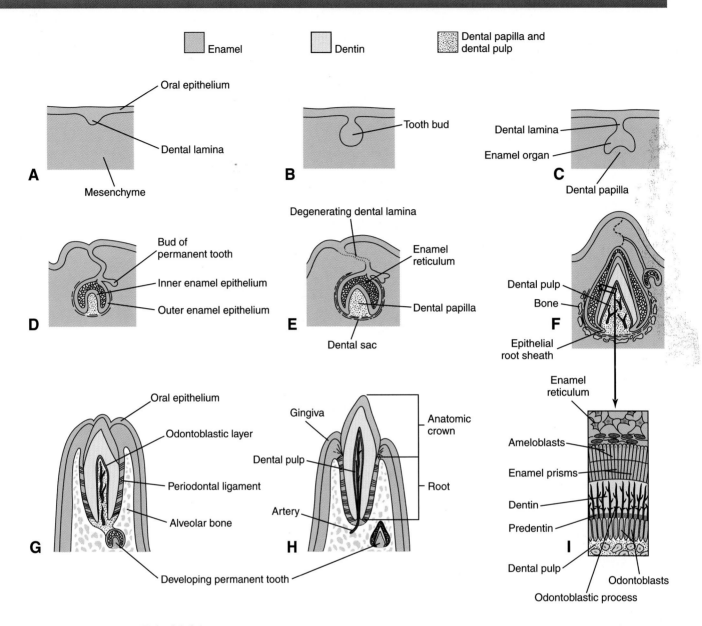

FIG. 15-16

Schematic drawings of sagittal sections illustrating successive stages in the development and eruption of an incisor tooth. **A,** 6 weeks, showing the dental lamina. **B,** 7 weeks, showing the tooth bud developing from the dental lamina. **C,** 8 weeks, showing the cap stage of tooth development. **D,** 10 weeks, showing the early bell stage of a deciduous tooth and the bud stage of a permanent tooth. **E,** 14 weeks, showing the advanced bell stage of tooth development. Note that the connection (dental lamina) of the tooth to the oral epithelium is degenerating. **F,** 28 weeks, showing the enamel and dentin layers. **G,** 6 months postnatal, showing early tooth eruption. **H,** 18 months postnatal, showing a fully erupted deciduous incisor tooth. The permanent incisor tooth now has a well-developed crown. **I,** Section through a developing tooth, showing ameloblasts (enamel producers) and odontoblasts (dentin producers).

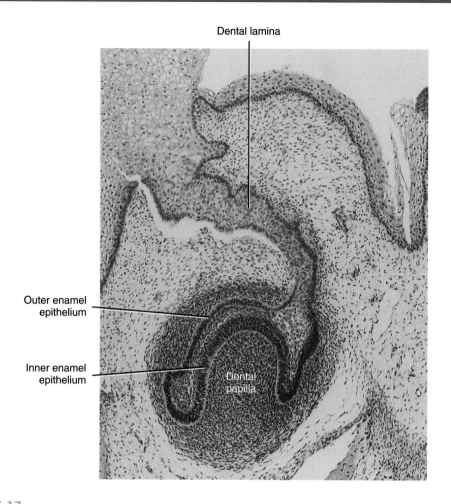

Dental lamina

Outer enamel epithelium

Inner enamel epithelium

Dental papilla

FIG. 15-17

Photomicrograph of the primordium of a lower incisor tooth in a 12-week fetus (early bell stage). A caplike enamel organ is formed and the dental papilla is developing beneath it.

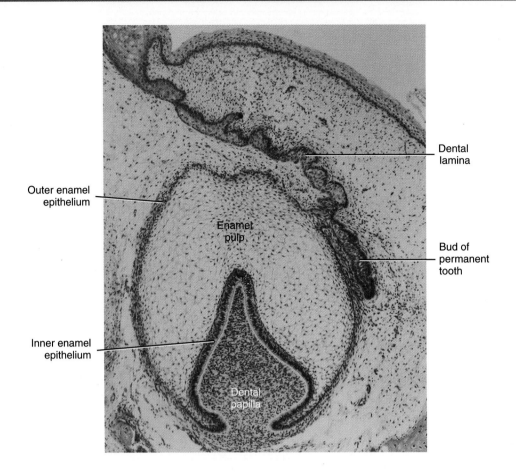

FIG. 15-18

Photomicrograph of a section of a primordial lower incisor tooth in a 15-week fetus (late bell stage). The bud of the permanent tooth is recognized.

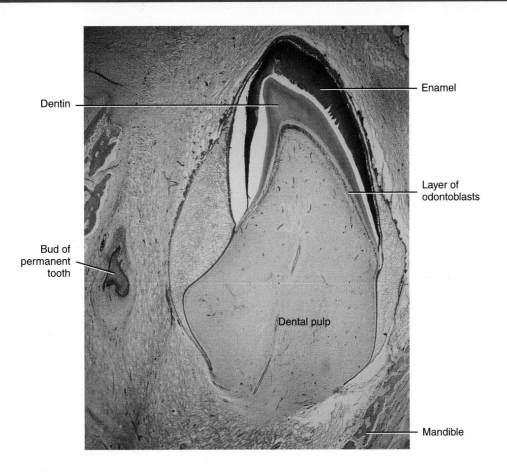

FIG. 15-19

Photomicrograph of a section of a lower incisor tooth in a term fetus. The enamel and dentin layers and the dental pulp are clearly demarcated.

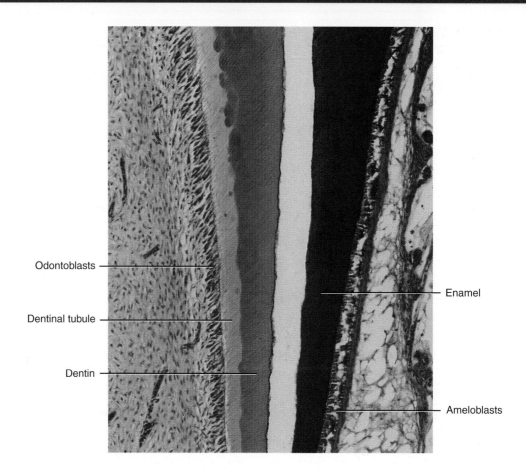

Odontoblasts

Dentinal tubule

Dentin

Enamel

Ameloblasts

FIG. 15-20

A higher magnification of part of Fig. 15-19. Odontoblastic cells form the dentin, and ameloblastic cells of the inner enamel epithelium form the enamel.

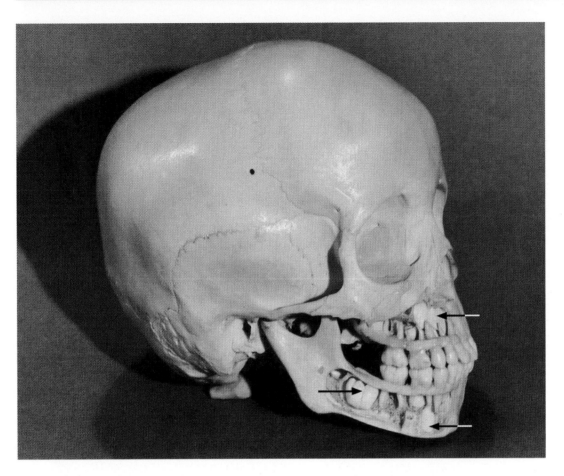

FIG. 15-21

Photograph of a 4-year-old child's skull. The bone has been removed to show the relations of the developing permanent teeth *(arrows)* to the erupted deciduous teeth.

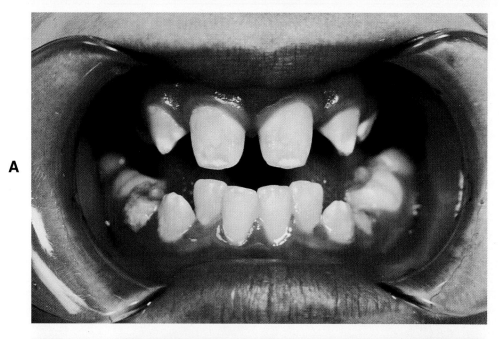

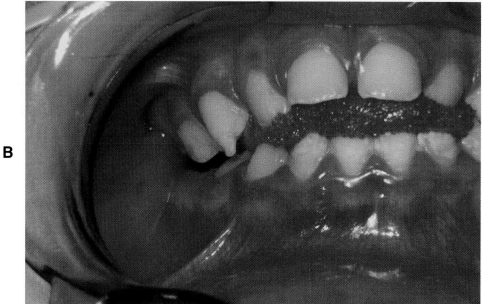

FIG. 15-22

Dental anomalies. **A,** Partial anodontia. Note congenital absence of maxillary lateral incisors. Other permanent teeth may be absent but such a diagnosis will require radiological examination. **B,** Defective amelogenesis (enamel formation). Enamel hyperplasia on maxillary right canine and lateral incisor teeth. Note enamel tubercles on mandibular incisors and hypermineralization. (Courtesy of Dr. A.E. Chudley, Department of Pediatrics and Child Health, University of Manitoba, Children's Hospital, Winnipeg, Manitoba, Canada.)

References and Suggested Reading

CHAPTER 1

Filly RA: Ectopic pregnancy. In Callen PW (editor): *Ultrasonography in obstetrics and gynecology,* ed 3, Philadelphia, 1994, Saunders.

Fleischmajer R, Timpl R, Werb Z (editors): *Morphogenesis: cellular interactions,* New York, 1998, New York Academy of Sciences.

Givens CR: Intracytoplasmic sperm injection: what are the risks? *Obstet Gynecol Surv* 55:58, 2000.

Hadlock FP: Ultrasound determination of menstrual age. In Callen PW (editor): *Ultrasonography in obstetrics and gynecology,* ed 3, Philadelphia, 1994, Saunders.

Jones EE: Abnormal ovulation and implantation. In Reece EA, Hobbins JC (editors): *Medicine of the fetus and mother,* ed 2, Philadelphia, 1999, Lippincott-Raven.

Kadar N: Ectopic and heterotopic pregnancies. In Reece EA, Hobbins JC (editors): *Medicine of the fetus and mother,* ed 2, Philadelphia, 1999, Lippincott-Raven.

Lundin K, Hanson C, Hamberger L: Are the new microfertilization techniques associated with an increased genetic risk to the offspring? *Acta Obstet Gynecol Scand* 77:792, 1998.

Moore KL, Persaud TVN: *The developing human: clinically oriented embryology,* ed 6, Philadelphia, 1998, Saunders.

O'Rahilly R, Müller F: *Developmental stages in human embryos,* Washington, 1987, Carnegie Institute of Washington.

O'Rahilly R, Müller F: *Human embryology and teratology,* ed 2, New York, 1996, Wiley-Liss.

CHAPTER 2

Dimmick JE, Kalousek DK (editors): *Developmental pathology of the embryo and fetus,* New York, 1991, Lippincott-Raven.

Durbin L, Brennan C, Shiomi K, et al: Eph signaling is required for segmentation and differentiation of the somites, *Genes Dev* 12:3096, 1998.

England MA: *Life before birth,* ed 2, London, 1996, Mosby.

Filly RA: Ultrasound evaluation during the first trimester. In Callen PW (editor): *Ultrasonography in obstetrics and gynecology,* ed 3, Philadelphia, 1994, Saunders.

Gasser RF: *Atlas of human embryos,* Hagerstown, 1975, Harper & Row.

Hay JC, Persaud TVN: Normal embryonic and fetal development. In Reece EA, Hobbins JC (editors): *Medicine of the fetus and mother,* ed 2, Philadelphia, 1999, Lippincott-Raven.

Holzgreve W, Flake AW, Langer JC: The fetus with sacrococcygeal teratoma. In Harrison MR, Golbus MS, Filly RA (editors): *The unborn patient: prenatal diagnosis and treatment,* ed 2, Philadelphia, 1991, Saunders.

Kalousek DK, Fitch N, Paradice BA: *Pathology of the human embryo and previable fetus: an atlas*, New York, 1990, Springer-Verlag.

Nishimura II (editor): *Atlas of human prenatal histology*, Tokyo, 1983, Igaku-Shoin.

Nishimura H, Semba R, Tanimura T, Uwabe C: Normal development of early human embryos: observation of 90 specimens at Carnegie stages 7 to 13, *Teratology* 10:1, 1974.

O'Rahilly R, Müller F: *Developmental stages in human embryos,* Washington, 1987, Carnegie Institute of Washington.

O'Rahilly R, Müller F: *Human embryology and teratology,* ed 2, New York, 1996, Wiley-Liss.

Shiota K: Development and intrauterine fate of normal and abnormal human conceptuses, *Cong Anom* 31:67, 1991.

Smith BR: Visualizing human embryos, *Sci Am* 279:77, 1999.

CHAPTER 3

Bowie JD: Fetal growth. In Callen PW (editor): *Ultrasonography in obstetrics and gynecology,* ed 3, Philadelphia, 1994, Saunders.

Campbell BA: Utilizing sonography to follow fetal growth, *Obstet Gynec Clin North Am* 25:597, 1998.

Collins VR, Webley C, Sheffield LJ, Halliday JL: Fetal outcome and maternal morbidity after early amniocentesis, *Prenat Diagn* 18:767, 1998.

Dimmick JE, Kalousek DK (editors): *Developmental pathology of the embryo and fetus,* New York, 1991, Lippincott-Raven.

England MA: *Life before birth,* ed 2, London, 1996, Mosby.

Evans JA, Hamerton JL: Limb defects and chorionic villus sampling, *Lancet* 347:484, 1996.

Filly RA: Sonographic anatomy of the normal fetus. In Harrison MR, Golbus MS, Filly RA (editors): *The unborn patient: prenatal diagnosis and treatment,* ed 2, Philadelphia, 1991, Saunders.

Filly RA: Ultrasound evaluation during the first trimester. In Callen PW (editor): *Ultrasonography in obstetrics and gynecology,* ed 3, Philadelphia, 1994, Saunders.

Filly RA: Sonographic anatomy of the normal fetus. In Callen PW (editor): *Ultrasonography in obstetrics and gynecology,* ed 3, Philadelphia, 1994, Saunders.

Haddow JE: α-Fetoprotein. In Harrison MR, Golbus MS, Filly RA (editors): *The unborn patient: prenatal diagnosis and treatment,* ed 2, Philadelphia, 1991, Saunders.

Hadlock FP: Ultrasound evaluation of fetal growth. In Callen PW (editor): *Ultrasonography in obstetrics and gynecology,* ed 3, Philadelphia, 1994, Saunders.

Harrison MR, Lipshutz GS: The fetus at surgery. In Reece EA, Hobbins JC (editors): *Medicine of the fetus and mother,* ed 2, Philadelphia, 1999, Lippincott-Raven.

Hauth JC, Merenstein GB (editors): *Guidelines for perinatal care,* ed 4, Elk Grove Village, Ill, 1997, American Academy of Pediatrics and American College of Obstetrics and Gynecology.

Hay JC, Persaud TVN: Normal embryonic and fetal development. In Reece EA, Hobbins JC (editors): *Medicine of the fetus and mother,* ed 2, Philadelphia, 1999, Lippincott-Raven.

Kleinman CS, Copel JA: In utero cardiac therapy. In Reece EA, Hobbins JC (editors): *Medicine of the fetus and mother,* ed 2, Philadelphia, 1999, Lippincott-Raven.

Kuliev A: Evaluation of chorionic villus sampling safety, *Prenat Diagn* 19:97, 1997.

Nimrod CA, Gruslin A: Biology of normal and deviant fetal growth. In Reece EA, Hobbins JC (editors): *Medicine of the fetus and mother,* ed 2, Philadelphia, 1999, Lippincott-Raven.

Robinson JS: Fetal growth and development. In Chamberlain G (editor): *Turnbull's obstetrics,* ed 2, Edinburgh, 1995, Churchill Livingstone.

Ross HL, Elias S: Maternal serum screening for fetal genetic disorders, *Obstet Gynec Clin North Am* 24:33, 1997.

Sauve RS, Robertson C, Etches P, et al: Before viability: a geographically based outcome study of infants weighing 500 grams or less at birth, *Pediatr* 101:438, 1998.

Simpson JL, Elias S (editors): *Essentials of prenatal diagnosis,* New York, 1993, Churchill Livingstone.

Terrone DA, Perry Jr KG: Ultrasound evaluation of the fetal central nervous system, *Obstet Gynec Clin North Am* 25:479, 1998.

Wagner RK, Calhoun BC: The routine obstetric ultrasound examination, *Obstet Gynec Clin North Am* 25:451, 1998.

Wapner RJ: Chorionic villus sampling, *Obstet Gynec Clin North Am* 24:83, 1997.

CHAPTER 4

Battaglia FC: Fetoplacental perfusion and transfer of nutrients. In Reece EA, Hobbins JC (editors): *Medicine of the fetus and mother*, ed 2, Philadelphia, 1999, Lippincott-Raven.

Brackley KJ: Twin-twin transfusion syndrome, *Hosp Med* 60:419, 1999.

Cohen WR: Normal and abnormal labor. In Reece EA, Hobbins JC (editors): *Medicine of the fetus and mother*, ed 2, Philadelphia, 1999, Lippincott-Raven.

Dimmick JE, Kalousek DK (editors): *Developmental pathology of the embryo and fetus*, New York, 1991, Lippincott-Raven.

Doubilet PM, Benson CB: Ultrasound evaluation of amniotic fluid. In Callen PW (editor): *Ultrasonography in obstetrics and gynecology*, ed 3, Philadelphia, 1994, Saunders.

England MA: *Life before birth*, ed 2, London, 1996, Mosby.

Filly RA: Ultrasound evaluation during the first trimester. In Callen PW (editor): *Ultrasonography in obstetrics and gynecology*, ed 3, Philadelphia, 1994, Saunders.

Finberg HJ: Ultrasound evaluation in multiple gestation. In Callen PW (editor): *Ultrasonography in obstetrics and gynecology*, ed 3, Philadelphia, 1994, Saunders.

Fox H: Normal and abnormal placentation. In Reece EA, Hobbins JC (editors): *Medicine of the fetus and mother*, ed 2, Philadelphia, 1999, Lippincott-Raven.

Francis ST, Duncan KR, Moore RJ, et al: Non-invasive mapping of placental perfusion, *Lancet* 351:1397, 1998.

Fung KFK: Ultrasound surveillance of twin pregnancy. I. Conception to mid-trimester, *J Soc Obstet Gynaecol Can* 20:641, 1998.

Fung KFK: Ultrasound surveillance of twin pregnancy. II. Mid-trimester to confinement, *J Soc Obstet Gynaecol Can* 20:1303, 1998.

Hutchinson KA, DeCherney AH: Endocrinology of pregnancy. In Reece EA, Hobbins JC (editors): *Medicine of the fetus and mother*, ed 2, Philadelphia, 1999, Lippincott-Raven.

Jessa EO: Twin pregnancy and perinatal deaths, *J Obstet Gynecol* 18:336, 1998.

Lewis SH, Gilbert-Barness E: The placenta and its significance in neonatal outcome, *Adv Pediatr* 45:223, 1998.

Lewis SH, Perrin E: *Pathology of the placenta*, ed 2, New York, 1998, Churchill Livingstone.

Lindsay DJ, Lovett IS, Lyons EA, et al: Endovaginal sonography: yolk sac diameter and shape as a predictor of pregnancy outcome in the first trimester, *Radiology* 183:115, 1992.

Lyons EA, Levi CS: Ultrasound of the normal first trimester of pregnancy. Syllabus. Special Course. Oak Brook, Ill, 1991, Ultrasound, Radiological Society of North America.

Moore KL, Persaud TVN: *The developing human: clinically oriented embryology*, ed 6, Philadelphia, 1998, Saunders.

Naeye RL: *Disorders of the placenta, fetus, and neonate*, St Louis, 1992, Mosby.

Nyberg DA, Callen PW: Ultrasound evaluation of the placenta. In Callen PW (editor): *Ultrasonography in obstetrics and gynecology*, ed 3, Philadelphia, 1994, Saunders.

Schwartz LB: Understanding human parturition, *Lancet* 350:1792, 1998.

Smith-Levitin M, Skupski DW, Chervenak FA: Multifetal pregnancies: epidemiology, clinical characteristics, and management. In Reece EA, Hobbins JC (editors): *Medicine of the fetus and mother*, ed 2, Philadelphia, 1999, Lippincott-Raven.

Spencer R: Theoretical and analytical embrology of conjoined twins. Part I. Embryogenesis, *Clin Anat* 13:36, 2000.

CHAPTER 5

Abel EL: What really causes FAS, *Teratology* 59:4, 1999.

Atanckovic G, Koren G: Young women taking isotretinoin still conceive, *Can Fam Physician* 45:289, 1999.

Beckman DA, Brent RL: Basic principles of developmental toxicology. In Reece EA, Hobbins JC (editors): *Medicine of the fetus and mother*, ed 2, Philadelphia, 1999, Lippincott-Raven.

Benshushan A, Brzezinski A, Ben-David A, Nadjari M: Early recurrent CMV infection with severe outcome to the fetus, *Acta Obstet Gynecol Scand* 77:694, 1998.

Bodéus M, Hubinont C, Goubau P: Increased risk of cytomegalovirus transmission in utero during late gestation, *Obstet Gynecol* 93:658, 1999.

Brent RL, Beckman DA: Prescribed drugs, therapeutic agents, and fetal teratogenesis. In Reece EA, Hobbins JC (editors): *Medicine of the fetus and mother*, ed 2, Philadelphia, 1999, Lippincott-Raven.

Briggs GG, Freeman RK, Yaffe SJ: *Drugs in pregnancy and lactation*, ed 5, Baltimore, 1998, Williams & Wilkins.

Burkett G, Gomez-Marin O, Yasin SY, Martinez M: Prenatal care in cocaine-exposed pregnancies, *Obstet Gynecol* 92:193, 1998.

Carmichael SL, Shaw GM: Maternal life event stress and congenital anomalies, *Epidemiology* 11:30, 2000.

Carr SR, Coustan DR: Nonprescription drugs and alcohol: abuse and effects in pregnancy. In Reece EA, Hobbins JC (editors): *Medicine of the fetus and mother*, ed 2, Philadelphia, 1999, Lippincott-Raven.

Chan L, Uerpairojkit B, Reece EA: Diagnosis of congenital malformations using two-dimensional and three-dimensional ultrasonography, *Obstet Gynecol Clin North Am* 24:49, 1997.

Cohen MM Jr: *The child with multiple birth defects*, ed 2, New York, 1997, Oxford University Press.

Dimmick JE, Kalousek DK (editors): *Developmental pathology of the embryo and fetus*, Philadelphia, 1992, Lippincott.

Dolk HM, Nau H, Hummler H, Barlow SM: Dietary vitamin A and teratogenic risk: European Teratology Society discussion paper, *Europ J Obstet Gynecol Reprod Biol* 83:31, 1999.

Dyer JJ, Strasnick B, Jacobson JT: Teratogenic hearing loss: a clinical perspective, *Am J Otol* 19:671, 1998.

Ebrahim SH, Luman ET, Floyd RL, et al: Alcohol consumption by pregnant women in the United Sates during 1988-1995, *Obstet Gynecol* 92:187, 1998.

Edwards MJ, Shiota K, Smith MSR, Walsh DA: Hyperthermia and birth defects, *Reprod Toxicol* 9:411, 1995.

Ford-Jones EL: An approach to the diagnosis of congenital infections, *Pediatr Child Health* 4:109, 1999.

Friedman JM, Kimmel CA: Teratology Society 1998. Public Affairs Committee Symposium: The new thalidomide era: dealing with risks, *Teratology* 59:120, 1999.

Friedman S, Ford-Jones EL: Congenital cytomegalovirus infection: an update, *Pediatr Child Health* 4:35, 1999.

Graham JM: *Smith's recognizable patterns of human deformation*, ed 3, Philadelphia, 1998, Saunders.

Gross C: Viral infections of the fetus and newborn. In Behrman RE, Kliegman RM, Arvin AM (editors): *Nelson textbook of pediatrics*, ed 15, Philadelphia, 1996, Saunders.

Gross SJ, Bombard AT: Screening for the aneuploid fetus, *Obstet Gynecol Clin North Am* 25:573, 1998.

Gupta GK, Bianchi DW: DNA diagnosis for the practicing obstetrician, *Obstet Gynecol Clin North Am* 24:123, 1997.

Hall JG: Chromosomal clinical abnormalities. In Behrman RE, Kliegman RM, Arvin AM (editors): *Nelson textbook of pediatrics*, ed 15, Philadelphia, 1996, Saunders.

Holmes LB: Teratogens. In Behrman RE, Kliegman RM, Arvin AM (editors): *Nelson textbook of pediatrics*, ed 15, Philadelphia, 1996, Saunders.

Hsu LYF: Chromosomal disorders. In Reece EA, Hobbins JC (editors): *Medicine of the fetus and mother*, ed 2, Philadelphia, 1999, Lippincott-Raven.

Jones KL: Dysmorphology. In Behrman RE, Kliegman RM, Arvin AM (editors): *Nelson textbook of pediatrics*, ed 15, Philadelphia, 1996, Saunders.

Jones KL, Fletcher J (editors): *Smith's recognizable patterns of human malformation*, ed 5, Philadelphia, 1996, Saunders.

Kliegman RM: The fetus. In Behrman RE, Kliegman RM, Arvin AM (editors): *Nelson textbook of pediatrics*, ed 15, Philadelphia, 1996, Saunders.

Kumar P, Angst DB, Taxy J, et al: Neonatal autopsies, *Arch Pediatr Adolesc Med* 154:38, 2000.

Lacombe D: Transcription factors in dysmorphology, *Clin Genet* 55:137, 1999.

Lindgren S, Ottenblad C, Bengtsson AB, Bohlin AB: Pregnancy in HIV-infected women, *Acta Obstet Gynecol Scand* 77:532, 1998.

Mahoney MJ: Single gene disorders. In Reece EA, Hobbins JC (editors): *Medicine of the fetus and mother*, ed 2, Philadelphia, 1999, Lippincott-Raven.

Martinez-Frias ML, Czeizel AE, Rodriquez-Pinilla E, Bermejo E: Smoking during pregnancy and Poland sequence: results of a population-based registry and a case-controlled registry, *Teratology* 59:35, 1999.

Martinez-Frias ML, Frias JL: VACTERL as primary polytopic developmental field defects, *Am J Med Genet* 83:13, 1999.

Mastroiacovo P, Mazzone T, Addis A, et al: High vitamin A intake in early pregnancy and major malformations: a multicenter prospective controlled study, *Teratology* 59:7, 1999.

Miller RW: Effects of prenatal exposure to ionizing radiation, *Health Physics* 59:57, 1990.

Milunsky JM, Milunsky A: Genetic counseling in perinatal medicine, *Obstet Gynecol Clin North Am* 24:1, 1997.

Milunsky JM, Milunsky A: Genetic counseling in prenatal and perinatal medicine. In Reece EA, Hobbins JC (editors): *Medicine of the fetus and mother,* ed 2, Philadelphia, 1999, Lippincott-Raven.

Moore KL, Persaud TVN: *The developing human: clinically oriented embryology,* ed 6, Philadelphia, 1999, Saunders.

Newman RB (editor): Prescribing in pregnancy, *Obstet Gynecol Clin North Am* 24:vii, 1997.

Ornoy A, Ratzon N, Greenbaum C, et al: Neurobehaviour of school age children born to diabetic mothers, *Arch Dis Child Fetal Neonatal Ed* 79:F94, 1998.

Persaud TVN: *Environmental causes of human birth defects,* Springfield, 1990, Charles C Thomas.

Phillips E: Toxoplasmosis, *Can Fam Physician* 44:1823, 1998.

Polifka JE, Friedman JM: Clinical teratology: identifying teratogenic risks in humans, *Clin Genet* 56:409, 1999.

Reece EA: Fetal diagnosis and therapy, *Obstet Gynecol Clin North Am* 24:1-217, 1997.

Ross HL, Elias S: Maternal serum screening for fetal genetic disorders, *Obstet Gynecol Clin North Am* 24:33, 1997.

Shepard TH: *Catalog of teratogenic agents,* ed 9, Baltimore, 1998, The Johns Hopkins University Press.

Simpson JL: Principles of human genetics. In Reece EA, Hobbins JC (editors): *Medicine of the fetus and mother,* ed 2, Philadelphia, 1999, Lippincott-Raven.

Sison AV, Sever JL: Teratogenic viruses. In Reece EA, Hobbins JC (editors): *Medicine of the fetus and mother,* ed 2, Philadelphia, 1999, Lippincott-Raven.

Smulian JC, Egan JFX, Rodis JF: Fetal hydrops in the first trimester associated with maternal parvovirus infection, *J Clin Ultrasound* 26:314, 1998.

Verma L, Macdonald F, Leedham P, et al: Rapid and simple DNA diagnosis of Down's syndrome, *Lancet* 352:9, 1998.

Webster WS: Teratogen update: congenital rubella, *Teratology* 58:13, 1998.

Wiedemann H-R, Kunze J (editors): *Clinical syndromes,* ed 3, London, 1997, Mosby.

Yip SK, Leung TN, Fung HYM: Exposure to angiotensin-converting enzyme inhibitors during first trimester: is it safe to fetus? *Acta Obstet Gynecol Scand* 77:570, 1998.

CHAPTER 6

Azarow K, Messineo A, Pearl R, et al: Congenital diaphragmatic hernia: a tale of two cities: the Toronto experience, *J Pediatr Surg* 32:395, 1997.

Glick PL, Irish MS, Holm BA (editors): New insights into the pathophysiology of congenital diaphragmatic hernia, *Clin Perinatol* 23:62, 1996.

Goldstein RB: Ultrasound evaluation of the fetal thorax. In Callen PW (editor): *Ultrasonography in obstetrics and gynecology,* ed 3, Philadelphia, 1994, Saunders.

Goldstein RB: Ultrasound evaluation of the fetal abdomen. In Callen PW (editor): *Ultrasonography in obstetrics and gynecology,* ed 3, Philadelphia, 1994, Saunders.

Hartman GE: Diaphragmatic hernia. In Behrman RE, Kliegman RM, Arvin AM (editors): *Nelson textbook of pediatrics,* ed 14, Philadelphia, 1996, Saunders.

Moore KL, Persaud TVN: *The developing human: clinically oriented embryology,* ed 6, Philadelphia, 1998, Saunders.

Quah BS, Hashim I, Simpson H: Bochdalek diaphragmatic hernia presenting with acute gastric dilatation, *J Pediatr Surg* 34:512, 1999.

Skandalakis JE, Gray SW: *The embryological basis for the treatment of congenital defects,* Baltimore, 1994, Williams & Wilkins.

Wilson JM, Lund DP, Lillehei CW, Vacanti JP: Congenital diaphragmatic hernia: a tale of two cities: the Boston experience, *J Pediatr Surg* 32:401, 1997.

CHAPTER 7

Benacerraf BR: Ultrasound evaluation of the fetal face. In Callen PW (editor): *Ultrasonography in obstetrics and gynecology,* ed 3, Philadelphia, 1994, Saunders.

Christensen K: The 20th century Danish facial cleft population: epidemiological and genetic-epidemiological studies, *Cleft Palate J* 36:99, 1999.

England MA: *Life Before Birth,* ed 2, London, 1996, Mosby.

Gorlin RJ, Cohen Jr MM, Levin LS: *Syndromes of the head and neck,* ed 3, New York, 1990, Oxford University Press.

Gürsoy MH, Gedikoglu G, Tanyel FC: Lateral cervical cleft: a previously unreported anomaly resulting from incomplete disappearance of the second pharyngeal (branchial) cleft, *J Pediatr Surg* 34:488, 1999.

Hinrichsen K: *The early development of morphology and patterns of the face in the human embryo: advances in anatomy, embryology and cell biology 98,* New York, 1985, Springer-Verlag.

Hunt P, Clarke JD, Buxton P, et al: Segmentation, crest prespecification and the control of facial form, *Eur J Oral Sci* 106(Suppl):12, 1998.

Jones KL, Fletcher J (editors): *Smith's recognizable patterns of human malformation,* ed 5, Philadelphia, 1996, Saunders.

Moore KL, Persaud TVN: *The developing human: clinically oriented embryology,* ed 6, Philadelphia, 1998, Saunders.

Niermeyer MF, Van der Meulen JC: Genetics of craniofacial malformations. In Stricker M, Van der Meulen JC, Raphael B, Mazzola R (editors): *Craniofacial malformations,* Edinburgh, 1990, Churchill Livingstone.

Nishimura H, Semba R, Tanimura T, Tanaka O: *Prenatal development of the human with special reference to craniofacial structures: an atlas,* Bethesda, 1977, US Department of Health, Education, and Welfare, National Institutes of Health.

Pfeifer G (editor): *Craniofacial abnormalities and clefts of the lip, alveolus and palate,* New York, 1991, Georg Thieme Verlag.

Sharma S: Ophthaproblem (congenital nasolacrimal duct obstruction), *Can Fam Physician* 44:2085, 1998.

Sperber GH: *Craniofacial embryology,* ed 4 (revised reprint), London, 1993, Butterworth.

Stricker M, Raphael B, Van der Meulen J, Mazzola R: Craniofacial growth and development. In Stricker M, Van der Meulen JC, Raphael B, Mazzola R (editors): *Craniofacial malformations,* Edinburgh, 1990, Churchill Livingstone.

Ueda D, Yoto Y, Sato T: Ultrasonic assessment of the lingual thyroid gland in children, *Pediatr Radiol* 28:126, 1998.

Van der Meulen J, Mozzola B, Stricker M, Raphael B: Classification of craniofacial malformations. In Stricker M, Van der Meulen JC, Raphael B, Mazzola R (editors): *Craniofacial malformations,* Edinburgh, 1990, Churchill Livingstone.

Vermeij-Keers C: Craniofacial embryology and morphogenesis: normal and abnormal. In Stricker M, Van der Meulen JC, Raphael B, Mazzola R (editors): *Craniofacial malformations,* Edinburgh, 1990, Churchill Livingstone.

CHAPTER 8

Chernick V, Boat TF (editors): *Kendig's disorders of the respiratory tract in children,* ed 6, Philadelphia, 1997, Saunders.

Evans JA, Greenberg CR, Erdile L: Tracheal agenesis revisited: analysis of associated anomalies, *Am J Med Genet* 82:415, 1999.

Finci V, Beghetti M, Kalangos A, Bründler M-A: Unilateral total and contralateral partial pulmonary agenesis associated with total anomalous pulmonary venous drainage, *J Pediatr* 134:510-1999.

Harrison MR: The fetus with a diaphragmatic hernia: pathology, natural history, and surgical management. In Harrison MR, Golbus MS, Filly RA: *The unborn patient: prenatal diagnosis and treatment,* ed 2, Philadelphia, 1991, Saunders.

Moore KL, Persaud TVN: *The developing human: clinically oriented embryology,* ed 6, Philadelphia, 1998, Saunders.

Nichols KV, Gross I: Fetal lung development and amniotic fluid analysis. In Reece EA, Hobbins JC (editors): *Medicine of the fetus and mother,* ed 2, Philadelphia, 1999, Lippincott-Raven.

Park WY, Miranda B, Lebeche D, et al: FGF-10 is a chemotactic factor for distal epithelial buds during lung development, *Dev Biol* 201:125, 1998.

Rapado F, Bennett JDC, Stringfellow JM: Bronchogenic cyst: an unusual cause of lump in the neck, *J Laryngol Otol* 112:893, 1998.

Reece EA: Fetal thoracic malformations. In Reece EA, Hobbins JC (editors): *Medicine of the fetus and mother,* ed 2, Philadelphia, 1999, Lippincott-Raven.

CHAPTER 9

Cobb RA, Williamson RCN: Embryology and developmental abnormalities of the large intestine. In Phillips SF, Pemberton JH, Shorter RG (editors): *The large intestine: physiology, pathophysiology, and disease,* New York, 1991, Raven Press.

England MA: *Life before birth,* ed 2, London, 1996, Mosby.

Herbst JJ: Development and function of the esophagus. In Behrman RE, Kliegman RM, Arvin AM (editors): *Nelson textbook of pediatrics,* ed 15, Philadelphia, 1996, Saunders.

Gabrielli S, Rizzo N, Reece EA: Gastrointestinal and genitourinary anomalies. In Reece EA, Hobbins JC (editors): *Medicine of the fetus and mother,* ed 2, Philadelphia, 1999, Lippincott-Raven.

Gonçalves LF, Jeanty P: Ultrasound evaluation of abdominal wall defects: In Callen PW (editor): *Ultrasonography in obstetrics and gynecology,* ed 3, Philadelphia, 1994, Saunders.

Kleigman RM: The umbilicus. In Behrman RE, Kliegman RM, Arvin, AM (editors): *Nelson textbook of pediatrics,* ed 15, Philadelphia, 1996, Saunders.

Moore KL, Persaud TVN: *The developing human: clinically oriented embryology,* ed 6, Philadelphia, 1998, Saunders.

Shandling B: Congenital and perinatal anomalies of the gastrointestinal tract and intestinal rotation. In Behrman RE, Kliegman RM, Arvin AM (editors): *Nelson textbook of pediatrics,* ed 14, Philadelphia, 1996, Saunders.

CHAPTER 10

Baskin LS: Society for fetal urology panel discussion: prenatal diagnosis and treatment of genital anomalies, *Urology* 53:1029, 1999.

Devesa R, Muñoz A, Torrents M, et al: Prenatal diagnosis of isolated hypospadias, *Prenat Diagn* 18:779, 1998.

England MA: *Life before birth,* ed 2, London, 1996, Mosby.

Gabrielli S, Rizzo N, Reece EA: Gastrointestinal and genitourinary anomalies. In Reece EA, Hobbins JC (editors): *Medicine of the fetus and mother,* ed 2, Philadelphia, 1999, Lippincott-Raven.

Gill FT: Umbilical hernia, inguinal hernias, and hydroceles in children: diagnostic clues for optimal patient management, *J Pediatr Health Care* 12:231, 1998.

Jimenez R, Burgos M: Mammalian sex determination: joining pieces of the genetic puzzle, *BioEssays* 20:696, 1998.

Limwongse C, Clarren SK, Cassidy SB: Syndromes and malformations of the urinary tract. In Barratt TM, Avner ED, Harmon WE (editors): *Pediatric nephrology,* ed 4, Baltimore, 1999, Lippincott Williams & Wilkins.

Mahony BS: Ultrasound evaluation of the fetal genitourinary system. In Callen PW (editor): *Ultrasonography in obstetrics and gynecology,* ed 3, Philadelphia, 1994, Saunders.

Moore KL, Persaud TVN: *The developing human: clinically oriented embryology,* ed 6, Philadelphia, 1998, Saunders.

Murcia NS, Woychik RP, Avner ED: The molecular biology of polycystic kidney disease, *Pediatr Nephrol* 12:721, 1998.

Parker LA: Ambiguous genitalia: etiology, treatment, and nursing implications, *JOGNN* 27:15, 1998.

Persaud TVN: Embryology of the female genital tract and gonads. In Copeland LI, Jarrell J, McGregor J (editors): *Textbook of gynecology,* ed 2, Philadelphia, 2000, Saunders.

Schafer AJ, Goodfellow PN: Sex determination in humans, *BioEssays* 18:955, 1996.

Stamilio DM, Morgan MA: Diagnosis of fetal renal anomalies, *Obstet Gynecol North Am* 25:527, 1998.

Woolf AS: Embryology. In Barratt TM, Avner ED, Harmon WE (editors): *Pediatric nephrology,* ed 4, Baltimore, 1999, Lippincott Williams & Wilkins.

CHAPTER 11

Belmont JW: Recent progress in the molecular genetics of congenital heart defects, *Clin Genet* 54:11, 1998.

Brumund MR, Lutin WA: Advances in antenatal diagnosis and management of the fetus with a heart problem, *Pediatr Ann* 27:486, 1998.

Chinn A, Fitzsimmons J, Shepard TH, Fantel AG: Congenital heart disease among spontaneous abortuses and stillborn fetuses: prevalence and associations, *Teratology* 40:475, 1989.

Creasy RK, Resnik R (editors): *Maternal-fetal medicine,* ed 4, Philadelphia, 1999, Saunders.

Feit LR: Genetics of congenital heart disease: strategies, *Adv Pediatr* 45:267, 1998.

Hess DB, Hess LW (editors): *Fetal echocardiography,* Stamford, 1999, Appleton & Lange.

Hess DB, Hess LW, Carter GA, et al: Obtaining the four-chamber view to diagnose fetal cardiac anomalies, *Obstet Gynecol Clin North Am* 25:499, 1998.

Leung MP, Tang MHY, Ghosh A: Prenatal diagnosis of congenital heart malformations: classification based on abnormalities detected by four-chamber view, *Prenat Diagn* 19:305, 1999.

Moore KL, Persaud TVN: *The developing human: clinically oriented embryology,* ed 6, Philadelphia, 1998, Saunders.

Pilu G, Jeanty P: Prenatal diagnosis of congenital heart disease. In Reece EA, Hobbins JC (editors): *Medicine of the fetus and mother,* ed 2, Philadelphia, 1999, Lippincott-Raven.

Schmidt KG, Silverman WH: The fetus with a cardiac malformation. In Harrison MR, Golbus MS, Filly RA (editors): *The unborn patient: prenatal diagnosis and treatment,* ed 2, Philadelphia, 1991, Saunders.

Silverman NH, Schmidt KG: Ultrasound evaluation of the fetal heart. In Callen PW (editor): *Ultrasonography in obstetrics and gynecology,* ed 3, Philadelphia, 1994, Saunders.

Sinning AR: Role of vitamin A in the formation of congenital heart defects, *Anat Rec (New Anat)* 253:147, 1998.

Stoll C, Alembik Y, Dott B, et al: Evaluation of prenatal diagnosis of congenital heart disease, *Prenat Diagn* 18:801, 1998.

Westmoreland D: Critical congenital cardiac defects in the newborn, *J Perinat Neonat Nurs* 12:67, 1999.

Yates R: Fetal cardiac abnormalities and their association with aneuploidy, *Prenat Diagn* 19:563, 1999.

CHAPTER 12

Brook CGD, deVries BBA: Skeletal dysplasias, *Arch Dis Child* 79:285, 1998.

England MA: *Life before birth,* ed 2, London, 1996, Mosby.

Francheschi RT: The developmental control of osteoblast-specific gene expression: role of specific transcription factors and the extracellular matrix environment, *Crit Rev Oral Biol Med* 10:40, 1999.

LeClair E, Bonfiglio L, Tuan RS: Expression of the paired-box genes Pax-7 and Pax-9 in limb skeleton development, *Dev Dyn* 214:101, 1999.

Mahony BS: Ultrasound evaluation of the fetal musculoskeletal system. In Callen PW (editor): *Ultrasonography in obstetrics and gynecology,* ed 3, Philadelphia, 1994, Saunders.

Maldjian C, Hofkin S, Bonakdarpour A, et al: Abnormalities of the pediatric foot, *Acta Radiol* 4:191, 1999.

Margulies EH, Innis JW: Building arms or legs with molecular models, *Pediatr Res* 47:2, 2000.

Maymon E, Nores J, Romero R: Fetal skeletal anomalies. In Reece EA, Hobbins JC (editors): *Medicine of the fetus and mother,* ed 2, Philadelphia, 1999, Lippincott-Raven.

Moore KL, Persaud TVN: *The developing human: clinically oriented embryology,* ed 6, Philadelphia, 1998, Saunders.

Riddle RD, Tabin CJ: How limbs develop, *Sci Am* 280:74, 1999.

Rust OA, Perry Jr KG, Roberts WE: Tips in diagnosing fetal skeletal anomalies, *Obstet Gynecol Clin North Am* 25:553, 1998.

Uhthoff HK: *The embryology of the human locomotor system,* New York, 1990, Springer-Verlag.

Wientroub S, Keret D, Bronshtein M: Prenatal sonographic diagnosis of musculoskeletal disorders, *J Pediatr Orthop* 19:1, 1999.

Zacksenhaus E, Jiang Z, Chung C, et al: pRB controls proliferation, differentiation, and death of skeletal muscle cells and other lineages during embryogenesis, *Genes Dev* 10:3051-3064, 1996.

CHAPTER 13

Abu-Heija AT, El-Sunna E: Neural tube defects in newborns, *Saudi Med J* 20:173, 1999.

Filly RA: Ultrasound evaluation of the fetal neural axis. In Callen PW (editor): *Ultrasonography in obstetrics and gynecology,* ed 3, Philadelphia, 1994, Saunders.

Goldowitz D, Hamre K: The cells and molecules that make a cerebellum, *Trends Neurosci* 21:375, 1998.

Jacobson M: *Developmental neurobiology,* ed 3, New York, 1992, Plenum Publishing.

Kerszberg M, Changeux J-P: A simple molecular model of neurulation, *BioEssays* 20:758, 1998.

Moore KL, Persaud TVN: *The developing human: clinically oriented embryology,* ed 6, Philadelphia, 1998, Saunders.

Müller F, O'Rahilly R: The development of the human brain from a closed neural tube at stage 13, *Anat Embryol (Berl)* 177:55, 1988.

Müller F, O'Rahilly R: Development of anencephaly and its variants, *Am J Anat* 190:193, 1991.

O'Rahilly R, Müller F: *The embryonic human brain: an atlas of developmental stages,* New York, 1994, John Wiley & Sons.

Persaud TVN: *Environmental causes of human birth defects,* Springfield, 1990, Charles C Thomas.

Pilu G, Gabrielli S: Prenatal diagnosis of central nervous system anomalies. In Reece EA, Hobbins JC (editors): *Medicine of the fetus and mother,* ed 2, Philadelphia, 1999, Lippincott-Raven.

Terrone DA, Perry Jr KG: Ultrasound evaluation of the fetal central nervous system, *Obstet Gynecol North Am* 25:479, 1998.

CHAPTER 14

Ars B: Organogenesis of the middle ear structures, *J Laryngol Otol* 103:16, 1989.

Bauer PW, MacDonald CB, Melhem ER: Congenital inner ear malformation, *Am J Otol* 19:669, 1998.

Cremers CWRJ: Hearing: cracking the code, *J Laryngol Otol* 114:6, 2000.

Dyer JJ, Stasnick B, Jacobson JT: Teratogenic hearing loss, *Am J Otol* 19:671, 1998.

Jean D, Ewan K, Gruss P: Molecular regulators involved in vertebrate eye development, *Mech Dev* 76:3-18, 1998.

Mathers PH, Grinberg A, Mahon KA, Jamrich M: The Rx homeobox gene is essential for vertebrate eye development, *Nature* 387:603-607, 1997.

Moore KL, Persaud TVN: *The developing human: clinically oriented embryology,* ed 6, Philadelphia, 1998, Saunders.

Nelson L: Disorders of the eye. In Behrman RE, Kliegman RM, Arvin AM (editors): *Textbook of pediatrics,* ed 15, Philadelphia, 1996, Saunders.

Parrish KL, Amedee RG: Atresia of the external auditory canal, *J La State Med Soc* 142:9, 1990.

Sevel D, Isaacs R: A re-evaluation of corneal development, *Trans Am Ophthalmol Soc* 86:178, 1989.

Sharma S: Ophthaproblem (congenital nasolacrimal duct obstruction), *Can Fam Physician* 44:2085, 1998.

Trigg DJ, Applebaum EL: Indications for the surgical repair of unilateral aural atresia in children, *Am J Otol* 19:679, 1998.

CHAPTER 15

Akiyama M: Severe congenital ichthyosis of the neonate, *Int J Dermatol* 37:722, 1998.

Cobourne MT: The genetic control of early odontogenesis, *Br J Orthod* 26:21, 1999.

Hirschhorn K: Dermatoglyphics. In Behrman RE, Kliegman RM, Arvin AM (editors): *Nelson textbook of pediatrics,* ed 15, Philadelphia, 1996, Saunders.

Horn TD: Developmental defects of the skin. In Farmer ER, Hood AF (editors): *Pathology of the skin,* Norwalk, 1990, Appleton & Lange.

Moore KL, Persaud TVN: *The developing human: clinically oriented embryology,* ed 6, Philadelphia, 1998, Saunders.

Shwayder T: Ichthyosis in a nutshell, *Pediatr Rev* 20:3, 1999.

Sperber GH: *Craniofacial embryology,* ed 4 (revised reprint), London, 1993, Butterworth.

Sturm RA, Box NF, Ramsay M: Human pigmentation genetics: the difference is only skin deep, *BioEssays* 20:712, 1998.

Verbov J: Dermatoglyphics in congenital absence of phalanges of the right hand, *Clin Exp Dermatol* 19:412, 1994.

Index

Note: Page numbers in *italics* indicate illustrations;
page numbers followed by t indicate tables.